MODERN DISPENSING PHARMACY

Dr. Atmaram Pawar
Professor, Department of Pharmaceutics
Bharati Vidyapeeth University,
Poona College of Pharmacy, Pune

Dr. R. S. Gaud
Dean, Pharmaceutical Sciences,
School of Pharmacy and
Technology Management,
NMIMS Deemed University, Mumbai.

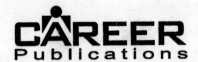

CAREER
Publications

MODERN
DISPENSING PHARMACY

First Edition	-	February	2004
Second Edition	-	April	2005
Second Edition Reprint	-	November	2005
Second Edition Reprint	-	September	2006
Second Edition Reprint	-	September	2007
Second Edition Reprint	-	February	2008
Third Edition	-	January	2009
Third Edition Reprint	-	August	2010
Third Edition Reprint	:	August	2012
Third Edition Reprint	:	March	2013

© Dr. A. P. Pawar

ISBN : 978-81-88739-66-0

Published by :
Career Publications

Communication Address :
Second Floor, Kaveri Smruti,
Ashok Stambh, Nashik - 422 001
Maharashtra, India.
Ph. : (0253) 2311210, 2310421, 2576175, 2311422
E-mail : info@careerandyou.com
Visit us : www.careerandyou.com

Pune Office :
First Floor, Gokhale
Building, Tilak Road,
Pune - 411 0030.
Maharashtra, India.
Phone : (020) 24497602
Email : careerpune@careerandyou.com

Typesetting :
Satish More
Career Publications

Illustrations :
Mr. Atul Bhalerao

Printer :
Replica Printers, Nashik

Price : ₹ 315/-

FOREWORD

I am extremely happy to have seen and critically gone through a book written by two Senior Pharmacists of this country. This type of book is the first of its kind in India. The authors have attempted to present a detail information on a subject which is normally given a low profile in the studies by teachers and students.

The "**MODERN DISPENSING PHARMACY**" has given us a proper insight of the subject in an interesting manner and the detailed information relevant to this country is presented in this book, which will generate interest of students and teachers in this subject.

The information given in this book not only contains the description of the dosage forms but also the way it is to be administered to patients and the precautions to be taken during therapy. This has been explained diagrammatically for better understanding of the subject. They have taken efforts to explain the principle and use of these dispensed products in a simple way. The book contains an information on common therapies like antacids, expectorants, skin diseases, etc.

The book has a unique feature of the detail information on how the controlled release drugs are to be administered to optimise their performance and to achieve maximum benefit to the patients which in itself is a major activity of properly trained community pharmacists.

For the first time an attempt has been made by the authors to present the information in a simple way by giving pictograms.

The posology chapter is of great help to students, teachers and practicing pharmacists which gives not only the doses of drugs, but also the care to be taken while administering these potent drugs to avoid their ill effects.

I trust that this book will be of great help to students, teachers and practicing pharmacists of this country.

I congratulate both the authors for presenting such a valuable book to those who are involved in patient care.

Date : 05 / 02 / 2004

Prof. S. G. Deshpande
Professor (Pharmaceutics),
School of Pharmacy and Technology Management,
NMIMS Deemed University, Mumbai.

OUR EARLIER PUBLICATIONS

For B.Pharm

1)	Inorganic Pharmaceutical Chemistry (Theory)	:Dr. H.P. Tipnis & Dr. A.S. Dhake
2)	Inorganic Pharmaceutical Chemistry (Practical)	:Dr. D.P. Belsare & Dr. A.S. Dhake
3)	Anatomy Physiology and Health Education (Including Sports & Practical Physiology)	:Rahul P. Phate
4)	Modern Dispensing Pharmacy	:Dr. A.P. Pawar & Prof. R.S. Gaud
5)	Experimental Pharmaceutical Organic Chemistry: A Benchtop Manual	:Dr. K.S. Jain, P.B. Maniyar & Mrs. T.S. Chitre
6)	Biostatistics	:Dr. Sai Subramanian
7)	Pharmaceutical Analysis - I (Practical)	:Mrs. Sonali Sheorey & Ms. Meera Honrao
8)	Pharmacology (Part I) For Pharmacy	:Dr. Vivek Bele
9)	A Handbook of Experiments in Pre-clinical Pharmacology	:Dr. Sanjay Kasture
10)	Pharmacognosy & Phytochemistry (Volume - I)	:Dr. Vinod Rangari
11)	Pharmacognosy & Phytochemistry (Volume - II)	:Dr. Vinod Rangari
12)	Pharmaceutical Microbiology (Experiments and Techniques)	:Dr. C. R. Kokare
13)	Pathophysiology for Pharmacy	:Dr. Prakash Ghadi
14)	Introduction to Clinical Biochemistry	:Dr. S. P. Dandekar
15)	Principles and Applications of Biopharmaceutics and Pharmacokinetics	:Dr. H. P. Tipnis & Dr.Amrita Bajaj
16)	Business Accounting	:Dr. Mahesh Kulkarni
17)	Managerial Economics	:S. D. Geet, V. V. Morajkar & M. P. Wagh
18)	Industrial Psychology and Sociology	:Dr.Milind Wagh
19)	Practical Physical Pharmacy	:Dr.H.N. More & A.A Hajare
20)	Textbook of Pharmaceutical Analysis III (As per RGTU,Bhopal)	:Narendra Pratap,Sengar, Agarwal & Mrs. Singh
21)	Introduction to Pharmaceutics (For B.Pharm)	:Dr. Atmaram Pawar
22)	Clinical Pharmacy	:Dr. H. P. Tipnis & Dr. Amrita Bajaj
23)	Hospital Pharmacy	:Dr. H.P. Tipnis & Mrs. Amrita Bajaj
24)	A Textbook of Pharmacy Practice	:Dr.K.G.Revikumar & Dr. B.D.Miglani
25)	Vesicular & Particulate Drug Delivery Systems	:Edited by Prof.R.S.R.Murthy.
26)	Illustrated Glossary of Mycology	:Prof.Jitendra Vaidya
27)	Community Pharmacy	:Dr.H.P. Tipnis
28)	Spectroscopy	:Dr. D.P. Belsare, Prof. V.S. Kasture

For D.Pharm

1)	Theory and Practice of Pharmaceutics - I	:Dr. A. P. Pawar
2)	Theory and Practice of Pharmaceutics - II	:Dr. A. P. Pawar
3)	Human Anatomy & Physiology	:Rahul Phate
4)	A Textbook of Biochemistry & Clinical Pathology	:Dr. Umekar, Lohiya & Kotagale
5)	Pharmaceutical Chemistry-II (for D.Pharm)	:Dr. A.S. Dhake, Dr. H.P.Tipnis
6)	Introduction to Pharmaceutical Chemistry	:S.K.Banerjee,Mashru & G. Banerjee
7)	Handbook for Community Pharmacists (Exclusively for Chemists & Druggists)	:Dr. Atmaram Pawar

For GPAT study...........

1)	GPAT : A Companion (For Pharmacy)	:N.N. Inamdar
2)	Pharmacy GATE Solved Question Papers	:N.N. Inamdar

Indian Reprints

1)	Managing Pharmaceuticals in International Health (Birkhauser)	:Anderson, Huss, Summers, Wiedenmayer
2)	Drug Metabolism (Springer)	:Caira, Mino R.; Ionescu, Corina (Eds.)
3)	Development and Manufacture of Protein Pharmaceuticals (Kluwer Academic/Plenum Publishers)	:Nail, Steve L.; Akers, Michael J. (Eds.)
4)	Liposomes Methods and Protocols (Humana Press)	:Basu, Subhash C.; Basu, Manju (Eds.)
5)	Drug Absorption Studies	:Carsten Ehrhardt
6)	Drug Delivery Systems	:Kewal Jain
7)	Polivinylpyrrolidone Excipients for Pharmaceuticals	:V.Buhler
8)	Chiral Separations	:G. Gobitz,Martin Schmid
9)	Optimization in Drug Discovery	:Zhengyin, Gary Caldwell
10)	Fundamentals of Clinical Research	:Bacchieri
11)	Modeling in Biopharmaceutics, Pharmacokinetics, and Pharmacodynamics	:Panos Macheras, Athanassios Iiiadis
12)	Biorelated Polymers	:Edited By: Emo Chiellini, Helena Gil, Gerhart Braunegg, Johanna Buchert, Paul Gatenholm and Maarten van der Zee
13)	Biopharmaceutical Drug Design and Development	:Edited By : Wu-Pong, Susanna, Rojanasakul, Yon
14)	New Approaches To Drug Development	:Edited By : P. Jolles

PREFACE TO THIRD EDITION

Pharmaceutical sciences and Pharmacy practice are the two main streams of pharmacy education worldwide. Pharmaceutical science has been taught in Indian universities since inception of the pharmacy education in 1930's. Due to industry-oriented curriculum, Indian Pharma sector has been growing in leaps and bounds and presently ranks fourth in the world. However, another equally important area Pharmacy Practice remained unopened. It is patient-oriented pharmaceutical service, which deals with patient care, placing emphasis on drug therapy. In developed countries, patient service has been the prime focus of this profession and consequently it has gained the status of topmost noble profession.

Publication of the patient-oriented book Modern Dispensing Pharmacy in February 2004, was an experiment based on the concrete logic and vision that not only resulted in a new pharmacy subject of pharmacy curriculum, but created a novel thought that can help Indian pharmacy graduates to keep pace with time. Due to the patient oriented view that is given to the dispensing pharmacy, during the period of its four years, Modern Dispensing Pharmacy has been accepted as a concept and included in the syllabi of many Indian universities. The valuable comments like '... Something was missing in the dispensing pharmacy due to which this subject was thought to be outdated from Pharmacy curriculum in India but this book has added value and now dispensing will never die...' have motivated us to give better.

In the changing global scenario, pharmacy curriculum in India is also focusing on patient care services. The introduction of six years Pharm.D programme by Pharmacy Council of India, from October 2008, is the vital step in this regard. We are fortunate that through Modern Dispensing Pharmacy we could contribute to the new pharmacy programme.

The Third edition is improved by adding more topics on patient care like, Good Pharmacy Practice, Art of dispensing, Therapeutic incompatibility, etc. The topics related to pharmaceutical sciences like extraction, sterilisation and unit operations have been deleted. This third edition will be more precise and an easy to elaborate concept of dispensing pharmacy.

We express thanks to all the teachers, students and professionals for their comments and suggestions. We offer sincere thanks to staff of Career Publications, specially Nishad Deshmukh and Mrs. Arundhati Jadhav for their technical support.

Date: 11/11/2008   Dr. Atmaram Pawar
Pune   Dr. R.S. Gaud

PREFACE TO FIRST EDITION

The scientific and technological advances in the development of drug and their dosage form, attempt to achieve self sufficiency to meet national need of medicines and vision to develop pharma industry, have led to tremendous growth in pharmaceutical industry in India. The diminished practice of compounding, coupled with ready-to-use manufactured formulations has changed the role of the pharmacist. However, the pharmacy profession is categorised mainly as manufacturers and traders of medicinal products. Besides several factors, negligence of the patient care as a part of curricula has increased the gap between the pharmacist and the patient. Till today, the dispensing pharmacy has been considered as just lab scale manufacturing of dosage forms and it is taught in view of production.

Over the last decade, pharmacy has become a focal point for global health policy framework. The pharmacist, by providing pharmaceutical health care, is serving the society. In addition to inclusion of hospital and community pharmacy, curriculum of dispensing pharmacy fortified with the concept of Patient Medication Record (PMR), Pharmacist Consultation and Patient Counselling can be used as a measure tool to turn the pharmacist from Pharma Trader to Health Care Provider. Modern Dispensing Pharmacy has been articulated by preserving the basics of art of compounding and adding modern concepts of dispensing pharmacy.

The main objective of the book Modern Dispensing Pharmacy is to guide the budding pharmacists to accept the challenge of transition of pharmacy profession from 'pharma traders' to 'pharmaceutical health care' approach, to provide a platform to pharma educators to teach dispensing pharmacy with a focus on the patient, to distinguish between industrial pharmacy and dispensing pharmacy and to co-relate the dispensing of compounded and the proprietary products.

Modern Dispensing Pharmacy has been organised in four distinct sections. The first section is an introductory part. It covers development of pharmacy, the role of the pharmacist as health care provider, prescription writing and prescription handling, art of compounding, concepts of dispensing pharmacy. Specific attention has been given to patient counselling and pharmacist consultation and use of pictograms. Concept of dosage form design highlights in brief the principle and methodology of formulation, including incompatibility, unit operations in compounding, selection of containers, etc. An attempt has been made to modernise the concept of incompatibility.

The second section is devoted to the various dosage forms. It includes compounding and dispensing of all non-sterile dosage forms, namely, liquid, semisolid and solid dosage forms. Special attention is given to dispensing pharmacy as patient oriented practice rather than just compounding oriented. Some of the features of Modern Dispensing Pharmacy are as follows:

- Method of compounding

  .Principle in depth to explain formulation, point wise method of compounding, selection of container, storage and label conditions and co-relation with proprietary preparations.

- Considers actual practice of dispensing

  Every dosage form is supported with instructions to the pharmacist explaining signs of instability of the product for proactive or corrective measures required, if any. The patient counselling and pharmacist consultation deals with indications – contraindications, method of administration and general advice for direction to use and storage conditions for both compounded and manufactured dosage forms.

- Diagrammatic presentation of principles, methods of compounding, methods for drug administration.

- Exclusive notes on common therapy such as antacids, expectorants, skin care, etc.

The third section is concerned with the dispensing aspects of novel drug delivery systems and sterile products. It considers the merits and demerits and in-depth method of drug administration. It includes oral CDDS, inhalers, rotahalers, TDDS, small volume parenterals, large volume parenterals. and insulin administration.

The fourth section is devoted to general pharmacy. It includes principle and methods to produce and preserve the galenical preparations such as extracts, aromatic water, etc. The 14th chapter deals with ligature and sutures.

In addition to point wise and schematic presentation, the description of every point is summarised under Concept Clear. It facilitates the subject understanding of the student.

The theory and practice of dispensing cannot be separated. The success of the practice of the compounding and dispensing of dosage form is real reflection of crystal clear understanding of the theory. Every dosage form is enriched with the maximum number of prescriptions for practical course. Every preparation is explained as : principle, compounding, container, storage, label, precaution during compounding and patient counselling. To promote use of pictograms, a sticker sheet of pictograms is enclosed herewith in the book.

The book Modern Dispensing Pharmacy is presented in a proper sequence, keeping pace for easy understanding of concept. To cover the syllabus of various universities, the number of prescriptions has reached high. Therefore, the prescriptions should be selected as per university syllabus. Some of the prescriptions are more logical to teach at a higher level of the course, e.g. as part of industrial pharmacy. Patient counselling and pharmacist consultation should be demonstrated during practical hours.

The authors would appreciate criticism, suggestions and comments, both from academic and professional pharmacists. Authors would be grateful if any deficiency or error is brought to their attention.

Authors wish to express their gratitude to Prin. Dr. Shivajirao Kadam, Pro-vice Chancellor and Dr. K.R. Mahadik, Dean, Bharati Vidyapeeth Deemed University, Pune for providing motivation and environment to Dr. Pawar for writing this book. Thanks are also due to Prof. A. R. Paradkar, who has shared his thoughts regarding patient focused teaching of dispensing pharmacy.

We are sincerely thankful to LiTaka Pharmaceuticals, Nu-Life Pharmaceuticals, T-Walker's Pharmaceuticals, Sanjivani Remedies, Miaami Pharma and Chemicals, all Pune, and Amrut Pharmaceuticals, Belgaum for permitting to mention photographs of their products in this book. We are also thankful to Suvida Medicals, Pune for their co-operation in selecting proprietary preparations.

We express our thanks to the team of Career Publications, specially Nishad Deshmukh, Milind Wagh and Mukesh for bringing out this book in its present form in a short period of time. We offer sincere thanks to Mr. Badodekar and Mr. Pradhan for editing this book and Atul Bhalero for drawing illustrations.

Thanks are also due to our colleagues and family members for the co-operation and patience during the process of book writing.

Date : 5.2.2004   Dr. R.S.Gaud

New Delhi   Dr. Atmaram Pawar

Contents

1 Pharmacist : A Health Care Provider

PHARMACIST

Pharmacists, as professionals, have been involved in many activities and thus perform multiple roles in the service of mankind in the way of producing and providing medicines. Some of these roles are:

Pharmacy Education

Any profession starts with a knowledge provider, a teacher, and the pharmacy profession is no exception. Pharmacy education is divided into different levels, viz., Diploma in Pharmacy (12th Science + two years), Bachelor of Pharmacy (12th Science + four years) and Master of Pharmacy (B.Pharm + two years). Pharm.D, a newer curriculum that focuses on pharmacy practice was recently introduced in India from the academic year 2008-09. This is a major step in pharmacy education that will help to change the image of the Indian pharmacists from 'traders' to 'health care providers'. The six-year professional course (12th Science + five year teaching and one year hospital training) will inculcate knowledge of clinical and community pharmacy. During the course the students have to learn therapeutics, clinical aspects of therapy, adverse drug reactions and interacting with physicians to know about managing diseases, diagnosis and treatment, prescription patterns and therapeutic drug monitoring both of in-patients and out-patients. Pharm.D (post-baccalaureate) programme will provide opportunity for B.Pharm students (B.Pharm + 3 years) to choose their career in pharmacy practice. The 4th, 5th and 6th year of Pharm.D. curriculum is common syllabus for post-baccalaureate programme.

Thus, pharmacy education can be divided in two classes, viz., pharmaceutical sciences and pharmacy practice. Bachelor of Pharmacy and Masters in Pharmacy are more industry and research oriented, whereas Diploma in Pharmacy, Pharm.D and M. Pharm and Ph. D in Pharmacy practice are patient oriented.

Role of Pharmacists

Many of the pharmacy graduates and postgraduates today, are serving society through this respected field.

1) Research and development : Research and development in pharmaceutical sciences in now not only confined to finding new drug molecules or to improve effectiveness of the existing drugs, but it has been expanded in various areas such as clinical research, novel drug delivery, drug targeting, nano pharmaceuticals, biotechnology, bioinformatics, etc. Pharmacists, owing to a blend of their biological and technical knowledge, can undertake a crucial role in R&D for better patient care.

2) Bulk drug manufacturing : Manufacturing of active pharmaceutical ingredients (API) from chemical, biological, synthetic or semi-synthetic sources.

3) Industrial pharmacy : It involves formulation development and conversion of active pharmaceutical ingredient (API) into suitable dosage form. This activity is further divided into production, packaging, storage, quality assurance and quality control.

4) Pharmaceutical marketing : It is an effort to reach the medicaments to the doorstep of patients, via a chain of distributors and retail pharmacies. Here marketing representatives act as liaison between physician and retail pharmacist. Their role cannot be counted in terms of sale only, but also by how they market concepts of bioavailability, bioequivalence, pharmacovigilance, patient compliance, safety and effectiveness of a medicine.

5) Wholesale distribution : Distribution of medicinal products is assured by wholesale distributors and recognised stockists. They distribute the medicines to retail pharmacists. They are required to contribute to the function of the public health services by complying with certain regulations ensuring reliability, safety, proper warehousing and rapidity of supply. However,in India, this business is mainly run by non-pharmacists. Pharmacists, due to their basic knowledge in storage and stability of drugs, can play a better role in this area.

6) Community pharmacy : Pharmacists directly interacting with the community are no other than retail pharmacists running medical stores. Almost 80 per cent of them serve the community through this profession.

7) Hospital pharmacy : It is that branch of pharmacy, where pharmacists are directly involved in in-patient care. Hospital pharmacists accompany doctors taking rounds in the hospital wards and help them in prescription writing and therapeutic drug monitoring. They get the opportunity to promote rational drug prescribing and can work as members of policy-making committees concerned with selection of drugs, use of antibiotics, controlling infections, recommending essential drugs, etc. Pharmacists also work as team members for clinical trails held in their hospitals.

8) Clinical pharmacy : It is a more specialised extension of community or hospital pharmacy, where pharmacists play a role in giving pharmaceutical advice on prescription writing, treatment strategies, treatment monitoring, checking the prescriptions on the basis of clinical aspects, monitoring for any adverse drug reactions, minimising potential drug interactions and patient counselling. There has been an alarming increase in cases of chronic diseases in India. Many of these co-exist and need multiple drug interventions and continued medical and pharmaceutical care. In developed countries, super-specialist pharmacists like paediatric pharmacists, pharmacists specialised in oncology or in respiratory care, and many others, are providing health care services.

9) Patient education : Presently, treatment of diseases is not only counted in terms of pharmacological response to drugs, but more emphasis is laid on patient compliance and proper use of drug delivery system or devices for drug delivery. Pharmaceutical companies involved in respiratory care, diabetic care and oncology have a separate team of representatives for patient education. It is an upcoming area in pharmaceutical marketing.

10) Clinical studies : Checking the quality of medicines on the basis of *in vitro* studies is no longer a reliable tool, but they should also have desirable pharmacokinetic properties, bioequivalence properties and safety. The clinical trials of a new drug and bioequivalence studies of new formulations are the two major activities in this regard.

11) Health insurance : Since pharmacists know about diseases, drugs, doses, drug delivery system and drug brands and their trade, they have been providing services for auditing health insurance claims.

12) Regulatory affairs : In the era of globalisation, the regulatory field is not restricted only to the drug inspectors and Food and Drug Administration (FDA), but every pharmacy unit has its own regulatory affair department (RAD), which looks after matters related to domestic licensing, patents and foreign regulations for exports.

13) Pharma journalism : Pharmacists can provide authentic and reliable information about drugs and diseases. Publishing relevant articles in various print media like journals, magazines, newspapers, etc., may play a crucial role in making the patients familiar and comfortable with drug use.

Concept Check : Role of Pharmacist

- Education : Pharmaceutical sciences : B. Pharm, M. Pharm, Ph. D.
- Practice of Pharmacy : D. Pharm, Pharm D., M. Pharm, Ph. D.
- Pharma education, R&D, Bulk drug manufacturing, Industrial pharmacy, Pharmaceutical marketing, Wholesale distribution, Health insurance, Hospital Pharmacist, Community Pharmacist, Patient education, Clinical studies, Regulatory affairs, Pharma Journalism.

PHARMACY PRACTICE IN INDIA

Good health is the requirement of all individuals, which is an added dimension to the commonly called basic needs, *'Anna, Vastra, Nivara'* (food, clothes and shelter). Secondly, a healthy community is the infrastructure of a nation, which is the key factor for its economical development. Fortunately, today's India is considered as 'A country of Youths', and since this is a state of healthiness, economists say that India is the one of the healthiest countries. However, if we study the social and health scenario of India, till date, people suffer from infectious diseases like tuberculosis, filariasis, etc. A class of population, that lives in modern and ultra modern townships, suffers diseases born from modern life-styles, like diabetes and hypertension. One class of society is deprived of the minimum health facility, whereas others are taking quality treatments in hospitals with state-of-art facilities. Wide disparities exist in public health facilities and health standards in different parts of the country and between inter- and intra-socio-economic groups.

Though health is a state of complete physical, mental and social well-being, and not merely absence of any illness, people confine its definition to illnesses only and consider a physician as the only community helper who can take care of them. Medical practitioners perform both,diagnosis of diseases and dispensing of medicines, where as the role of pharmacists is overlooked. As a result, access to medicines is nominal and drug treatments are grossly inadequate.

Chemists and Druggists, Medicals, Medical Stores or Pharmacy, and recent names like Medicine Shoppe, are the places where patients get medicines. These are commonly known as retail pharmacies, where all the licensed medicines, health care products and surgical items are stocked, exhibited and sold to consumers or patients by a professionally qualified person, that is, a registered pharmacist, on prescription and without prescription, when legally permitted.

Depending on the qualification, we have three types of registered pharmacists, viz., a) those registered before enforcement of the Pharmacy Act with only experience as the criterion, b) 10th + 2 years diploma or 12th + directly second year of diploma followed by training and c) according to ER 91, (12th science) + 2 year diploma followed with practical training in a community pharmacy or a hospital pharmacy. Pharmacy graduates rarely opt for the profession of community pharmacists.

The registration of pharmacists and professional health related activities of pharmacies are under the control of Pharmacy Council of India. India has nearly 7,00,000 registered pharmacists with 30,000 per year being added. We have about 5.6 pharmacists per 1000 people and approximately one pharmacist per physician. In 1940, when the Drugs and Cosmetics

---

Pharmacist : A Health Care Provider

Act was enacted, there were a lot more of compounding and dispensing activities in retail pharmacies than today. Nowadays, the basic job performed by the retail pharmacists is just prescription filling (dispensing). They are not required to maintain patient medication records. Information on drugs is provided only on patient's request. Pharmacies and hospitals do not provide patient counselling in the usual situation.

Pharmaceutical care is an evolutionary way of practicing pharmacy, but it requires considerable rethinking about what they have been practicing. In one of the reports, WHO states, "Effective medicine can be practiced only where there is efficient drug management." The complete health care would not be complete unless all healthcare partners, such as pharmacists, nurses and the social groups, which are directly, or indirectly, involved in the community health, make their contribution.

PHARMACEUTICAL HEALTH CARE

'Pharmaceutical Care', A new philosophy of pharmacists is based on two fundamental aspects, i.e., dispensing pharmaceutical products and services ensuring maximum benefit and minimum risk to the patient; and accepting the total responsibility of drug therapy outcomes. According to this philosophy, a pharmacist should as certain all the medicines that a patient is taking, from whatever sources, and assess them for reasonableness and effectiveness in the light of the patient's condition, develop a care plan and follow up the progress of the patient on regular basis (Adepu, et al., 2002).

In developed countries, community pharmacists are a basic unit of health care, which acts as liaison between patients and physicians. Unlike Indian pharmacists, they not only concentrate on trade, but also represent a readily available health care resource for helping medical problems including therapeutic drug monitoring related to long-term treatment of chronic diseases. They do not merely read and supply medicines, but also understand the prescription and the patient. As a part of patient counselling, the pharmacists provide drug related information, identify and solve drug-drug and drug-food interactions and adverse drug reactions. They ensure dosage compliance and support the treatment with clinical inputs. In summary, they take overall responsibility of the outcome of the drug therapy. Therefore, Pharmacists are most accepted among the professionals and have been receiving very high social and monitory rewards. More surprisingly, majority of these pharmacists have graduated from Indian universities and grown in Indian culture.

The pharmacies are established for definite populations. All patients and consumers of OTC drugs and cosmetics, purchase their items from that pharmacy. Pharmacies maintain the medical history of every patient and also his address, phone number and e-mail ID. In emergency, it helps a lot to serve an individual within a couple of minutes. In case of any adverse reaction, the patient calls the pharmacist before the physician. The system of communication, called as 'HOT LINK', is so rapid, that the information of any new adverse drug reactions reaches every corner of the country within few minutes.

Seven Star Pharmacists : The WHO in a report of its consultative group on Preparing Future Pharmacist (1997) identified 'Seven Star Pharmacist' concept that explains the endless activities of pharmacists. They are as follows:

i)   Care-giver to provide caring services to an individual and the population.

ii) Communicator to establish proper link between the physician and the patient, closer support for prescribers and medicine management.

iii) Manager to manage health resources and information effectively.

iv) Decision-maker for the appropriate, efficacious and cost effective use of health resources.

v)   Leader to lead multi-disciplinary team including other health care providers.

vi) Life-long learner, undergoing continuous education and keeping himself updated with recent developments in health care, to perform his task. He should be involved in research and development taking place in the field of pharmacy.

vii) Teacher to educate next generation pharmacists and train other professionals, like nurses.

Concept Clear :   Pharmaceutical Care

- Health: Complete physical, mental and social well-being of an individual or group.
- Pharmacy profession is expanding rapidly in areas like dispensing of medication, home care services, health screening, patient counselling, etc., and are also recognised as health care providers.
- Pharmaceutical Care, a new philosophy based on dispensing of pharmaceutical products and providing services for the maximum benefit of the patient, and accepting the total responsibility of drug therapy outcomes.
- Seven Star Pharmacist concept: Care-giver, Communicator, Manager, Decision–maker, Leader, Life-long learner and Teacher.

ROLE OF COMMUNITY PHARMACISTS

According to the changed scenario, the expanded functions of community pharmacists as health care provider in India are as follows :

1. Architecture of the modern dispensing pharmacy : The schedule N of the Drugs and Cosmetics Act 1940, gives information about architecture and working of pharmacy. The minimum space requirement to run a pharmacy as per the Act is about 12 m².

Adequate area should be available for providing full-fledged dispensing services. In the absence of privacy, patients often hesitate to discuss their health problems. A separate consultation cabin in the pharmacy is sufficient to serve as a confidential area. A space for display of health promotion information should be provided and kept-well maintained and updated regularly. A suitable layout, with ramps for easy access for disabled customers should be taken care of. A safe policy, with instruction of 'no smoking', should be adopted.

2. Family pharmacists : The concept of Family Physician is not new to the Indian community. Going one-step ahead, pharmacists have to develop their image as Family Pharmacist. The Patient Medication Record (PMR) is one of the keys to initiate this and PMR should be maintained for each individual. This is beneficial to avoid drug-drug interactions that are possible due to multi-therapy from two or more physicians or simultaneous administration of OTC and prescription drugs. Information about health history, allergic reactions, etc., help to make pharmacists Family Pharmacist, where patients take all their medicines from the same shop. Employing women pharmacists is advisable because women patients hesitate to state their problems to male pharmacists.

3. Dispensing of medication : Pharmacists should thoroughly evaluate the prescription. Instructions related to use and storage of medicines help the patients to adhere to their medication and in turn get maximum benefit from their medicines. Use of patient information leaflets in vernacular language, with pictograms, is an effective way to educate them. The pharmacist can also develop a handy and useful patient information leaflet using his therapeutic knowledge and available drug information from various sources. The PMR should be updated by noting patient's current progress.

4. Patient counselling : Patient counselling is the most widely recognised function of the pharmacist while dispensing medication. One-to-one interaction with the patient can thoroughly assess the patient's knowledge and improve understanding about the therapy. Patients with chronic conditions such as heart diseases or asthma should have formal regular reviews with the pharmacist. This improves pharmacists' responsibility for issuing repeat prescriptions.

5. Avail clinical services : In developed countries, about 28 per cent of hospital admissions are due to drug-induced reactions. In India such data is not available, but definitely the figure would be many times more. Retail pharmacists can play a key role in improving the patient's medication adherence, identifying the possible drug interactions and monitoring and reporting adverse drug reactions.

Modern Dispensing Pharmacy

6. Health screening services : The qualified and trained pharmacists should have liaison with medical practitioners for providing health-screening services to patients. Such services include blood glucose estimation, recording blood pressure, estimation of cholesterol and calculating body mass index in obese patients and advising them to reduce weight. Pharmacists can advice on following healthy lifestyles and provide tips for the same. Providing health-screening services will enhance the image of the pharmacist as a professional.

7. Treating common ailments : As and when possible and permissible, the pharmacists can give basic treatment, such as providing OTC drugs in case of common cold and headaches or contraceptives, etc.

8. Individualisation of Drug Therapy (IDT) : The general classification of patients as infant, paediatric, adult and geriatric will not be sufficient in the near future for deciding drug therapy. Every individual is unique with different lifestyles, mental status, stress and strain experienced and uniqueness in functioning of organs and secretions of different glands. Though today it is a dream, the progress made in Information Technology (IT) and stem cell and gene therapy will enable physicians and patient counsellors to achieve the implementation of IDT.

9. Home care services : Pharmacists should extend their services to geriatric patients and bed ridden patients. Here they should supply medicines, advise and develop dosing protocol to improve the quality of life and outcomes of treatment. Such services are also beneficial to patients who have been recently discharged from hospital.

10. Access to medicine : Since the pharmacist is involved right from the birth of medicine, i.e., manufacturing, to distribution, dispensing, and even administration, his services can be better utilised in this respect. Better patient advice, round the clock services and efficient procurement and distribution systems would definitely improve the access to medicine. With the help of medication reviews in nursing homes, especially these of high-risk groups, pharmacists can develop a treatment protocol, especially for therapy of chronic cases, and review patients on multiple therapy.

11. Reduce substandard medicines : A transparent procurement procedure, assurance to purchase high quality medicines, reduction in time period required to transport medicines from manufacturers' quarantine to a medical shop and the right inventory control, are the different ways to reduce substandard medicines. Development of drug formulary with consultation of prescribers in that area, developing PACT (prescribing analysis and cost) report and guiding doctors for cost-effective prescribing, can also indirectly reduce substandard medicines.

12. Professional relationship : The lack of scientific knowledge, failure to keep oneself updated with advances in drug therapy and the very big number of formulations (about 90,000) available in the Indian market, are the main reasons of irrational prescriptions. The medical practitioners do not generally have access to unbiased information, and rely heavily upon the pharmaceutical industry for prescribing information. The practicing pharmacists should extend their professional role by helping the physician in selection of the proper brand of drug. Pharmacists are best positioned to support cost-effective prescribing. As the pharmacists have necessary knowledge of quality and cost of medicines, at a strategic level, they can appraise the evidence and make recommendations for the medicines, which account for 80 per cent of all prescriptions in primary care.

13. Drug information services : The pharmacist should have complete information regarding the standard therapeutic procedures, alternative therapies and adverse drug reactions. Printed literature, different database systems and on-line information are the main sources of current information. CIMS is widely used drug index in Indian medical stores. State pharmacy councils also run drug information centers. The USP-DI is an official drug index that can be used by pharmacists. Drug related information should be provided to physicians and patients for betterment of health. Millions of people visit a Pharmacy each day, thus the Pharmacist is one of the best professionals to improve access of people to medicine and to provide them health promotion information.

14. Nutrition Counsellor : Food pharmacy is emerging as a new branch of pharmacy, where community pharmacy can make significant contributions by advising patients about basic food needs, suggesting special diet instructions for diabetics and people with food allergies. On the other hand, foods can also have pharmacological action and hence can be used as supplementary to drugs. For example, Onion is useful in lowering blood pressure, preventing the platelets sticking together, or dissolving blood clots.

15. Women welfare and infant care : Women go through different stages throughout their lives and many changes also occur during the initial 5 years of a child's age. Pharmacists who understand the normal course of pregnancy and infancy and who know about drug actions and toxicity, can guide them in matters of drug use. Community pharmacists can encourage breast feeding and can guide mothers to properly immunise children according to schedule. In addition, they can counsel patients about family planning and prevention of sexually transmitted diseases.

16. Health Insurance Adviser : With improved lifestyles, the Indian population is becoming health conscious. Knowledge about diseases, drug therapy, pharmacology, drug delivery systems and trading of medicines make pharmacists ideal professionals for health insurance business. This role of pharmacists is not only beneficial for insurance companies to settle the bills, but positive input by pharmacists would definitely assure proper and essential drug treatment.

17. Continuing education : Continuing professional development programmes will help pharmacists learn the pharmaceutical care concepts and train them to offer better services to the patients. Since a single Pharmacist will not be able to sell items, as well as counsel the patients, in a busy shop, all the staff should be adequately trained. Pharmacists have to organise and attend seminars on various issues like drug therapy, adverse effects, etc.

18. Participation in social work and in national health programmes : To ensure rational use of medicines, pharmacists should organise educational activities for health care providers. In addition to this, they should actively participate in health promotion campaigns such as tobacco cessation, alcohol quitting, family planning, vaccination, diabetic therapy, asthma therapy, AIDS prevention, etc.

Concept Clear : **Role of Community Pharmacists**

- Architecture of Modern Dispensing Pharmacy.
- Dispensing of medication.
- Pharmacists' consultancy
- Pharmacist consultation
- Treating common ailments.
- Individualisation of drug therapy.
- Drug information services.
- Health Insurance Adviser
- Continuous education.
- Women welfare and infant care

- Family Pharmacist
- Patient counselling.
- Avail clinical services.
- Health screening services.
- Home care services.
- Professional relationship.
- Access to medicine.
- Reduce substandard medicines.
- Nutrition counsellor
- Social and national health programmes.

Reasons for Poor Development of Community Pharmacy in India

The integration of pharmacists in dispensing and counselling has not yet been achieved. Drug counselling, drug information, labelling systems and pharmacy therapeutic committees do not exist even in large hospitals. The community services offered in small hospitals and chemist shops is still questionable. The reasons and remedies for poor development of dispensing practices in India are as follows:

---

1. Role of pharmacists : Patient, health care providers and the government have not recognised the role of the pharmacist. They are not aware of what services the pharmacist might or should provide beyond trading of medicines. In hospitals also persons other than pharmacists look after the purchase and inventory of drugs under the supervision of the medical officer of the hospital. The standing committee report of Ministry of Chemicals and Fertilisers in 2002 has already threatened pharmacists, it says "there is no need for pharmacists to sell drugs, but any educated person can be given permission to run the drug store".

2. Continuing education and training : The poor recognition of the role of the pharmacists in health care has been linked with insufficient education and a lack of their professional functioning. The standard of education and or curricula must be upgraded for each level of training to ensure that appropriate and relevant knowledge is imparted. Recently, many universities, after realising the concept of pharmacy practice, have introduced pharmacy practice subjects like clinical pharmacy, hospital pharmacy and community pharmacy. Besides, modernising the curriculum, upgradation in teaching methods and professionalism of the educator is a major contributing factor for the pharmacist to perform his role as health care provider. For instance, though the ER 91 for D.Pharm is a modern syllabus comprising of modern concepts of dispensing, health care and community pharmacy, it is still taught theoretically and in an old fashion (IJPER 40 (4), 2006). A pharmacist who holds a diploma, runs almost all retail pharmacies in India.

Whether the pharmacist is diploma or degree holder, there is no patient-focused training and compulsion for continuous professional development for the practicing pharmacists. Recently, PCI made it mandatory for pharmacists to complete at least two refresher courses within a period of five years. Indian Pharmaceutical Association (IPA) has setup Community Pharmacy Division to train the working pharmacists and to propagate the functioning of Community Pharmacy. In most of the developed countries, basic qualification to practice pharmacy is six years university degree (Pharm.D) and upto two years internship before registration. Periodically, they have to undergo refresher courses to upgrade knowledge.

3. Motivation : Retail pharmacists are the most trusted and most available health care professionals. They have the opportunity to provide one-to-one health care. But today's pharmacists are more interested in trading. They have to take the initiative to implement all kinds of innovations and interventions to change their professional behaviour.

4. Isolation of pharmacist : At both, the government and the public levels, the pharmacy profession is isolated. Though pharmacists are in direct contact with the patient, the patient and administrators are not aware of the role of the pharmacists in improving his health. As part of the curriculum, the degree pharmacists mostly take industrial training and industry related jobs,

---

whereas diploma pharmacists take training in running private medical shops or working in hospital pharmacies.

5. Remuneration for pharmaceutical services : Pharmacists around the world are providing remunerated services such as drug information, medication reviews, medication management, dosage administration, health screening services, immunisation, etc. In 1987, Dr. Vijay Kelkar's committee proposed some fee, 50p and Re.1 per prescription, for day and night, respectively, as service charges. As patient counselling and other services are not legalised in India, pharmacists cannot charge any professional fee. The pharmacists should upgrade their professional image and also simultaneously discuss details of the Kelkar Committee report with the Government. The patient should feel that he is being offered the services he is paying for. A suitable professional fee will motivate the pharmacists to offer pharmaceutical health care to the full extent.

6. Population : In India, 80 per cent of the population lives in rural areas and 80 per cent of the doctors live in urban areas. This is the main reason of poor health care. Large population, low literacy, poor communication between the prescriber and the patient and patient's fear of asking questions, are some of additional public related problems. The training of pharmacists alone is not sufficient for effective functioning of pharmaceutical care. The benefits that can be gained by pharmaceutical care should make the population aware of services that can be offered by Pharmacists. In addition to counselling, pharmacists should take every opportunity to educate a patient. They should encourage patients to ask questions and to speak up during dispensing; more especially, when unusual circumstances occur. In developed countries, majority of patients use one Pharmacy as a Family Pharmacy for their medicines. Thus, Pharmacists have computerised Patient Medication Record to check the accuracy of the new prescription. Therefore, not only prescription drugs, but also OTC medicines must be purchased under the guidance of a particular registered pharmacist.

7. Product focused practice : The pharmacy is the only health profession that is estimated by its sale of product, rather than its contribution towards the society's health.

8. Regulatory control : Pharmacists, as per the prescription of the medical practitioner, dispense the schedule H drugs. The number of OTC products is also not small, but there is no special drug index for such medicines, so these can be dispensed safely for minor ailments. The label or product information leaflet of OTC products should bear information such as – strength and category of medicines, route of administration, maximum dosing period, possible side effects, drug-drug and drug-food interactions, warnings, etc. This information, plus the pharmacist's advice will definitely contribute to proper dispensing of OTC medicines. To encourage the treatment of common ailments, regulatory authorities should increase and monitor OTC drugs. On the contrary, a large number of prescriptions of medicines are stocked and dispensed by medical practitioners. To a larger extent, this practice has escaped strict regulatory controls.

9. Government : The Government's role should ideally, be Thus:

i) Health has top priority on the agenda of any country. In developed countries, 12-14 per cent of GDP is spent on health care; whereas in India, it is just 0.9 per cent. Recently, the Government of India has set up National Commission on Micro Economics and Health to assess the cost and to ensure that the poor get free treatment for 80 per cent of their ailments.

ii) The aim of National Health Policy (NHP) is to take the health services to the doorsteps of the people. As the pharmacist is the only health professional in direct public contact, his role needs to be considered in designing NHP.

iii) Worldwide, the governments of different countries are encouraging further development of the professional role of pharmacists in the field of health promotion and disease prevention. The same should happen in India.

iv) In India, the registration authority, the PCI, has no role in evaluating current knowledge of pharmacists other than their educational qualifications at the time of registration. Though recently, there is a compulsion for continuous professional development for the practicing pharmacists, which includes two refresher courses every five years. But this may not be enough to keep pace with the rapidly growing pharmaceutical technology.

v) Doctors should not be permitted to hold stock of medicines. But, if a pharmacy is not at an approachable distance, then doctors should dispense the medicines. Though, in such cases also, they should purchase only dispensing packs from medical shops and not hold the stock of medicines. In UK, the current legislation states that, when a pharmacy is at a minimum distance of 1.5 km from the patient, then only he can register his name for dispensing from doctors; otherwise, he has to take all the medicines from a pharmacy.

The 'off label' dispensing is another practice that highly contributes for errors in dispensing. To keep the medication 'secret', a doctor dispenses the medicines without any label. Ideally, doctors should disclose the name of the drug and its strength to the patient and it should be mandatory to write the information on the dispensing pack.

vi) USP mentions general chapters such as Good Dispensing Practices, giving guidelines for storage and stability of products for dispensing. According to *USP-24*, the dispensing pharmacists should be qualified and competent persons, who can monitor dispensing procedures, environmental conditions, testing procedures, stability evaluation and documentation during compounding and dispensing of medicines. There is need to take steps to initiate official procedures for its implementation.

- No recognition of pharmacists.
- Lack of motivation.
- No remuneration for pharma services.
- Product focused practice.
- No involvement in NHP and proper utilisation of pharmacist by Government.
- No continuing education.
- Isolation of pharmacists.
- Population and low literacy.
- Regulatory control.

●●●●●

2 Prescription

INTRODUCTION

The prescription (pre = before, *scribo, scriber* = to write) is a requisition written by a registered medical practitioner, requesting the pharmacist to compound and dispense medicines or dispense prefabricated medicines to the patient under his treatment. Prescription is a combined process between the prescriber and the pharmacist, to provide treatment to the patient, utilising their expertise and skill. A Registered Medical Practitioner (Doctor, Dentist, Veterinarian) writes a prescription only after diagnosis of the patient. The Pharmacist interprets the written prescription and makes medicines available to the patient. Prescribing follows a definite pattern in order to facilitate its interpretation and its subsequent noting on a special form, called a prescription blank.

a) Pre-fabricated Product

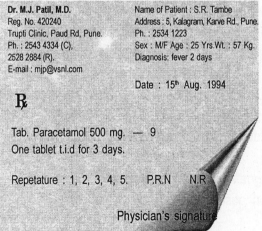

b) Product to be Compounded

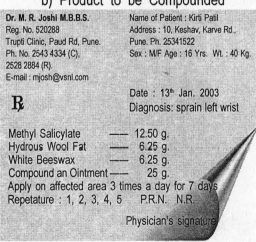

Figure 2.1: Typical Prescriptions

Parts of Prescriptions

The major seven elements of a model prescription are as follows:

1) Patient information: Name, address and age of the patient are necessary so as to avoid delivering the medication wrongly to any other patient. Age and weight of the patient help in checking the dose of the prescribed drugs, especially in the case of paediatric and geriatric patients.

2) Superscription: The symbol ℞, which is the abbreviation of the Latin world *recipe*, meaning 'You take'. Initially it was believed to be the sign of Jupiter, ♃, the God of healing.

3) Inscription: The main part, or the body, of the prescription contains the names and quantities of each ingredient required to compound and dispense products, or the name and quantity of the dosage form. The quantity of ingredients to be compounded in dosage form is expressed in metric system. A physician may ask the pharmacist to dispense an official preparation, without giving its formula in detail.

Prescriptions for compounding contain drug and non-drug components. When a physician prescribes only the name of an active ingredient and asks to compound a dosage form of a particular strength, the pharmacist has to utilise his knowledge to select proper additives and the vehicle.

4) Subscription: It includes directions to the pharmacist by the physician, regarding the dosage form and the number of doses to be compounded and dispensed.

5) Signature (Signa): It is that part of the prescription, which consists of directions to the patient, regarding the dose, route of administration, frequency and time of administration and the vehicle to be used for administration. If the prescriber writes the world 'Label' in the signa, it is an instruction to the pharmacist to mention the name and strength of the prescribed drug on the label. It helps in rapid identification of the medication in emergency, such as, overdose.

6) Refill instruction: It consists of the directions to the pharmacists regarding repetition of the prescription. A physician may advice the pharmacist to re-dispense the medicines against the same prescription when he judges that the patient needs another course of same treatment after particular interval of time. This practice avoids purchasing of large quantities of medicines by the patients and thus their possible misuse of the medication. Though it is beneficial to write refill instructions, especially for chronic therapy, doctors are not familiar with it. The refill directions may be given as:

"repetature - 1 2 (3) 4 5 : Repeat upto a designated number (three times in this case)

"p.r.n." (pro renata)   : Repeat when occasion arises.

"n.r." (non-repetature)   : Do not refill.

The prescription with refill instruction should be given back to the patient. When prescription does not mention any such instructions or mentions n.r., pharmacists should not dispense medicines for more than once against the same prescription. It is legal binding on pharmacists. The refilled prescription must be stamped with the date after each refill.

For example, when a doctor has to prescribe Glimepiride (oral antidiabetic) tablet, to be taken once a day for three months, total making 90 tablets, then he can prescribe for 30 tablets and twice refill. Another interesting example is of Iron preparation for a child of age 3 years for a treatment of three months period.

Restoration of body iron requires a prolonged iron therapy. Therefore, the prescription bears initial dispensing plus two refills. The patient need not visit the physician every month for new prescriptions. The prescriber could have prescribed total dose of 900ml for three months' therapy. But to avoid complications, such as misuse of the drug and chances of improper handling of medicines, he can order two refills. Secondly, the compounded products should be used within one month. The pharmacists have to dispense 300ml of prescribed solution per month for 3 months therapy (300ml × 3 times). But, due to its poor chemical stability, ferrous sulphate solution should be used within two weeks. Therefore, only 150ml of the solution should be dispensed and repeated after every two weeks (150ml × 6 times) instead of 300ml × 3 times. This typical prescription handling involves two refills but six times dispensing.

Prescription

℞

Ferrous Sulphate Solution, BPC.
5 ml b.i.d. for 1 month. — 300 ml
Repetature : 1 (2) 3 4 5 p.r.n n.r

For an infant, the dose of ferrous sulphate solution is 5ml per day, eg. 2.5ml b.i.d. When the dose is less than 5ml, the liquid should be compounded and dispensed after dilution, making a 5ml dose. The diluted preparations also should be used within two weeks. This means that, 150ml of the diluted solution (75ml ferrous sulphate solution diluted to 150ml) should be dispensed for every two weeks. Alternatively, spoon or syringe measuring a 2.5ml dose can be provided.

7) Date and prescribers' signature: The prescription must be dated at the time of writing and also when it is received and filled in the pharmacy. Signature of the prescriber gives authenticity to the prescription. In the case of a prescription for a controlled drug, it must be signed with full name.

Occasionally, pharmacists may have to substitute another brand for the one specified by the physician, if they do not have the prescribed brand in stock. In such cases, pharmacists should consult the concerned physician before dispensing. Sometimes the physicians write 'ARB' (any reliable brand) and the pharmacists can ethically dispense a substitute. The generic prescriptions should be prescribed with manufacturer's name. If no manufacturer is specified, the pharmacists are expected to dispense only a high quality and efficacious brand.

8) Note on diagnosis: Writing a brief note on diagnosis has both, a positive and negative side to it. Most of the prescriptions do not bear this information, it is to avoid self-medication by patients. On the other hand, information about diagnosis helps pharmacists to dispense right medicine in right dose and also give patient counselling. For example, adult dose of albendazole for the treatment of ascariasis, hookworm infections or trichuriasis is 400mg once daily; but in treatment of cystic echinococcosis it may be given in 400mg twice a day for 30 days. Thus, information about diagnosis not only increases confidence of dispensing pharmacists, but also provides opportunity to understand patients, helping better counselling. But noting the diagnosis on prescriptions is not legally mandatory.

Concept Clear : Prescription

Prescription is an order written by a registered medical practitioner, directing the pharmacist to compound and/or dispense a pharmaceutical product to a patient.

Parts of Prescription

- Patient information : Name, address, age, wt.
- Inscription : Formula or dosage form
- Sign : Direction to patient
- Date and sign of Prescriber
- Superscription : Symbol
- Subscription : Directions to pharmacist
- Refill instruction : Repetature, p.r.n., n.r

Types of Prescription

1) Central Government Health Scheme prescription (CGHS): These prescriptions are for those who come under the health scheme of the government. These are not charged, but levy charges may be taken. After dispensing the medicines, prescriptions are sent to the accounts section for pricing. The prescription bears common information, and a column for pricing.

2) Private prescription: Prescriptions are fully charged. These bear the same format as Figure 2.1. Except for drugs of controlled class, these prescriptions are returned to the patient.

3) Hospital prescription: a) Inpatient prescription: Prescriptions for inpatients are written on the physician's order form. The physician order forms are prepared in multiple copies for utilisation in the pharmacy, in the nursing station and to attach to the patient medication record. The prescription bears information regarding hospital name, ward number, period of stay, date and time of admission and discharge of patient. The prescription should provide space to note the

---

time of drug administration and a column to keep record of change in therapy with the prescribers' initials. After discharge of the patient, these prescriptions are filed with the patient medication records.

Prescriptions are fully charged, or not charged, depending on the provision of the health scheme. The charges may be included in hospital charges at the time of discharge. Medicines are usually prescribed in one week or for 15 days doses.

b) Outpatient prescriptions: Format of prescription is the same as that of private prescriptions. These are charged or uncharged prescriptions as per health scheme. Usually, medicines are supplied in quantities sufficient up till the next appointment. Record of prescriptions should be included in the patient's medication record.

4) Veterinary prescription: The prescription written for an animal should state the type of animal, weight, breed and colour along with name and detailed address of the owner. For example-

Animal: Dog   Breed: Alsatian

Name of owner: Miss Riti Khanna   Weight: 20 Kg

Address: 12 Raj Heights,

Thakur Chal, Mumbai.

Language of Prescription Writing

Today prescriptions are preferably written in English with metric system of measures. Some Latin abbreviations are still used in prescribing the dose because:

1) It is the language of medical sciences throughout the world and therefore it is well understood by both the physicians and the pharmacists.

2) The meaning of the pharmaceutical Latin terms remains the same in any part of the civilised world with very negligible chance of misinterpretation.

3) It assures some secrecy regarding the medication prescribed, which is necessary to avoid self medication by the patient.

4) It is very convenient for the busy practitioner to use abbreviated Latin terms.

However, in current practice, it is outdated to use Latin and imperial systems to write prescriptions. It is considered as a minimum knowledge so that if anyone looking at old formulae may need at least a rudimentary understanding of the prescription.

The most frequently used Latin terms and abbreviations are summarised in Table 2.1.

Table 2.1: Latin Terms and Abbreviations

Abbreviation	Latin Term	Meaning	Abbreviation	LatinTerm	Meaning
a	*ante*	Before	a.a.	*ana*	Of each
a.j.	*ante jentaculum*	Before breakfast	a.c.	*ante cibos*	Before meals
a.p.	*ante pronium*	Before dinner	d.	*dies*	A day
i.c.	*Inter cibos*	During meal	in. d.	*In dies*	Daily
p.c.	*Post cibos*	After meal	n.	*nocte*	At night
h.s.	*Hora somni*	At bed time	m.	*Mane*	Morning
a.m.	*ante meridium*	Before noon	stat.	*statim*	Immediately
p.m.	*post meridium*	After noon	b.i.d.	*bis in die*	Twice a day
s.o.s.	*si opus sit*	If necessary	t.i.d.	*Ter in die*	3 times a day
p.r.n.	*Pro re nata*	when necessary	q.i.d	*Quarter in die*	4 times a day
alt.hrs.	*alternis horis*	Alternate hours	omn.	*Omni*	Every
dol. urg.	*Dolore urgente*	When pain is severe	tuss. urg.	*Tussi urgente*	In troublesome cough
Rx	*Recipe*	Take	co.	*compositus*	Compound
ft.	*Fiat*	To make	mitt.	*Mitte*	Send
div.	*Divide*	Divide	p.aeq.	*partes aequales*	Equal parts
ss	*Semis*	Half	c	*Cum*	With
ad.	*ad*	Up to	sum.	*Sumendus*	To be taken
Capiend	*Capiendus*	To be taken	m. dict.	*Modo dicto*	As directed
aq.	*aqua*	Water	m. pres.	*Modo prescripto*	As prescribed
aq. bull.	*aqua bulliens*	Boiling water	e. lacte	*E. lacte*	With milk
aq. dest.	*aqua destillata*	Distilled water	u. utend.	*Utendus*	To be used
ex. aqua.	*ex aqua*	In water	cap.	*Capiat*	Let him take
n.r., non rep	*Non repetature*	Do not repeat	app.	*applicandum*	To be applied
sec.art.	*Secundum artem*	With pharmaceutical skill	agit	*agita*	Shake, stir.
			p.o.	*Per os*	By mouth
coch.	*cochlear*	A spoonful	q.s.	*Quantum sufficiat*	As sufficient
coch. amp.	*cochlear amplum*	one table-spoonful (15 ml)	coch. med.	*cochlear medium*	one desert-spoonful (8 ml)
coch. mag.	*cochlear magnum*		coch. mod.	*cochlear modicum*	
coch. min.	*cochlear minimum*	one tea spoonful (4 ml)	gtt.	*guttae*	A drop
			o.	*octarius*	A pint.
coch. parv.	*cochlear parvum*		gr.	*grana*	A grain

Honour of Prescription

In India various systems of medicine exist viz., Allopathic, Homoeopathic, Ayurvedic, Siddha and Unani. As per the law, a medical practitioner from one system of medicine can neither practice, nor prescribe, medicines from another system of medicine. Therefore, registered pharmacists should not honour/dispense allopathic medicines prescribed by doctors of any other system of medicine and medicines of other system prescribed by allopathic practitioners.

Concept Clear : Prescription

Types of Prescription: Central Government Health Scheme prescriptions, private prescriptions, hospital prescriptions, inpatient prescriptions and outpatient prescriptions and veterinary prescriptions.
Language of Prescription: Latin is language of medical sciences, no misinterpretation, easy to use abbreviations, avoids self-medication. Nowadays frequently replaced by English.
Honour of Prescription: Prescriber should recommend medicines only from that system of medicine in which he is expert.

3 Art of Compounding of Medicines

Dispensing Pharmacy is the branch of pharmacy, which is concerned with compounding and distribution of medicaments. It involves reading the prescription, checking it, compounding, packing, labelling and dispensing the products, filing the prescription, patient counselling and preparing and maintaining documents. Thus dispensing pharmacy mainly works in two fields, compounding and dispensing.

Compounding is extemporaneous preparation of a pharmaceutical product according to formula prescribed in the prescription or in the pharmacopoeia. The pharmacist evaluates the formulation for incompatibility, toxicity and stability in the final container.

Dispensing of medication is accurate supply of medicine(s) directly to a patient, checking that the medicines are appropriate for a patient and counselling them on their appropriate use.

Pharmaceutical Manufacturing is large-scale production of pharmaceutical products. The Food and Drug Administration (FDA) must approve the formula of products to be manufactured and the premises for manufacturing. These formulations are thoroughly studied for physicochemical stability. The expiry date on the product indicates the period of drug stability, and it varies from formulation to formulation. A particular industry manufactures and markets their own products, or products are manufactured by one agency and marketed by some other agency. The manufactured products travel through a link of stockists, wholesalers and retailers. Then, in accordance with the prescription, the retail pharmacists dispense medicaments to the consumers.

Today, relatively few prescriptions involve compounding, but the pharmacists must still possess the knowledge and skills of compounding that they formerly did, so that they can prepare special formulations that are called for. Secondly, it helps in understanding of the concepts of dosage forms and its way of administration. The prescription handling for compounded products involves compounding as additional step in the dispensing methodology described in the chapter 'Art of Dispensing of Medicines'.

Concept Clear: Scale of Production

Compounding is extemporaneous preparation of a pharmaceutical product.
Dispensing is the supply of pharmaceutical products to patients.
Manufacturing is large-scale production of pharmaceutical products.

COMPOUNDING

Compounding is extemporaneous preparation of dosage form on receipt of prescription, which involves issuing the raw material, weighing, mixing, filling and finishing of dosage form. Only one prescription should be compounded at a time, paying full attention to the details. Filling more than one prescription at a time may lead to crossover of drugs. Some pharmacists first prepare labels and then compound the prescription; this helps prevent dispensing of an excessive dose, but can also increase chances of misplacing the label.

Steps in compounding:

During compounding, the following steps should be observed:

a) Issue of ingredients

i) Assemble all the ingredients on the left side of a balance in the order of their use.

ii) Pharmacists should read the label on every container at least three times, once while taking the bottle from the shelf, secondly, when the contents are removed during compounding and finally, while returning the bottle to the shelf.

iii) After weighing or measuring each ingredient, the container should be kept on the right side of the balance, which will maintain the mechanical check on the ingredients.

iv) To maintain cleanliness, a white paper is placed under the balance before weighing. While pouring liquid ingredients, care must be taken not to stain the label on the bottle.

v) For greasy or waxy constituents, greaseproof paper should be used. If beaker or dish is used as weighing vessel, the total weight should not exceed 50g.

b) Mixing of Ingredients

i) The ingredients must be handled in such a manner as to prevent their loss during compounding.

ii) Prescription should always be kept with the pharmacist during compounding.

iii) The type of product and the general order of mixing must be clear in the pharmacists' mind before beginning the compounding of prescription.

iv) Pharmacists should always use their technical knowledge and skill to prepare quality medicines in required quantity.

v) In case of prescriptions to be refilled at a later time, certain information should be written on the prescription for guidance. A refilled medication should have the same appearance as that originally dispensed. This avoids any doubts on the part of the customer regarding possibility of an error.

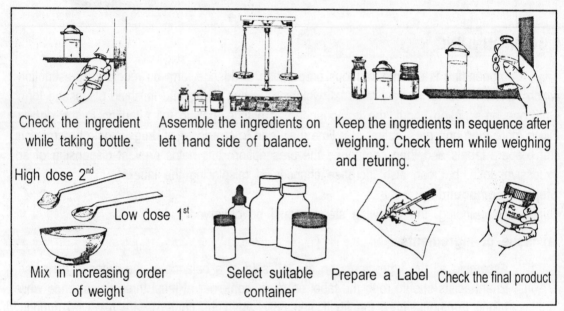

Check the ingredient while taking bottle.

Assemble the ingredients on left hand side of balance.

Keep the ingredients in sequence after weighing. Check them while weighing and returing.

High dose 2nd

Low dose 1st

Mix in increasing order of weight

Select suitable container

Prepare a Label

Check the final product

Figure 3.1: Steps involved in Compounding of Medication

c) Finishing the prescription

The completed prescription represents the highest skill of pharmaceutical profession. The product should be dispensed in a pack that should convey its value to the patient. Finishing of prescription includes (i) selection of container (ii) preparation of label and (iii) checking of the products.

i) **Selection of the container:** The container and closure should not only hold the product, but should also maintain the quality of the filled product and create confidence in the patient regarding its purity. Pharmaceutical containers should protect the contents from contamination with extraneous solids, moisture and microorganisms and maintain the quality, safety and stability of the medicinal product. The design and colour of containers and closures should also serve as a means of identification of the product.

The commonly used containers for compounded dosage forms are summarised in Table 3.1.

Table 3.1: Containers for Compounded Dosage Form

Sr.No.	Dosage Form	Type of Containers
1	Oral liquids, Pediatric drops with calibrated dropper, Draught	Plain, amber, screw-capped, round, glass or plastic bottles.
2	Viscous liquids, honey.	Wide mouthed, screw-capped, plain white glass bottles.
3	Gargles, Mouthwashes, Inhalations, Irrigations, Sprays, Liniments, Lotions, Enemas, Paints.	Fluted, amber, screw-capped, glass or plastic bottles.
4	Ear drops, Nasal drops	Hexagonal, amber, fluted, screw-capped, glass or plastic bottles, supplied/fitted with suitable dropper.
5	Tablets, Capsules, Lozenges, Pills, Bulk powders, Granules, Compressed suppositories, Pessaries.	Screw capped, plain or coloured, glass or plastic jar, or internally-lacquered aluminium jar.
6	Powders containing hygroscopic or volatile ingredients, suppositories.	Double wrapped using wax paper or aluminium foil; stout cardboard boxes with bonded plastic membrane; plastic boxes.
7	Dusting powders	Plastic squeeze bottles, closures should be covered with readily breakable seal.
8	Ointments, Creams, Pastes, Jellies.	Wide-mouthed, screw-capped, plain glass or plastic jars or metal or plastic, flexible tubes, screw caps.
9	Moulded suppositories	Wrapped in foil and packed in amber glass jar/ partitioned boxes.

ii) **Making the label:** A label judges the quality of the dispensed product; therefore it should have an aesthetic appearance and should be selected carefully in relation to the size of the container. Generally, black ink should be used to make labels of preparations for internal use and red ink for preparations for external use.

Label is also source of errors in dispensing. An erroneous label (non-readable, confusing, different name, strength, direction, storage, etc.) or labelling the wrong container, are two major factors which lead to errors. Therefore, labels should always be prepared immediately after reading the prescription and should be applied to the container as soon as it is prepared. The unused labels should be discarded. Same pharmacist should do prescription reading, checking and label preparation.

The compounded preparations must be used within one month. Transfer from original pack to dispensing container, or dilution of product, will reduce its shelf life, which is usually two weeks (recently prepared preparations). Most unstable preparations are freshly prepared and should be used within 24 hours. The compounded products should be labelled with actual date of compounding 'DD-MM-YY' and 'Use before 'DD-MM-YY.'

A label should have the following information:

i)   Type of dosage form (i.e., Mixture, Emulsion, Tablet, or official name of product).
ii) Quantity dispensed (ml/g/units).
iii) Prescription identification number (instead of it, a slip may be attached).
iv) Name of the prescriber.
v)   Name of the patient.
vi) Compounded by (in the case of prefabricated dosage form: Repacked by).
vii) Date of compounding (DD/MM/YY. If needed, time of compounding).
viii) Shelf life (Use before DD/MM/YY).
ix) Direction to use (dose, method of administration).
x)   Storage conditions.
xi) Name and address of the pharmacy.

The content of active ingredients may appear on the label when the prescriber writes 'Label' in signa part of prescription. The auxiliary or cautionary label conditions for various dosage forms are summarised in Table 3.2. The typical labels for compounded dosage forms are shown in Figure 3.2.

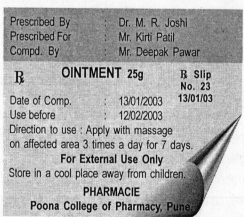

Figure 3.2: Typical label for compounded product

Table 3.2: Label conditions for Pharmaceutical dosage forms

No.	Dosage Form	Auxiliary Label Condition
1	Mixtures	Dilute Well Before Use (If applicable). Shake Well Before Use (If suspensions).
2	Emulsions	Shake Well Before Use.
3	Linctus	To be sipped and swallowed slowly without addition of water.
4	Throat Pain	For External Use Only. Not to be swallowed in large quantity.
5	Gargles and Mouthwashes	For External Use Only. Not to be swallowed in large quantity. If appropriate : Dilute well before use.
6	Inhalation	For External Use Only. To be added to hot water and inhale the vapours whenever necessary. If appropriate: Dilute well before use.
7	Application	For External Use Only. If appropriate: Shake Well Before Use.
8	Liniments	For External Use Only. Apply without friction. Not to be applied on broken skin. If appropriate : Shake Well Before Use.
9	Lotion	For External Use Only. Apply without friction. Not to be applied on broken skin. If appropriate : Shake Well Before Use.
10	Collidion	For External Use Only. Flammable. Apply with brush.
11	Enema	For Rectal Use Only. If appropriate: Shake Well Before Use. When large volume to be administered : Warm to body temperature before use.
12	Eye Lotion	For Ophthalmic Use Only. If unpreserved : Discard 24 hours after first opening.
13	Eye Drops	For Ophthalmic Use Only. Avoid contamination during use. Discard 30 days after first opening. If irritation persists contact physician.
14	Nasal drops	For Nasal Use Only. For decongestant preparations : Avoid prolonged or excessive use.
15	Ointment	For External Use Only. If appropriate : Sterile.
16	Creams, Paste, Jellies	For External use only.
17	Suppositories	For Rectal Use Only. To be unwrapped before insertion. If appropriate : Dip in water just before insertion.
18	Pessaries	For Vaginal Use Only. If appropriate : To be unwrapped before insertion. If appropriate : Dip in water just before insertion.
19	Tablets	Soluble or dispersible tablets : Dissolve or disperse in water before administration. Chewable Tablets : Chew before swallowing. Sustained release, enteric coated, unpleasant tasting tablets : Do not crush or chew.

20	Cachets	Buccal tablets : Keep in the buccal pouch or under the upper lip. Sublingual Tablets : To be placed below the tongue. Immerse the cachet in water for a few seconds, place on the tongue and swallow with a draught of water.
21	Granules	To be dissolved or dispersed in water before administration or to be placed on the back of the tongue and swallowed with a draught of water.
22	Insufflations	Not to be swallowed. Blown in nasal cavity.
23	Pastilles and Lozenges	To be sucked.
24	Dusting Powder	For External Use Only. If non-sterile : Not to be applied on broken skin. If sterile : Sterile.

iii) Checking the Product: There should be a proper checking system at the pharmacy. The pharmacists, other than the compounding pharmacists, must check the following parameters:

   i) Safety and legality of prescription.

   ii) Colour, odour and other symptoms of physical instability of the product to be dispensed.

   iii) Neatness, completeness and legality of the label.

      Pharmacists should write on the prescription 'Checked by', followed by their initials.

d) Pricing the Prescription: Pricing of the prescription must be systematic and should cover the cost of ingredients and container, time required for compounding and dispensing, professional services, and overhead expenses. In addition to this, it should yield a net profit. Cost of an ingredient should be based on the regular wholesale cost of usual package size, but discounts or advantages due to cash payment, larger orders or special offers should not be considered, as they are compensation for additional investment. Cost of container is the average cost of all the containers. Cost of time required for compounding and dispensing is obtained by calculating average time required for compounding the products. The professional service charge is the amount that covers cost for knowledge, professional skills and time required for duties other than compounding and dispensing. These related duties include consulting with physicians, discussion with patients and time required for filling the prescriptions, arranging stock, etc. It is considered that one-third time of pharmacists is spent in related duties. Overhead expenses include rent, electricity, taxes, insurance, depreciation, delivery service and degradation or expiry of drugs. Average overhead cost should be charged. A number of methods are proposed for pricing, but, in summary, it is cost of all the parameters discussed above. The cost of prescription can be calculated as:

     Prescription Price = Cost of ingredient + Minimum professional fees

     The minimum professional fees include profit plus all expenditures other than cost of ingredients. The cost of ingredients varies from drug to drug.

WEIGHING AND MEASUREMENT

Weighing and measuring the ingredients have a direct effect on the quality and effectiveness of the product, therefore it is considered to be an important fundamental skill of a pharmacist. Dispensing balances are of class B type, which comply with the prescribed limits of error. The minimum and maximum weighable quantities for these balances is 100mg and 50g respectively. These balances have accuracy of ± 10mg. Therefore, when amount of substance to be weighed is less than 150mg, it is advisable to use an electronic balance, which has an accuracy of ± 1mg.

Before weighing any ingredient, the working formula of the product should be written out in full. The balance must be set on flat solid surface. With the help of tweezers, the correct weights should be placed on the left hand side metal pan. If the right hand side pan is of metal, butter paper should be used to hold solid substances and if it is of glass, solid substances can be directly placed on pan. However, greasy/sticky substances should be weighed using greaseproof paper. Paper used to hold substances should not touch the sides of the balance or bench. When quantity of a liquid in the formula is mentioned in grams or milligrams, a small lightweight pot can be used to hold it. Putting the same type of paper/pot/watch-glass in the left hand side pan, counterbalances the weight of sample holder put in the right hand side pan. Using an electronic balance, makes it very easy to tare weight of sample holder. Setting the balance display back to zero will ensure that only the weight of the substance placed in the sample holder will be displayed. The weight of viscous sticky substances is noted by Weighing by Difference (Figure 3.4).

Conical dispensing measure is used to measure liquids. This has many advantages like, easier to fill and drain without spilling liquids on the sides. It is also easier to rinse out residual liquid and clean up after use. However, it is harder to read the meniscus accurately, using a conical measure. Some important points for proper use of conical measures are as follows:

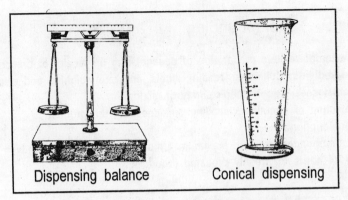

Dispensing balance   Conical dispensing

Figure 3.3: Balance and Conical measure

Place weighing dish on right pan (RP)

↓

Place weights in left pan (LP) to set balance

↓

Place required weights (Xg) in LP

↓

Add excess substance in dish placed on RP

↓

Balance RP and LP by putting some weights in LP

↓

Remove (Xg) form LP

↓

Remove substance from weighing dish till RP balances with LP

Figure 3.4: Weighing by Difference

- Use smallest possible measure.
- Rest measure on flat stationary surface.
- To measure a liquid, the bottom of the meniscus should be in line with the desired graduation mark and if needed, move your head down to the correct level but do not lift the measure to the level of your eye.
- While measuring coloured liquids, if it is difficult to see the bottom of the meniscus clearly, placing a white card paper behind the measure may help to view the meniscus.

Art of Compounding of Medicines

Dark coloured, or very viscous, liquids are measured by difference (Figure 3.4 and 3.5). If a liquid is less than 1ml, then a graduated pipette is used. In case of suspensions or emulsions, final volume adjustment is done in a tared container. The pourable liquid is transferred to the tared container, and after rinsing the mortar and pestle with the remaining vehicle, the final volume is adjusted (Figure 3.6).

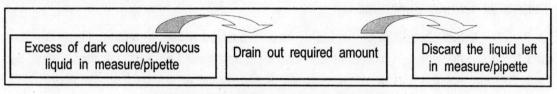

Excess of dark coloured/visocus liquid in measure/pipette	Drain out required amount	Discard the liquid left in measure/pipette

Figure 3.5: Measurement by Difference

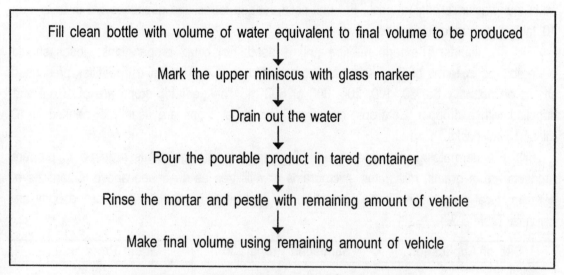

Fill clean bottle with volume of water equivalent to final volume to be produced

↓

Mark the upper miniscus with glass marker

↓

Drain out the water

↓

Pour the pourable product in tared container

↓

Rinse the mortar and pestle with remaining amount of vehicle

↓

Make final volume using remaining amount of vehicle

Figure 3.6: Measurement using Tared Container

To incorporate small amounts of ingredients, especially in less than minimum recommended weighable quantity of a balance, aliquot or trituration method is preferred. A known excess of the drug, equal to multiples of the quantity needed, is weighed or measured and then diluted to a convenient weight or volume. The part of the dilution, which represents the desired quantity of drug, is used in the prescription. The limitation of the trituration method is, wastage of potent drug as well as the additive used, for example:

Prescription 3.1

R
Powder Digitoxin — 1.5 mg
send single dose.

Digitoxin is prescribed for rapid digitalisation. The initial dose is 1.5 mg and maintenance dose is 200 mg daily. The 1.5 mg quantity is not directly weighable using dispensing balance. The powder can be compounded by trituration method as follows:

i) 100 mg of digitoxin + 900 mg of starch = 1000 mg of Ist triturate, which contains 10 mg of drug per 100 mg of triturate.

ii) 150 mg of Ist triturate + 850 mg of starch = 1000 mg of IInd triturate, which contains 1.5 mg of digitoxin per 100 mg of triturate.

Pattern of writing quantities

i)   For solids: Quantities of 1 gram or more should be written in unit 'g'. Quantities less than 1g should be written in milligrams and less than 1mg should be written in micrograms, eg. Write 300 mg, not 0.3 g. The terms micrograms and nanograms should not be abbreviated. Quantities of solids prescribed should normally be 15, 25, 50, 100, 200, 300 or 500 grams or as in manufacture's original pack. For unit solid dosage forms, the quantities are in units, i.e., 10 tablets, 6 suppositories, etc.

ii)   For liquids: The term millilitre (ml) is used. For liquid preparations, doses should preferably be in terms of 5 ml spoonful, or in multiples of it. The liquid quantities prescribed should be normally 30, 60, 100, 200, 300 or 500 ml. The pediatric drops are of 10 ml and supplied with a dropper. Eardrops, eye drops and nasal drops are usually dispensed in 10 ml or 15 ml packs.

iii) For dermatological preparations: The quantities of ingredients required to prepare products are in grams, milligrams, micrograms or millilitres as described above. Quantities of dermatological preparations to be prescribed for application on specific area of the body are given in Table 3.3.

Site of Application	Semisolid Preparation	Liquid Preparation
Face	5 – 15 gm	100 ml
Hands	25 – 50 gm	200 ml
Legs or Arms	100 – 200 gm	200 ml
Scalp	50 – 100 gm	200 ml
Body	200 gm	500 ml
Dusting powders	50 – 100 gm	
Paints	10 – 25 ml	

Table 3.3 : Quantities of dermatological preparations

Sensitivity and Precision :

The sensitivity of the balance may be defined as the magnitude of deflection produced by one unit of weight and an error is the excess or deficiency at full load. For example, if 100 mg is weighed on a balance having a sensitivity of 2 mg, the actual weight will be between 98 mg to 102 mg, and a possible error of ± 2 per cent. During dispensing, such an error should not be more than ± 5 per cent. Sensitivity is inversely proportional to the mass of the system.

Precision or reproducibility of results is connected with agreement in a series of observations, where accuracy refers to closeness of measurement to the true magnitude. For example, sample of 100 mg on repetitive measurement shows weight within the range 95 to 105 mg. It is precision or reproducibility. Any other balance, which gives value for the same sample in the range of 98–102 repetitively, has more precision and accuracy.

SYSTEMS OF WEIGHTS AND MEASURES

Nowadays, all the dispensing work is required to be carried out in the metric system. The imperial system is considered illegal almost all over the world.

Metric system:

Units of mass: The standard unit of mass is Kilogram.

1 kilogram (kg) = 1000 g

1 gram (g) = 1000 mg

1 miligram (mg) = 1000 μg

1 microgram (μg) = 1000 ng

1 nanogram (ng) = 1000 pg

1 picogram (pg) = 1/1000 ng

Units of volume: The standard unit of volume is Litre.

1 litre (l) = 1000 ml

1 mililitre (ml) = 1000 μl

1 microlitre (μl) = 1/1000 ml

Units of length: The standard unit of length is Metre.

1 centimetre (cm) = 1000 mm

1 millimetre = 1000 μm

1 micrometre (μm) = 1000 nm

1 nanometre (nm) = 1/1000 mm

Avoirdupois (AV) system: The standard unit of mass is Pound.

Imperialweights and Its Conversion into Metric System:

1 pound (lb) = 7000 grains / 16 oz (Av) = 450 g

1 Kg = 2.2lb

Apothecaries: It is known as troy system. The standard unit of mass is Grain.

1 grain (gr) = 64.8 mg (65 mg)

1 scruple (∋j) = 20 gr = 1.296 g

1 ounce (troy) ($\frac{Z}{\partial}$j) = 480 gr = 30 g

1 pound (troy) (lb) = 5760 gr = 370 g

15.43 gr (15 gr) = 1 g

1 drachm ($\frac{Z}{\partial}$j) = 60 gr = 4 g

1 ounce (Av) (oz) = 437.5 gr = 30 g

1 pound (Av) (lb) = 7000 gr 450 g

Imperial measures and their conversions into metric system:

1 minim (m) = 0.0592 ml (0.06 ml) = one drop

15 m = 1 ml

1 Fluid ounce ($\frac{Z}{\partial}$j) = 437.5 gr = 30 ml

1 gallon (C) = 8 pints = 4.5 l

1 pint (O) = 20 fl oz = 500 ml

1 quart = 1000 ml

1 Fluid drachm (fi$\frac{Z}{\partial}$) = 60 m = 4 ml

Table 3.4 : Conversion for Domestic Measures

Domestic measure	Metric system	Imperial system
1 drop	0.06 ml	1 minim
1 teaspoonful	4.00 ml	1 fluid drachm
1 desert spoonful	8.00 ml	2 fluid drachm
1 tablespoonful	15.00 ml	4 fluid drachm
2 tablespoonful	30.00 ml	1 fluid ounce
1 wine glassful	60.00 ml	2 fluid ounce
1 teacupful	120.00 ml	4 fluid ounce
1 tumblerful	240.00 ml	8 fluid ounce

In current practice, teaspoonful and desert spoonful are respectively considered as 5 and 10 ml

Imperial measures of length and their conversions into metric system:

1 inch (in) = 25.40 mm (2.54 cm),   1 yard (yd) = 3 ft = 0.914 m

1 foot (ft) = 12 in 30.4 cm,   1 mile = 1760 yd = 1.609 km

4 Art of Dispensing of Medicine

DISPENSING OF MEDICATION

Medicines are dispensed to an individual patient, his representative, in case of veterinary medicines,or to the owner of the animal, in response to a prescription written by a medical practitioner. Patient counselling by the pharmacist is an integral activity of dispensing. Dispensing of medication can be categorised as follows:

i) According to the level of production

a) Compounding and dispensing: Here dosage forms are fully or partly compounded according to the prescription.

b) Count-out or pour-out dispensing: In civil and municipal hospitals, or primary health centers, the common medicines such as expectorant mixtures or tablets/capsules are purchased in institutional packs. As per the prescribed dose, these dosage forms are measured or counted from bulk containers. The prescription handling involves repacking (filling the dispensing pack) and dispensing.

c) Dispensing as manufactured: Modern medicines, dispensed by chemists and druggists, in the original packs in which they are packed after manufacturing, are the examples of this class. Prescription handling involves only dispensing. Original pack dispensing facilitates ease of identification, improved patient compliance, reduced contamination and better physicochemical stability. But, it reduces flexibility in dispensing small units.

d) Generic dispensing: Medicines are manufactured by brand name and also with the title of the active ingredient, eg. Crocin Tablet containing paracetamol 500 mg, is brand product and Paracetamol tablet, I.P., 500 mg, is generic product. Generic dispensing is dispensing of product from among the generically equivalent drugs. Pharmacists should accept the responsibility and practice high morals and ethics to dispense generic products. If a doctor has prescribed a brand drug, then as per code of ethics, pharmacists cannot substitute the brand.

ii) According to drug regulations

Pharmacists dispense medicines from two major classes, prescription and non-prescription drugs. For this purpose, the Drugs and Cosmetics Act, 1940, classifies medicines under different schedules. Drugs coming under schedule H, including schedule C and C1, schedule G and Narcotic Drugs and Psychotropic Substances (NDPS) are prescription drugs. The Schedule K lists some safe medicines as non-prescription medicines. Schedule X drugs are list of drug, that are strictly controlled. The new drug under clinical studies is handled differently, which is out of scope of this book.

a) Prescription drugs: The prescription drugs are dispensed only against the prescription of a registered medical practitioner. The prescription must be handled by registered pharmacists, or under their direct supervision. These medicines carry mandatory warning on the label "Schedule H drug: Warning- To be sold on retail, on the prescription of a registered medical practitioner only." The labels of such products bear symbol of ℞ for Schedule H drugs, N℞ for Narcotic drugs and Psychotropic substances (NDPS), and X℞ for schedule X drugs. The bills of purchase and sale of these drugs should be retained in the pharmacy for a period of at least 3 years. The medicines come under NDPS are neither refilled nor substituted.

The manufactured drugs such as Paracodine and Pethidine that come under NDPS are purchased after special permission and stored under lock and key. Quarterly report of purchases and sales should be submitted to the FDA.

The schedule G drugs are to be taken under direct supervision of doctors. The label of such drugs also carries the warning "Caution: It is dangerous to take this prescription except under medical supervision".

b) Non-Prescription drugs: In the above mentioned type, consultation with the concerned physicians before dispensing, and patient counselling during dispensing, are the two main activities involved. A physician may not prescribe Over the Counter (OTC) medicines; in such cases, its safety to the user is of prime importance. The pharmacists should interact with the patients in a professional manner, to ascertain their intention and guide them in selection and use of the product.

The D & C Act does not clearly mention about OTC drugs. The schedule K drugs is a list of safer drugs that are needed for common ailments such as headache, acidity, common cold, etc. Schedule K drugs require sales license in form 20A, which permits the sale of the medicines (excluding prescription drugs) only in villages where there is no licensed medical shop. Non-pharmacy personnel can sell these. These medicines include aspirin tablets, paracetamol tablets, antacid tablets, syrups, pills, tablets and lozenges for cough, pain balms, inhalers, eucalyptus oil, castor oil, liquid paraffin, gripe water, liniments, skin ointments for burns, absorbent cotton, tincture iodine, tincture benzoin, tablets of quinine sulphate and iodochlorohydroxy quinoline. The other non-prescription drugs include paracetamol 500mg, calamine lotion, clotrimazole cream, chlorhexidine solution 5 per cent, lindane lotion 1 per cent, povidone iodine solution/ointment 5 per cent, xylometazoline 0.1 per cent.

Since there is no authentic list of OTC medicines, this practice is confusing and has many loopholes. The medicines with labels not bearing the symbol ℞, N℞ and X℞ are considered as OTC medicines. Government must notify the list of OTC medicines to the public, and pharmacists should be held responsible for outcome of the OTC therapy.

c) Cosmetics: Cosmetics are considered as safe formulations for topical application and non-professionals can sell these. However, many of the cosmetics cause milder irritation, skin redness or keratolytic activities, eg. depilatories and antidandruff cosmetics. The perfumes used in the cosmetics may cause allergic reactions. Keeping this in mind, pharmacists should provide his consultancy differently and scientifically, for selection of cosmetics.

d) Alternative medicines: Drug license is not required for sale of Ayurvedic, Siddha and Unani drugs. These medicines can be stocked and sold by pharmacists or any person, shop or outlet. But these medicines must be manufactured under the license issued by FDA.

It is compulsory to obtain a license from the state drug licensing authority to stock and sale homeopathic drugs. Homeopathic pharmacies are run under the supervision of persons who have a qualified homeopathic degree.

Concept Check : Dispensing of Medication

Dispensing of Medication is defined as the supply of a pharmaceutical product to an individual patient.
- Compounding and dispensing
- Count-out or pour-out dispensing
- Dispensing as manufactured
- Generic dispensing
- Prescription drugs
- Non-Prescription Drugs
- Cosmetics
- Alternative medicines

HANDLING THE PRESCRIPTION

The activities performed during dispensing of prescribed medicines are termed as handling or responding of the prescription. The prescription may be for compounding and dispensing of medicine, or just dispensing of manufactured medicine. The modern dispensing practice mainly involves dispensing of manufactured medicines. Except the compounding procedure, all the steps of prescription handling are identical for dispensing of manufactured medicine. Dispensing of manufactured medicines is discussed below. The process of prescription handling is summarised in Fig. 4.1.

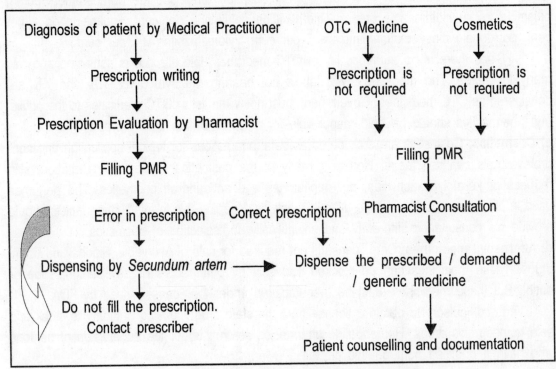

Figure 4.1 : Dispensing Methodology

i) Receiving the prescription: Pharmacists should receive the prescription with a smile, eye-to-eye contact and friendly welcome, creating a feeling of caring. A dialogue initiated by pharmacists should encourage the patients to speak about their health problems and ask for advice. Firstly, pharmacists should check patient's name, age and whether the patient in person is handling it. The second important aspect is checking legality of the prescription. A prescription must be written and signed by a registered medical practitioner and should have all the required information as mentioned in the parts of prescription. Pharmacists should politely request a patient to wait while his prescription is being filled. While receiving the prescription, the pharmacists should in no way, either verbally or through facial expression, express doubts, which may shake the faith of the patient in the physician.

To avoid wrong delivery of the compounded preparation, in large dispensaries, a prescription slip (token) system can be adopted. Three prescription slips bear the identification number. Out of these three, one is given to the patient, second is attached to the prescription

     Art of Dispensing Medicine

and the third is attached to the outer wrapping of the product ready for dispensing.

ii) Checking the prescription: Pharmacists should read the prescription carefully and thoroughly in privacy. If necessary, they can consult with another pharmacist or a physician without arousing doubts or fears in the patients' mind. Before removing the medicines from shelves, the pharmacists must understand the prescription and the intention of the prescriber. The basic rule that should be strictly followed is 'Never Dispense Guesswork'.

Secondly, the prescription is checked for pharmaceutical quality such as physical, chemical or therapeutic incompatibility in the prescription. It can be judged by checking the product details such as name of medicine, dosage form, strength, correctness of dose according to the age or weight of patient and quantity dispensed. The frequency of administration and way of administration should be checked for its simplicity of clear understanding. Pharmacists should identify any drug-drug or drug-food interaction. They can assess Patient Medication Record (PMR) so as to check for allergy, contraindications, parallel drug therapy and lifestyle of patients. As an expert, he has to correct it, if necessary, after consultation with the prescriber.

iii) Pre-dispensing activities: Dispensing of product in its original pack ensures high standards of pharmacy practice. For the dispensing by count-out or pour-out from bulk containers high level of cleanliness and hygiene is required. Pharmacists have to select suitable dispensing containers and make a label for it.

iv) Removal of medicines: Pharmacists should remove the required medicines from the shelves confidently, with attention and concentration. While removing medicines, pharmacists should be attentive about dosage form, strength and expiry date. The medicines should be placed on a separate table, where they are processed for billing and entries in PMR. According to the prescription, the number of units of medicines should be separated and placed in a plastic tray. While cutting strips, preferably the unlabelled portion should be cut first so that the portion of strip having expiry date and batch number will remain at the pharmacy.

Good inventory management is the art of stock management of any pharmacy and it should be such that, at any given time, the pharmacy should hold a minimum stock of every medicine. If any medicament is not in stock, pharmacists should make it available to the client after a period of time. In such cases, pharmacists can make home delivery of the medicine.

v) Labelling : The labels for products prepared on large scale are different from those of the repacked or compounded products. Products that are manufactured on a large scale are not made for a particular patient. Such preparations move through a long distribution link: Manufacturer ⟶ Distributor ⟶ Wholesaler ⟶ Retail Pharmacy ⟶ Patient.

The general format for label of proprietary product is as follows:
i)   Brand name, Generic name.
ii)   Quantity dispensed: (ml/g/units).
iii) Composition: (Each 5 ml contains/per cent/g/ml)
iv)   Schedule:
v)   Mfg. Lic. No. :
vi)   Mfg. Batch No.:
vii) Mfg. Date: (MM/YY)
viii) Exp. Date: (MM/YY/No Exp. date)
ix)   Direction to use
x)   Storage conditions.
xi)   Manufactured By & Marketed By.
xii) If medicine is schedule H drug, it should bear a warning in rectangle. Such labels should bear symbol R$_X$ on left side top corner of a label and vertical red line on left side of the label.

Warning: To be sold by retail on the prescription of a registered medical practitioner only.

Small size dispensing labels or stickers mentioning number of units dispensed, dosing schedule, date of dispensing and name of pharmacy should be prepared and stuck on strips, boxes or containers while dispensing.

vi) Dispensing loose from bulk packs: The pre-fabricated dosage forms such as tablets and capsules are available in both, unit dose packs (blister/strip pack) or in the form of bulk containers. The former are dispensed in required units without repackaging. When a pharmacy purchases bulk packs, then the required number of tablets/capsules have to be counted and

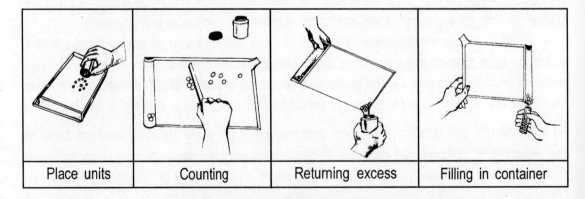

| Place units | Counting | Returning excess | Filling in container |

Figure 4.2: Counting of solid unit dosage forms

repacked in a suitable container. Number of units is counted without touching the tablets by hand. Clean and dry counting devices are preferable to avoid any cross contamination.

Tablets and capsules are usually dispensed in paper envelopes. The plastic coated paper envelopes are impermeable to environmental humidity and provide good protection, especially for capsules. Tablets with their coat cracked or tacky and tablets with variation in colour shade, should not be dispensed. As much as possible, dispensing of loose liquids should be avoided; otherwise the bottles should be of highest possible cleanliness and completely dry.

The pharmacist should make two labels. The dispensing label is affixed on the container and bulk pack label is filed to patient medication record. The bulk pack label should mention the of strength of product, name of manufacturer, batch number and manufacturing and expiry date. In addition to common parameters, the dispensing label should highlight the number of units, repacked and/or dispensed by, safe period for use, etc. The repacked solid dosage

a) Bulk pack	b) Dispensing pack
Mfg : 4 / 99 Exp : 3 / 2002	**PARACETAMOL TABLETS 9 Tabs.**
	Prescription ID No. : 75
	Prescribed By : Dr. V. R. Patil
TAB PARACETAMOL 500 mg	Prescribed For : Mr. Kaushal Patil
	Repacked By : Mrs. Deepti Choudhari
	Date of Comp. : 15 /08/1994
Get.Rid Pharma Ltd, Pune	Use before : 14 /10/1994
Pack size : 1000 tabs	Dose : 1 tablet three times a day with water, after meal, for 3 days.
Batch No. 009.	Store in cool place away from children.
	PHARMACIE **Poona College of Pharmacy, Pune.**

Figure 4.3: Label for Repacked product a) Bulk Pack   b) Dispensing Pack

forms should be used within one month. Pharmacists should maintain a record of dispensing, in the following form:

i)   Name of patient.
ii) Name of prescriber.
iii) Name and strength of dosage form.
iv) Manufacturer, batch no., mfg date, expiry date.

v) Bulk pack size.

vi) Pre-packed and or dispensed by.

vii) Date of repacking.

viii) Dispensing pack size.

ix) Dispensing container.

x) Dose, direction to use and storage.

xi) Patient counselling.

xii) Checked by.

vii) Checking of medicines for dispensing: The pharmacists should check whether the product to be dispensed is as per the prescription. The dispensing pharmacist should recheck the calculation done by the compounding pharmacist, dose and directions about administration. Special attention should be paid to observe the physical symptoms for instability of product. The pharmacists should dispense the prescription immediately on receiving it. During dispensing of medicines the pharmacists should ask for a prescription slip to identify the product. When a prescription is delivered directly to the patient, it provides an excellent opportunity for the pharmacists to ensure that the patient has understood as to how the medicine is to be used.

viii) Billing and Filling the PMR: Chief pharmacist must do the billing. While billing, the pharmacists have an additional opportunity to recheck the medicines for dosage form, strength, quantity and expiry date. Computer billing is the best alternative to make single entry of medicines both for billing as well as PMR updating. The pharmacists should check and sign the bill. Recently manufactured medicines are priced with MRP inclusive of all taxes.

Pharmacists should maintain Patient Medication Record (PMR) for each individual patient and make appropriate entries during each dispensing.

ix) Patient counselling: Patients have the right to know everything about the treatment that they are undergoing. Patient counselling is a professional activity, which deals with providing information to the patient about their illness and medicines. Pharmacists should act as advisers to patients regarding use of medicines, method of administration, dose and time of administration, precautions to be taken during therapy and possible side effects. They should demonstrate the use of devices and storage conditions of medicines. Pharmacists should also provide consultation for use of cosmetics and beauty products. It can be either verbal or written, but the former provides more opportunity to understand the patient and his basic knowledge about medicines.

Experienced pharmacists with good knowledge of clinical aspect of the prescribed drugs, drug interactions and stability and storage of dosage forms, as well as good communication skills, should do patient counselling. It can be done either while billing and filling the PMR or if detailed information or advice is needed, it can be done in an isolated place at the end of the billing process. An effective use of pictograms and product information leaflet (PIL) is a convenient and easy way of patient education. Patient counselling should be practiced positively, keeping in mind that 'misuse of drugs by educating people, would never be more than the misuse occurring due to wrongly prescribed and dispensed medicines'.

Counselling patients about the proper way of drug administration, is the main task while dispensing, which is explained in depth under individual dosage forms. In addition, dispensing pharmacists should focus attention of patients and physicians on commonly occurring drug interactions, storage conditions and contraindications. Following are some general points for patient counselling that can be done at the time of dispensing medicines:

1) Check understanding of instructions: Pharmacists should ensure that patients have understood the instructions given by their doctor, mainly the time for taking the medicines, i.e., whether before or after food, how frequently and for how long, etc. Eg. B complex vitamin should be taken on full stomach, whereas paracetamol shows fast onset if taken on empty stomach with glass of water.

2) Explain reason for prescription: Evaluating a patient's social and intellectual level, pharmacists may explain the reason for prescribing a particular drug and what benefits and side effects to expect. When they are not sure about the reason or when such information can develop fear in the minds of patients or lead to self-medication, pharmacists should give such information tactfully.

3) Ask about parallel treatment: It helps to avoid drug-drug interactions as well as to minimise chances of re-dispensing of a drug or drugs from same therapeutic class. For example, patients asking for paracetamol as OTC drug may be taking the same drug as a component of cough formula. Cephalosporins (antibiotic) have therapeutic drug interactions with coumarins (anticoagulants), where Cephalosporins may increase anticoagulant effect of coumarins, which may lead to an increased risk of bleeding.

4) Ask about allergic history: Many drugs, including antibiotics, sulpha drugs and non-steroidal anti-inflammatory drugs (NSAID) cause allergic reactions in some patients. Some individuals are also allergic to colours used in formulations. For example, NSAID should be prescribed/ given with caution to asthma patients.

5) Warn about habits: Taking alcohol, or smoking during drug therapy, may adversely affect drug action. Alcohol increases gastric ulceration caused by NSAID and depresses the effect of antihistaminic drugs. Metronidazole (antimicrobial) taken with alcohol, may cause flushing, headache, nausea, vomiting, abdominal pain, fall in blood pressure or fainting.

6) Alert about side effects: Pharmacists should alert the patients to report if any new symptoms develop, especially if it is persistent and troublesome. Make patients aware not to perform skilled tasks like driving, if a drug causes side effects like drowsiness, dizziness, blurred vision, etc. Regular use of aspirin prolongs bleeding and hence may need to be stopped about a week before menstrual cycle of women or before any medical or dental surgery.

7) Counsel for long term treatments: If patients are taking medicines for long term treatments, instruct them that abruptly stopping certain medicines may lead to worsening of the underlying condition, or develop other complications. At the same time inform them that periodic checkup by their physician is necessary and that they should have new prescriptions written. For example, long term administration of olanzapine (antipsychotic drug) without consulting the physicians may lead to weight gain, which in turn may cause complications like diabetes and hypertension.

8) Counsel pregnant and breast-feeding women: Many drugs are contraindicated in pregnant women especially in the first three months and during breast-feeding. For example, Aspirin, which is a commonly used analgesic, can cause bleeding in pregnant women and in case of nursing mothers, it may pass into the baby, via milk.

9) Counsel paediatric and geriatric patients: Paediatric dose of a drug is usually a fraction of the adult dose, secondly both paediatric and geriatric patients face difficulties in drug administration. Therefore, pharmacists should pay more attention while dispensing medicines to such patients. For example, aspirin should be avoided in children below age of 16 years because it may cause Reye's syndrome. Geriatric patient may have difficulty in removing tablet from strips, or from child resistant containers, or they may have difficulty in synchronising the actuation and inhalation of the puff while using metered dose inhalers.

10) Guide about missed dose: A missed dose is generally taken as soon as possible but should be skipped if it is almost time for the next regular dose. Patients should not take a double dose. They should never exceed the recommended dose; and if pharmacists suspect an overdose, seek immediate medical attention.

11) Prove role in OTC medication: Patients should take over-the-counter medicines after consultation with pharmacists. Though OTC drugs are comparatively safe, taken individually, they may affect adversely in the presence of other drugs, or cause therapeutic complications. Eg. antacids should not be taken with enteric-coated formulations; otherwise enteric polymers dissolve in the alkaline content, in the stomach itself. Sodium bicarbonate-based antacids may increase sodium level of blood, which is contraindicated for hypertensive patients.

12) Explain hazards of self-medication: Many times, in different patients, symptoms of diseases appear same, but they may be suffering from two entirely different diseases. In such instances, intimate patients that they should neither share prescription drugs with each other, nor take their own left over medicines from earlier prescriptions.

13) Carry warning cards: Sometimes patients may need emergency medical help, eg. hypoglycemia in diabetic patients, epileptic patients, etc. Pharmacists should insist that patients

---

carry warning cards bearing information about the disease, with name of the doctor and contact numbers.

14) Guide about storage condition: Drugs require being stored at particular storage conditions, otherwise it may affect their physicochemical stability, eg. insulin and nicorandil should be stored in refrigerator at 2-8°C.

15) Handling of medicines: Patients should never keep medicines within reach of children and should not mix the contents of one container with another.

16) Expiry medicines: Pharmacists should explain the importance of the expiry date to the patient. Patients should take complete dose of medicines and should not store the left over medicines for a prolonged time period. The expired/left over medicines should be put in the dustbin and should be flushed down the toilet.

17) Maintain PMR: Pharmacists should prepare and maintain patient medication record and create the patients' interest in doing it.

18) Disease management: In addition, pharmacists can play a crucial role in the management of diseases such as asthma, hypertension, tuberculosis, etc. Special meeting with patients, giving pre-appointment for this purpose, are more effective.

x) Endorsement: All prescriptions should be stamped, dated and signed by the pharmacists. For refill prescriptions, the number of times and dates of refill should be noted on the prescription. When only part of the prescription is dispensed, the pharmacists should write down the quantity dispensed against each medicine and stamp the prescription. Since medicines are dispensed and not supplied, the stamp should have the word "Dispensed".

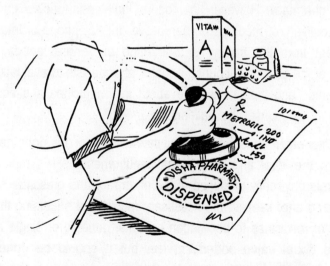

Figure 4.4: Endorsement of Prescription

xi) Filing of prescription: The original prescription must be kept as record in the pharmacy or in wards in the hospital, or returned back to the patient as per the type of prescription. The prescriptions containing NDPS drugs must be filled separately and should be documented in the pharmacy for at least three years. The bills of purchases and sales of all medicines should be retained for a period of at least three years.

xii) Documentation: All the activities performed during dispensing of prescription should be documented and such records should be retained for three years. The different records include stock record, bills, patient medication record (PMR) and compounding and dispensing record (CDR).

Concept Clear : Handling the prescription

- Receiving Prescription
- Checking Prescription
- Pre-dispensing activities
- Removal of Medicines
- Dispensing loose from bulk packs.

- Checking medicines for dispensing
- Billing and filling the PMR
- Patient counselling
- Endorsement of prescription.
- Filling of prescription
- Documentation

HOME DELIVERY OF MEDICINES

Dispensing of medicines at the counter against the prescription or dispensing of OTC medicines, is main activity of the pharmacy. However, in modern India, pharmacists can extend their services such as home delivery of medicines ordered over the telephone or internet. The sale of medicines is different from the trading or marketing of general goods and is called 'dispensing'. Dispensing at the pharmacy counter enables pharmacists to evaluate prescriptions, judge condition of patients and their knowledge about the medicines and accordingly, they can utilise this opportunity to counsel the patients.

i) Home delivery: Like other household items, medicines can be door delivered to the client/patient, preserving the legal and professional requirements.

    a)   If a prescription is physically produced at the pharmacy, the prescribed medicines can be home-delivered after keeping the necessary record and endorsing the prescription.

    b)   Home delivery of medicines to bed-ridden patients, geriatric or single member family patients, is no doubt value added service, but it should be done after proper prescription handling procedures. For that the prescription can be kept at the pharmacy, and

---

                Art of Dispensing Medicine

whenever required, patients can call pharmacists to deliver medicines. Long-term therapy may need periodic supply of medicines, for which pharmacists can refer PMR for refilling the prescription.

c) Non-prescription medicines can be home-delivered, but it is better to enter the information in PMR.

ii) Telephonic orders: Prescription drugs cannot be dispensed against telephonic order unless the prescription is physically present before the pharmacist.

iii) Internet Pharmacy: In the world of e-marketing, one can log-on and order any household item, clothes or electronic items, but no prescription medicines. Some important aspects of this concept are as follows:

a) The pharmacy must have a physical address and it should be licensed and authorised.
b) Medicines are only dispensed against actual prescription of a RMP.
c) Cosmetics can be purchased via the internet.
d) To sell medicines to foreign patients, pharmacies must have export license from drug-controller of India.
e) At present, internet pharmacies are not authorised in India.

STATUS OF DISPENSING PRACTICE IN INDIA

Most of the modern medicines are company manufactured and hence dispensed in original packs by the retail chemists. This demands not only accurate supply of medications, but also checking that the medication is appropriate for the patient.

Many strong-acting medicines have been developed recently, which has resulted in many unexpected side effects. Other drug related problems, such as duplication of therapy, drug-drug/drug-food interactions, or misuse of drugs also occurs with great frequency. The information available at the finger tips for the common man, is most of the times either incomplete or misinterpreted, which is the main cause of misuse of medicines. Recent withdrawals of potent, but dangerous, medicines, indicate that our drug awareness system is increasingly growing incapable of assuring patients that they will be treated in the best way. After proper selection of a drug and its dose, instructions for their correct use should be given. Effects of drugs, during and after use; and their side effects should be evaluated. Pharmacists, both, in hospital and community pharmacies, should develop and practice standard operating procedures (SOPs) of dispensing processes. All these elements contribute to good and safe use of drugs. The pharmacists, the ultimate medical professionals that are supplying medicines to the patients, can monitor it. Dispensing medicines professionally, perfect patient counselling and attitude of pharmacists' is observed by the society and all these judge pharmacists either as 'Drug Trader' or as 'Professional Health Provider'. In practice, Indian pharmacies are not community pharmacies; they work as Medical Shops for sale of medicines. Salesmen and consumers discuss much more during shopping of household items than during dispensing of medicines.

The main reasons of poor dispensing practices in India include:

Education:
- As compared to developed countries, India is fifty years late in commencing pharmacy education.
- Insufficient education imparted, due to minimum qualification required to open and run a medical store.
- Teaching outdated concepts such as compounding, Latin terms, imperial systems of weights and measures.
- Reluctance on the part of the teachers to accept modern practice; and student's attitude to study minimum in view of examinations.
- Limited theoretical and practical exposure during pharmacy education.

Continuous Education:
- Lack of motivation and inadequate training to pharmacists.
- Lack of instant information sources.
- Poor utilisation of information technology and computer technology.

Patient:
- Large number of patients due to poverty and illiteracy.
- Consulting different doctors each time for treatment.
- Using multiple therapies simultaneously from two or more doctors.
- Lack of concept of 'Family Pharmacist'.

Physician:
- No identified role of pharmacists in health care.
- Limited involvement and motivation of pharmacists by physicians.

Government Policy:
- Industry and commercial oriented policies.
- No separate ministry to look after pharmaceutical products and the pharmaceutical profession. At present it is part of Ministry of Chemicals and Fertilisers, the objectives of which are very different from objectives of pharmacy practice.
- Unproven and irrational drugs and their combinations.

5 Good Pharmacy Practices

Medicines are required for correcting abnormal body conditions caused when individuals are physically, physiologically and/or psychologically weak. The use of incorrect medicines is more dangerous in such cases and only quality medicines can serve the purpose. They should be suitable for the patient and the patients should know the proper way of their storage and administration. Good Pharmacy Practices (GPP) is a way to practice community pharmacy in a professional way. GPP is a comparatively broader term that also includes dispensing of medication as main activity, with other pharmaceutical services such as clinical services, health screening services, drug information services, continuing education, etc.

In 1993, International Pharmaceutical Federation (FIP) adopted international guidelines for GPP. Developed countries have already implemented the concept of GPP. Indian pharmaceutical industries have been following GMP (Good Manufacturing Practices), but concept of GPP is still to come in practice. Though, Indian Pharmaceutical Association (IPA) developed first GPP manual in 2005, it will not be fully implemented unless and until it is made compulsory.

Safe practices do not come about by chance, but by positive attitudes of personnel; safe procedures and a conducive working environment have to be developed. The successful application of GPP is not complex if the systems governing the various activities of personnel, equipment, building and documentation are properly planned and controlled. For convenience and understanding GPP is categorised as dispensing practices and compounding practices.

GOOD COMPOUNDING PRACTICES

1) **Personnel:** People are the actual judges to decide quality of practice. In addition to the qualification and attitude of compounding pharmacists, they must have skills of weighing and

mixing. They should have thorough knowledge about physicochemical incompatibilities between active ingredients and additives and selection of containers.

2) Building and Equipment: Building should be constructed as per acceptable standards of ventilation, lighting, plumbing and electrical systems, refreshment and cloak room facilities, etc. Rooms used for compounding, packaging, counselling and storage should provide a logical workflow and should be maintained in a clean and orderly manner. Equipment must be of adequate size, and suitably located according to its intended use. Equipment should be as simple as possible to allow easy cleaning and they should not contaminate the product, eg. filters should not release fibers into the product.

3) Housekeeping: In general, raw materials are classified into two groups: active ingredients and additives. These should be purchased from authentic suppliers and the information written on the label of the containers must be noted. Using clean equipment and observing good housekeeping practices can avoid cross-contamination of raw material. The material of containers should be non-reactive with products, eg. methyl salicylate causes softening of plastics, iodine preparations should be stored in iodine resistant containers. The raw materials should be properly stored to maintain their physicochemical stability, eg. volatile oils and methyl salicylate should be stored in cool places, ferrous sulphate in airtight containers and paraldehyde in dark, cool places and airtight containers.

4) Documentation: The Compounding and Dispensing Record (CDR) comprises information about patients and the products dispensed, in a particular pharmacy. This information includes:

i)   Patient: Name, age, sex, address, phone number.

ii) Product: Name, information source, formula (official or unofficial).

iii) Raw material: Name, manufacturer, batch no., manufacturing and expiry date.

iv) Procedure: Apparatus and equipment used, order of mixing, and physical and chemical incompatibility, which is observed and corrected.

v)   Container, closure selected and storage condition.

vi) Label format.

vii) Name of the compounding pharmacist, date of compounding, expiry date, checked which pharmacist it.

viii) Patient counselling note.

ix) Prescription disposal and fee charged.

x)   Name of the dispensing pharmacist and person who rechecked.

xi) In addition, the pharmacies should develop and maintain the following Standard operating procedures (SOP).

Any deviation from SOP must be investigated and recorded and approved before dispensing of a product.

---

a) SOP for receipt of raw material, identification, testing, storage, rejection, etc.

b) SOP for compounding of most frequently prescribed formulations.

c) SOP for drug distribution and dispensing.

d) SOP for cleaning and disinfecting procedures.

Concept Clear : Good Compounding Practices

- Personnel: Skills of weighing and mixing, knowledge of selection of additives & incompatibilities.
- Building and Equipment: Design, construction, flow of activity, cleanliness.
- Housekeeping: Purchase, storage, cross-contamination, cleanliness.
- Documentation CDR, SOP.

GOOD DISPENSING PRACTICES

Dispensing practices include planning and implementation of a group of activities logically and ethically to provide quality medicines to the person in question, which are needed and suitable for him.

1) Personnel: Being a component of health care unit, the role of the pharmacist is to ensure patient safety during drug use, which can be achieved by delivering quality products, setting standards and procedures, performing self assessments, committing to life long learning and demonstrating leadership. According to Dr. Peter Kielgast, Ex-President of International Pharmaceutical Federation (FIP), the most powerful maps we got since Columbus discovered the new world, are computer chips and genome. Learning to read these maps and combining them will lead to a new paradigm in health care. But it needs knowledge of biology and technology, hence there is no profession better positioned to initiate the leadership, than Pharmacy. Pharmacists know drugs and drug delivery systems, the way they work, their vast benefits, dangers, costs and complexities of their distribution and use.

Proper selection, training, motivation and attitudes of individuals are vital to produce quality products and services. Neatness, accuracy and speed are the qualities that must be developed by the individual. Attention should be paid on hygiene, protective clothing and a ban imposed upon food consumption and smoking in the dispensary. The pharmacists should involve themselves in many activities, eg. discussion with physicians, providing drug information, participating in case studies of therapeutic incompatibility and counselling patients.

Unfortunately in India, a country of 1 billion people, pharmacy education is industry oriented. Medical practitioners are mainly considered to be responsible for health care. To upgrade the functionality of the Indian pharmacists, with the help of WHO and Pharmacy Council of India, a number of institutes are arranging training courses for the working pharmacists. More emphasis is laid on using advanced techniques for acquiring knowledge of latest medicines and communication skills, so as to discuss with physicians about advances in drug therapy, and with patients, about their health. To play role of a 'patient-centered pharmacist' and not a 'trade centered' one, the pharmacists should be familiar with the patients' language. The computer systems have already been introduced in pharmacy practice and a number of softwares and web sites are accessible to the pharmacists. Nonetheless, these developments are insignificant, considering the present status of pharmacy, overall health standard and size of the country.

2) Building and Equipment: The dispensing section should have a prescription counter, waiting area, patient counselling room and shelves or racks of suitable size. The prescription counter should be easily accessible to the clients. It should be clean and orderly. The waiting area should have comfortable sitting arrangement and it should display general guidelines about handling of medicines, pictograms and popular health magazines. Wooden shelves, metal racks and drawers are the different means of storage of medicines. Shelves with sliding glass doors and drawers are ideal to prevent entry of dust. However, it hampers speed in removing the medicines, hence an air-conditioned pharmacy with a closed entrance, is the modern approach. Patient counselling during billing can serve the purpose, but, for detailed discussion, a pharmacy should have a separate cabin with pleasant environment.

An adequate number of refrigerators should be kept to store medicines requiring cold storage. Preferably, frost-free refrigerators should be used. It not only provides large area but also avoids damage that is caused by water falling from trays below the freezer of conventional refrigerators. A separate door to each compartment does not disturb the storage temperature in other compartments. Ice-packs should be available, which can be used for transporting medicines requiring cold conditions.

During dispensing, an un-interrupted process should be carried out, without confusing the orderly sequence, right from receiving a prescription, to filling it and checking the stock. The pharmacy should be a peaceful place with no radios and televisions. These can divert the attention of the pharmacists during dispensing and lead to dispensing errors.

3) Housekeeping: In a pharmacy, medicines are arranged in various ways, the commonly employed ways are: a) alphabetical arrangement, b) according to manufacturer, c) according to type of dosage form and d) according to frequency of sale of product. The new items must always be placed behind previous ones and medicines having an earlier expiry date should be sold first; this is also termed as FEFO (First Expiry First Out) system. A small shelf should be labeled as "Quarantine" and exclusively used to receive stock from wholesalers. The stock should be kept on this shelf, until they are checked. A separate area should also be designed to store expired products. It should be labeled as "Expired Medicines, Not For Sale". The stock should be checked regularly for out-dated items. Veterinary medicines should be stored in separate racks and should be adequately marked as "For Veterinary Use Only'.

4) Documentation: Since pharmacists are the ultimate health providers who come in contact with the patients, they cannot deny moral and legal responsibility for any wrong drug therapy. Documents prepared and maintained by the pharmacists may work as the key evidence to save a patient's life if such an occasion arose.

Concept Check : Good Dispensing Practices

GDP: Planning and implementation to dispense quality medicines to patient.
- Personnel: Knowledge of biology and technology, know about drugs and drug delivery systems. Training, motivation and attitude, communication and computer.
- Building: Accessible to patients, waiting area, storage area, counselling cell. A.C., Frost free refrigerator. Quarantine, Expired and veterinary medicines.
- Housekeeping: Alphabetical arrangement, manufacturer, type of dosage form and frequency of sale of product. FEFO concept.
- Documentation : Prescription related, Stock records, Application forms.

RECORD KEEPING

Prescription related records

1) Prescription Slips: The prescription slip is a typical token system. A prescription slip has three parts, one part is given to the patient, the second is attached to the prescription and the third is attached to the final pack containing medicines. At the time of dispensing, the patient's slip is collected from him and the corresponding medicines are handed over. This system prevents wrong delivery of medicines, prevents mix-up of parcels and thus reduces errors in dispensing. A typical prescription is shown in Figure 5.1.

Deo Pharmacy, Pune Token No. 25 Date: 14/09/2006 Name of Patient: Puja Bhat Please bring this token when you come to collect medicines. **To the Patient**	Deo Pharmacy, Pune Token No. 25 Date: 14/09/2006 Name of Patient: Puja Bhat **Attach to prescription**	Deo Pharmacy, Pune Token No. 25 Date: 14/09/2006 Name of Patient: Puja Bhat **Attach to dispensing pack**

Figure 5.1: Typical prescription slip

Good Pharmacy Practices

2) Patient Medication Record (PMR): The success of dispensing medicines is governed by accurately checking the suitability of prescribed medicines to treat the specific health problem. Pharmacists utilise their skill to collect factual information about the illness and overall life style of a patient. An interview of a patient, reviewing of prescription and case paper and discussion with other health care professionals are the commonly utilised sources for correct drug dispensing, among which patient history and prescription reading is mostly utilised. During the first visit of any new patient, pharmacists have to do the tough job of making a detailed Patient Medication Record (PMR). PMR is nothing but systematic medical history of a patient along with his life style and medical background of the family; it contains information about his disease condition, past medication record, present prescribed/OTC drugs, their interactions, allergic reactions, signs of improvement and record of prescriptions and whether given by one or more prescribers (Fig. 5.2).

Patient Medication Record								
Patient No. :			Disease/Clin. Condition : _____					
Name : _____			Allergies/Reactions : _____					
Sex : M/F Age : Wt. : kg. :			Note (Past medication, : drug, dosage form, strength, dose, actual dose taken etc.)					
Address : _____			_____					
Telephone :			_____					
Date	R #	Physician	Age/Wt.	Drug/Strengh/Qty	Signa	Refill	Charge	Pharmacist Sign

Figure 5.2: Patient Medication Record

In India, mostly medical practitioners retain the case paper as patient history. However, not all of them prepare case papers. Therefore, when a patient visits any other doctor, it is difficult to analyse the medical history of the patient. It increases chances of duplication of drugs or prescribing incompatible drugs. In developed countries, pharmacists maintain PMR, and if required, provide this information to physicians also.

Pharmacists, with their judgement and skill, review the PMR for subsequent dispensing. The review of PMR against the current prescription is helpful to identify the possibility of adverse drug reactions, allergic and hypersensitivity reactions and patient's failure to respond to a therapy. Pharmacists could assess the patient's view regarding the therapy, beliefs, perceptions, expectations, experience and his understanding about way of medications. It is not wrong to say that PMR creates openness in the relationship of patients with pharmacists. This would not only count as a benefit for patients, but also as an addition of value in the business. The use of computer in pharmacies serves the simultaneous billing and entries of current medication in the PMR. Maintenance of prescription files and diary are the other ways of maintaining records. PMR includes almost all the information about the patients' dispensed drugs and can be also used as a record for dispensed drugs.

Benefits of PMR in Pharmacy

1) Pharmacists could assess the patient's knowledge regarding the medication, beliefs, perceptions and experience of medicines.
2) Helpful to identity medication risk factor and efficacy of medicines on the basis of adverse drug reactions, allergic and hypersensitivity reactions and patient's failure to respond to therapy.
3) Minimise drug interactions especially when patient is simultaneously taking medical advice from two or more doctors (multi-therapy).
4) Helps in selection of OTC products and cosmetics that suit the patient and have no drug interactions.
5) Helpful to monitor the therapy in pregnant and critical patients.
6) For better understanding about way of administration of medication.
7) It can be used as a tool to check medication adherence by patients.
8) Pharmacists can provide patient information to prescribers.
9) It will not only increase the business, but also develop the image of the pharmacists as professional pharmacists.
10) It is the first step to becoming a 'Family Pharmacist'.

Preparation of PMR

a) Prior requirements

- PMR should be designed by competent pharmacists having sufficient knowledge of clinical pharmacy and good communication skills to extract the required information.
- They should be able to judge the appropriateness of dose, route and frequency of administration.
- Pharmacists should be able to correlate weight and age of a patient and his pathological conditions with effectiveness of therapy.
- Structured interview forms should be ready.
- Execute good conducive environment and privacy, especially in case of women patients.
- Patient's interest and availability should be given due preference.

b) Steps involved in design of PMR.

- Explain to the patient the purpose of PMR.
- Discuss and judge the knowledge, understanding and beliefs of patients regarding disease and medication.
- Fix the level and language of interview.
  - i) Use specific words that avoid misinterpretation.
  - ii) Sympathies with patient's situation and acknowledges what he is explaining.
- Review the case paper and/or ask about current and previous medical history.
- Ask about habits such as alcohol, smoking and general food habits and life style.
- All important points should be highlighted.
- Note the address and contact numbers of family physician and consultants of the patient.

3) Product Information Leaflet (PIL)

The Product Information Leaflet (PIL) is common literature provided with medicines. It bears information about the chemical nature of active drug, composition of formulation, pharmacology, indications, contraindication, precautions, symptoms and treatment of overdose, use, dosage and direction to use. (A typical PIL for paracetamol suspension is shown in fig. 5.3)

Paracetamol Suspension :			पॅरासेटामोल सस्पेन्शन		
Category : Analgesic in mild to moderate pain, antipyretic.			उपयोग : सौम्य ते मध्यम वेदनानाशक व ज्वरनाशक		
Composition : Each 5 ml contains paracetamol 120 mg.			घटक : प्रत्येकी ५ मिली मध्ये १२० मिलीग्राम पॅरासेटमोल.		
Dose : Take each dose 3 to 4 times a day.			मात्रा : प्रत्येकी एक मात्रा दिवसांतून ३ ते ४ वेला घेणे.		

Age	Average weight	Dose	वय सरासरी	शारीरिक वजन	मात्रा
Under 3 months	4 kg	1 to 1.5 ml	३ महिन्यापर्यंत	४ कि. ग्रा.	१ ते १.५ मिली
3 months to 1 yr.	7 kg	5 ml	३ महिने ते १ वर्ष	७ कि. ग्रा.	५ मिली
1 yr. to 3 yr.	12 kg	7 ml	१ वर्ष ते ३ वर्ष	१२ कि. ग्रा.	७ मिली
3 yr. to 5 yr.	17 kg	10 ml	३ वर्ष ते ५ वर्ष	१७ कि. ग्रा.	१० मिली
6 yr. to 12 yr.	25 kg	15 ml	६ वर्ष ते १२ वर्ष	२५ कि. ग्रा.	१५ मिली

- Minimum interval between two successive doses 4 hours.
- Maximum dose 60 mg / kg body weight in divided doses.
- Not to be taken for more than 48 hours without doctor's advice.
- Shake well before use.

Patient advice : It should not be administered along with other paracetamol-containing medicines.
- **Overdose may be injurious to liver.**
- Take doctor's advice if patient is suffering from liver and kidney impairment.
- Contraindicated in patients with known paracetamol hypersensitivity.

Storage : Store at 15 to 30°C. Protect from direct sunlight.
For further information please contact :
   Mr. U. R. Sathi, D.Pharm.
Jeevan Pharmacy, Pune. E-mail : jeevanph@cda.com

- दोन मात्रा मध्ये किमान ४ तासांचे अंतर ठेवा.
- कमाल मात्रा ६० मिलीग्राम प्रत्येक किलोग्रॅम शारीरिक वजनासाठी विभागुन घेणे.
- डॉक्टरांच्या सल्ल्याशिवाय सलग ४८ तासांपेक्षा जास्त वेळ औषध घेऊ नका.
- बाटली हलवून औषधाची मात्रा घ्यावी.

पेशंट सल्ला: पॅरासेटामोल घटक असलेले दुसरे कोणतेही औषध या औषधाबरोबर घेण्याचे टाळावे.
- **अतिमात्रा यकृतास हानिकारक आहे.**
- यकृता किंवा मुत्रपिंडाचा विकार अरोत तर डॉक्टरांच्या सल्ल्याने औषध घ्यावे.
- पॅरासेटामोल घेतल्याने ऑलर्जीक किंवा हायपरसेनसेटिव्ह परिणाम होत असेल तर हे औषध घेऊ नये.

साठवण:१५° ते ३०° डि.से. तापमानामध्ये व प्रत्यक्ष सुर्यप्रकाशापासुन औषध दुर ठेवा.
आधिक माहितीसाठी कृपया भेटा: श्री.यु. आर. साथी, डी. फार्म.
जीवन फार्मसी, पुणे. दूरध्वनी: (020)२५२८६८२१

पॅरासेटामॉल — सस्पेन्शन (Hindi)

पॅरासेटामॉल		सस्पेन्शन
उपयोग :	सौम्य से मध्यम वेदना नाशक व ज्वरनाशक	
घटक :	प्रत्येकी ५ मिली मे १२० मिलीग्राम पॅरासेटामोल.	
मात्रा :	हर एक मात्रा दिन मे ३ से ४ बार लेना.	

उम्र	औसत वजन	मात्रा
३ महिने तक	४ कि. ग्रा.	१ ते १.५ मिली
३ महिने से १ साल	७ कि. ग्रा.	५ मिली
१ साल से ३ साल	१२ कि. ग्रा.	७ मिली
३ साल से ५ साल	१७ कि. ग्रा.	१० मिली
६ साल से १२ साल	२५ कि. ग्रा.	१५ मिली

- दोन मात्रा मे कमसे कम ४ घंटो का अंतर रखे ।
- अधिकतम मात्रा ६० मिलीग्राम प्रत्येक किलोग्रॅम शारीरिक वजना के लिए अलग कर ले ।
- डॉक्टर की सलाह के बिना ४८ घंटे से ज्यादा सलघन दवा का प्रयोग ना करे ।
- उपयोग पूर्व बाँटल अच्छी तरह मिलाएँ ।

मरीज को सलाह: जिन दवाओं मे पॅरासेटॉमॉल हो ऐसी दवाओं के साथ इसका सेवन न करे ।

- **अतिमात्रा** यकृत के लिए हानिकारक है ।
- यकृत या मुत्रपिंड का मरीज हो तो डॉक्टर की सलाह ले ।
- पॅरासेटामोल के सेवन से एलर्जी या हाप सेंसिटिव्ह तो दवा का प्रयोग ना करे ।

रखरखाव : इस औषध को १५°० ते ३०° डि.से. तापमाने रखीए । प्रत्यक्ष सुर्यप्रकाश से दुर रखे ।

आधिक जानकारी के लिए संपर्क करे: श्री.यु. आर. साथी, डी. फार्म.
जीवन फार्मसी, पुणे. दूरध्वनी: (020)२५२८६८२१

પૅરાસેટામોલ સસ્પેન્શન (Gujarati)

ઉપયોગ :	ધીમે થી મધ્યમ દર્દનાશક અને જવરનાશક
ઘટક :	દરેક ૫ મિલી માં ૧૨૦ મિલીગ્રામ પૅરાસેટામોલ
માત્રા :	રોજ એક માત્રા ૩ થી ૪ વખત

વય	સરાસરી શારીરિનો વય	માત્રા
૩ માસ સુધી	૪ કિ. ગ્રા.	૧ થી ૧.૫ મિલી
૩ માસ થી ૧ વરસ	૭ કિ. ગ્રા.	૫ મિલી
૧ વરસ થી ૩ વરસ	૧૨ કિ. ગ્રા.	૭ મિલી
૩ વરસ થી ૫ વરસ	૧૭ કિ. ગ્રા.	૧૦ મિલી
૬ વરસ થી ૧૨ વરસ	૨૫ કિ. ગ્રા.	૧૫ મિલી

- બે માત્રા માં ૪ કલાકનો અંતર રાખવા જરૂરી છે.
- વધરામાં માત્રા ૬૦ મિલી ગ્રામ દરેક કિલોગ્રામ શારીરિક વજન માટે જુદા-જુદા કરાવજો.
- ૪૮ કલાક સુધી ઔષધનો વાપર થાય તો ડૉક્ટર નો સલ્હા જરૂરી છે.
- દવાની બાટલી - હલાવીને દવાની માત્રા લો.

પેશંટ માટે સલ્લા :
- પૅરાસેટામોલ સાથે બીજી દવા લેવાની નહી.
- વધરામાં ચુકત માટે હાનિકારક છે
- પૅરાસેટામોલ લેવાથી એલર્જી તથા હાયપરસેંટિવનો વિકાર થાય તો દવા લેવી નહી.
- સંરક્ષણ : ૧૫ થી ૩૦૦ ડિ.સે. તથા સુર્યપ્રકાશ થી દવા દૂર રાખવો.
- વધારે ની જાનકારી માટે સંપર્ક :
શ્રી. યુ.આર. સાથી, ડી.ફાર્મ.
જીવન ફાર્મસી, પુણે (020) ૨૫૨૮૬૮૨૧.

பெராசிட்டாமால் திரவம் (Tamil)

வகை :	மிதமான, மத்திய ஜ்வரம், உடல் வலி போன்றவற்றிற்கு
அளவு :	ஒவ்வொரு 5 மிலி பேராசிட்டாமால் 120 மிலி கலந்துள்ளது.
டோஸ் :	ஒவ்வொரு நாளைக்கு 3 முதல் 4 முறை எடுத்துக் கொள்ளலாம்.

வயது	தோராயமான எடை	டோஸ்
3 மாதங்களுக்குட்பட்டு	4 கிலோ	1 முதல் 1.5 மிலி
3 மாதம் முதல் 1வருடம்	7 கிலோ	5 மிலி
1 வருடம் முதல் 3 வருடம்	12 கிலோ	7 மிலி
3 வருடம் முதல் 5 வருடம்	17 கிலோ	10 மிலி
6 வருடம் முதல் 12 வருடம்	15 மிலி	15 மிலி

- ஒவ்வொரு முறை மருந்து உட்கொள்ள போதுமான கால இடைவெளி 4 மணி நேரம் இருக்க வேண்டும்.
- அதிகபட்சமாக 60மிலி டோஸ் உடல் எடையை கொண்டு தீர்மானிக்கப்படும்
- 48 மணி நேரத்திற்கு மேல் இந்த மருந்தை உட்கொள்ள வேண்டுமானல் டாக்டர் அதிகாரமாய கேட்கவும்.
- சிறுநீரகம் நன்கு பாட்டிலை குலுக்கி உபயோகிக்கவும்.

நோயாளிகள் கவனிக்க : இங்கு குறிப்பிட்டுள்ள மருந்துக்கு வேறு பாராசிட்டாமால் மருந்துடன் ஏற்படையது அல்ல.

- அதிகபடியான மருந்து குடலை பாதிக்கும்
- சிறுநீரக, குடல் பண் உள்ளவர்கள் டாக்டரின் ஆலோசனைக்கு பிறகே இம்மருந்தை உட்கொள்ள வேண்டும்.
- இம்மருந்தை உட்கொண்டோர் இதனால் ரத்த அழுத்தம் போன்றவை ஏற்பட்டால் சாப்பிடுவதை உடனே நிறுத்திவிட வேண்டும்.

பத்திரப்படுத்துதல் : 15 முதல் 30° உள்ள இடத்தில் வைக்க வேண்டும் சூரிய வெளிச்சம் நேரடியாக படும் இடத்தில் வைக்க கூடாது.

மேலும் விபரங்களுக்கு
திரு. U.R. சத்தி, D. Pharm.,
ஜீவன் பார்மஸி, பூனா டி மெயில்: jeevanph@cda.com
Ph. : (020) 25286821

ಪ್ಯಾರಾಸಿಟಮೋಲ್ ದ್ರಾವಣ (Kannada)

ವರ್ಗ : ಮಂದ ಹಾಗು ಮಧ್ಯಮ ನೋವು ನಿವಾರಕ ಮತ್ತು ಜ್ವರನಿವಾರಕ
ಸಂಕಲನೆ : ಪ್ರತೇ5 ಮಿ ಲೀ ದ್ರಾವಣ 120 ಮಿ ಗ್ರಾಂ. ಪ್ಯಾರಾಸಿಟಮೋಲ್ಸ್ ಹೊಂದಿರುತ್ತದೆ.
ಪ್ರಮಾಣ : ದಿನಕ್ಕೆ 3-4 ಬಾರಿ ನಿಗದಿತ ಪ್ರಮಾಣದಲ್ಲಿ ಸೇವಿಸಿ.

ವಯಸ್ಸು	ಸರಾಸರಿ ತೂಕ	ಪ್ರಮಾಣ
3 ತಿಂಗಳ ಒಳಗೆ	4 ಕೆ.ಜಿ	1-1.5 ಮಿ ಲೀ
3 ತಿಂಗಳಿಂದ 1 ವರ್ಷ	7 ಕೆ.ಜಿ	5 ಮಿ ಲೀ
1 ವರ್ಷದಿಂದ 3 ವರ್ಷ	12 ಕೆ.ಜಿ	7 ಮಿ ಲೀ
3 ವರ್ಷದಿಂದ 5 ವರ್ಷ	17 ಕೆ.ಜಿ	10 ಮಿ ಲೀ
6 ವರ್ಷದಿಂದ 12 ವರ್ಷ	25 ಕೆ.ಜಿ	15 ಮಿ ಲೀ

- 2 ಪ್ರಮಾಣಗಳ ನಡುವೆ ಕನಿಷ್ಠ 4 ಗಂಟೆಗಳ ಅಂತರವಿರಬೇಕು.
- ಗರಿಷ್ಠ ಪ್ರಮಾಣ 60 ಮಿ ಗ್ರಾಂ. ಪ್ರತ್ಯೇಕ ಕೆ.ಗ್ರಾಂಗೆ ದೇಹತೂಕಕ್ಕೆ ಅನುಗುಣವಾಗಿ ಪ್ರಮಾಣವನ್ನು ವಿಭಾಗಿಸಿ.
- ವೈದ್ಯರ ಸಲಹೆಯಿಲ್ಲದೆ 48 ಗಂಟೆಗಳನ್ನು ಮೀರಿ ಔಷಧಿಯನ್ನು ಸೇವಿಸಬಾರದು..
- ಸೇವಿಸುವ ಮೊದಲು ಚೆನ್ನಾಗಿ ಕುಲುಕಿ.

ರೋಗಿಗೆ ಸಲಹೆ :
- ಪ್ಯಾರಾಸಿಟಮೋಲ್ಹೊಂದಿರುವ ಇತರ ಔಷಧಿಗಳೊಂದಿಗೆ ಸೇವಿಸಬೇಡಿ.
- ಅಧಿಕ ಪ್ರಮಾಣ ಸೇವನೆ ಯಕೃತ್ತಿಗೆ ಹಾನಿಕರಕ.
- ಯಕೃತ್ತು ಮತ್ತು ಮೂತ್ರಪಿಂಡ ರೋಗಿಗಳು ವೈದ್ಯರ ಸಲಹೆಯನ್ನು ಪಡೆಯಬೇಕು.
- ಅಧಿಕ ಪ್ಯಾರಾಸಿಟಮೋಲ್ ಸೇವನೆಯಿಂದ ಅಲರ್ಜಿ ಅಥವಾ ಹೈಫರ್ಪೆನ್ಸಿಟಿವಿಟ ಉಂಟಾದವರೆ ಸೇವನೆಯನ್ನು ನಿಲ್ಲಿಸಿ.
- ಸಂಗ್ರಹಣೆ : 15c ದಂದ 30°c ತಾಪಮಾನದಲ್ಲಿ ಡಿ. ಸೂರ್ಯನ ನೇರ ಕಿರಣಗಳಿಂದ ಸಂರಕ್ಷಿಸಿ.

ಹೆಚ್ಚಿನ ಮಾಹಿತಿಗಾಗಿ ಸಂಪರ್ಕಸಂಬೇಕಾದ ವಿಳಾಸ
Mr. ಯು. ಆರ್. ಸಾಥಿ D. Pharma
ಜೀವನ ಫಾರ್ಮಸಿ ಪುಣೆ ಈ ಮೇಲ್ – jeevanph@cda.com
ಫೋನ್ : (020) 25286821

Figure 5.3: PIL for Paracetamol suspension

In developed countries, pharmacists have a legal obligation to provide a PIL each time a medicine is sold. In India also, this type of literature is considered for proper use of medication, most of these are printed in English and these are mainly for use of Registered Medical Practitioner. For the common man the PIL should be in his language. Unfortunately, to minimise the cost, manufacturers avoid inserting a PIL with the product. Therefore, in addition to pictograms, the pharmacists should prepare PIL in the local language. Experienced pharmacists should prepare a PIL. It must be authentic and unbiased. The optimum and easy to understand information along with pictograms serve better for understanding. However, PILs should not encourage self-medication.

4) Medication Card: Pharmacists can routinely use PIL, pictograms and medication records as patient counselling aids. Medication card is the tabular abstract explaining information about timing of administration of medication. It is useful when many medicines are prescribed simultaneously, for long-term treatments and in case of bed-ridden patients, where somebody else is administering the medicines to them. It should be handy, explained in the patient's language and easy to understand. It may be handwritten or computer generated. The computer-generated card will be easy to produce and it can be part of PMR. Single computer entry of medicines along with its cost and dosing schedule will produce a bill, PMR and medication card. Medication card is one of the best ways to achieve medication adherence.

Jeevan Pharmacy, Pune MEDICATION CARD							Ph. 2528 6434
Patient Name: Yogesh Gandhi **Address :** 11A Surajbag, Elphinston Rd, Mumbai				**Doctor Name:** Dr. S.Jejurkar **Address :** Shivsadan, Vashi			
Drug	**Strength**	**Brand & Dosage form**	**Breakfast**	**Lunch**	**Dinner**	**Bedtime**	**Specific Advice**
Omeprazole	20mg	Cap. Omezol		1			1 hr Before food
Antacids	-	Liq. Gelusil		5 ml	5 ml		2 hrs after food

Figure 5.4: Medication Card

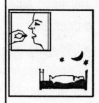 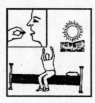

Take at bed time Take in the morning

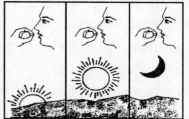

Take 2 times a day   Take 3 times a day

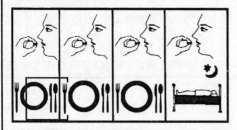

Take 4 times a day, with meals and at bedtime

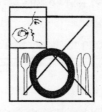

Do not take with meals

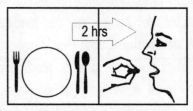

Take 2 hours after meals

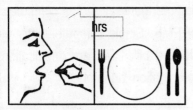

Take 3 hours before meals

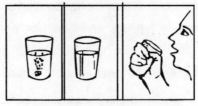

Dissolve in water and drink

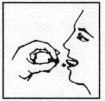

Dissolve under the tounge

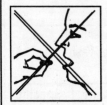

Do not swallow

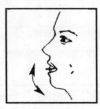

Chew

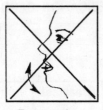

Do not chew

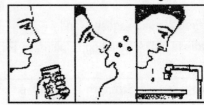

Use this medicine as a gargle

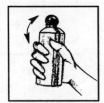

Shake well before use

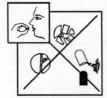

Do not break or crush tablets or open capsules

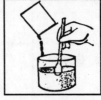

Dilute with water

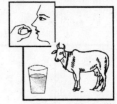

Take with milk

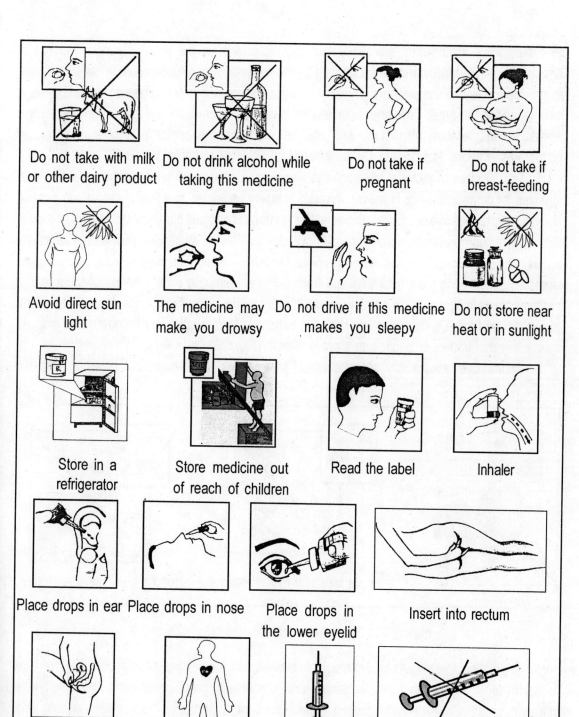

Figure 5.5: Pictograms used in Pharmacy

5) Pictograms: Pictograms are the schematic information in the form of simple pictures of directions for use or precautions to be taken by the patients during medication. When information is provided orally to the patients, there are many chances of them forgetting the information over a period of time. The pharmacists can develop handy and useful pictograms, which should be in the form of stickers that can be stuck on the container's label. The use of pictograms is more appropriate for counselling of illiterate patients. (Fig.5.5).

The success of pictorial messages is determined by the ability to create and use visual symbols for communicating. However, this skill is totally neglected in a formal curriculum existing in India. This results in a poorly developed ability to interpret pictorial conventions and visual media. Secondly, pictograms are based on general knowledge, intellectual quality and social and educational status of an individual. The images used in pictograms must be simple, clear, familiar and culturally acceptable, reflecting local traditions and habits. For example, in rural sections of India milk is neither packed in bottles nor in bags, whereas in urban areas packed milk is distributed. Therefore, to explain the term 'Do not take with milk', it is better to show the picture of a cow and a glass of milk, instead of bottles or bags, with a cross over it. (Fig. 5.6).

To improve applicability of pictograms, they should be designed with input from the

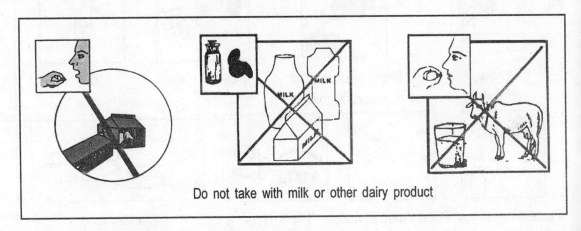

Do not take with milk or other dairy product

Figure 5.6: Pictograms for: Do not take with milk

target population and should be rigorously evaluated and modified until an acceptable outcome is achieved. It means, in India, no single and similar pictogram could serve the purpose in different areas. Chemist and druggist associations of a particular district/state should take initiative to design pictograms for patients in that region. No doubt, pictograms serve better for illiterate people, but they should not be used alone as the sole substitute for text instructions.

Stock Records

1) Purchase Record: Purchase record is made according to daily purchase bills. It should contain information about date, bill no., name of distributor and amount. If record is computer generated, then pharmacists can feed details about batch no., expiry date and name of the manufacturer also. The computer is becoming part and parcel of modern pharmacy and a single entry of medicines can be enabled to generate different data sheets, for example entries of purchase can be automatically used by computer for billing and to generate PMR and stock records. Thus computerisation avoids duplication of work.

2) Cash Memo: To sell medicines against the bill is ideal procedure of good pharmacy practice. The bill should be legible enough to be understood and a duplicate/carbon copy of it should be kept as record for at least three years. The cash memo should include the following particulars:
About Pharmacy :

   i)   Name, address, telephone number and e-mail of pharmacy.
   ii) Drug license number.
   iii) Serial number of bill and date of billing.
   iv) Tax identification number.
   v)   Name of Chief Pharmacist should appear under the head signature and should be signed by him/her.

About Patient and Prescriber:

   i)   Name and address of the patient.
   ii) Name and address of the prescriber.

About Medicine:

   i)   Name of the product and quantity.
   ii) Schedule of drug.
   iii) Name of manufacturer.
   iv) Batch number.
   v)   Expiry date.

---

vi) Price in Rupees.

Advantages of sale of medicines against the bill:

i) A proof of sale of medicine and its quality.

ii) Automatic generation of PMR of patient.

iii) Easier to find expiry date of medicine even if expiry date is part of the strip/loosely packed medicine is missing or difficult to trace.

iv) It helps in accepting return medicines/defective medicines.

v) The cash memo and PMR would be strong legal documents if anything goes wrong during therapy.

3) Expired Medicine Record: The expired medicines or medicines showing signs of instability, damaged containers and containers with smeared labels should be stored in separate shelves specially meant for expired products and marked as "Expired Medicines Not For sale". Such products need to be sent back to the supplier or manufacturer for appropriate disposal. Care should be taken to ensure that no human or animal consumes any expired product. Guidelines for disposal of expired medicine:

i) Pour liquids into sink and wash away properly.

ii) Tablets, capsules or powders are removed from packs and completely dissolved in buckets of water.

iii) Burying deep into the ground whenever suitable.

iv) Proper record of such disposed medicines must be maintained.

- Name of the disposed product.
- Details of the product: Mfg. date, Batch No., Exp. date and manufacturer.
- Stock details: Name of distributor, Bill No., Number of units expired.
- Disposal method: Returned to distributor/manufacturer/disposed in Pharmacy.
- Details of disposal in pharmacy to be recorded: date of disposal, method of disposal and signature of disposer.
- Name and signature of the pharmacist.

4) Returned Medicine Records: Sometimes patients may return the purchased medicines to the pharmacy or medicines may have to be recalled as per instructions of manufacturer or regulatory agency. Dispensing practice takes a different turn when the medicines are returned by patients or recalled/withdrawn from the market. Pharmacies should have standard procedure for such practices. Patients return the medicine for three reasons:

- Defective medicines: Physical defects like leakage, missing tablets/ capsules in strip/blister, defective labels.
- Unused medicines: When a doctor changes medicines and when patients

experience side effects.
- Expired medicines.

Guidelines to accept returned medicines:

i)   To accept the returned medicine or not, is the discretion of the pharmacy.

ii)   Only stable medicines whose package and container is not damaged can be accepted by pharmacies and equivalent money is reimbursed to the patient.

iii) The damaged, defective or expired medicines can be received by the pharmacy but these should be stored separately and appropriately labeled as "Expired Medicines Not For Sale". This practice will minimise the misuse of drugs and ensure proper disposal, but such items cannot be reimbursed.

iv)   The returned medicines should be verified whether they were purchased from this pharmacy. Proper billing system and entry in the PMR are immediate sources to check.

v)   Patients should be asked for storage conditions adopted for storage of the returned medicines. Only medicines that were properly stored should be accepted. The medicines requiring refrigeration are usually not accepted.

vi)   Appropriate adjustment in stock, entry in the records, as well as PMR of the patient, should be done.

The content of Returned Medicine Record:
- Name and signature of the pharmacist. Name of patient and patient number.
- Name of product, batch no., expiry date.
- Date of purchase and bill no.
- Condition of the product: Suitable For sale ☐ Not for sale ☐
- Amount returned.
- Name and signature of pharmacist.

5) Recalled Medicine Record: Procedure for recall or withdrawal of medicines from market is more complicated and is usually most urgent for safety purposes. The common reason for recall of medicines is, they are thought to be unsafe or unstable and can be categorised into three types:

Class I: Medicines that may cause serious adverse reactions or irreversible damage to life and may prove fatal.

Class II: Medicines that can cause potential health hazards and severe damage and can prove to be life threatening.

Class III: Medicines with minor defects or physicochemical instability, but are not life threatening and may not pose immediate health hazards.

The FDA issues the recall order, and immediately after receiving the order, a particular medicine or batch of the medicine is suspended. The existing stock of the medicine in question should be isolated and handed over to the wholesaler or company representative. For Class I type of recall, FDA should issue recall order within 24 hours of the submission of report of defective product. Authority can take help of media, chemists and druggists association to take corrective measures on war footing to avoid fatal cases. For recalling Class II type medicines, time frame to issue orders may be 48 to 60 hours after assessment of faulty product and for class III medicines, time frame to collect product is appropriately decided by authority considering the seriousness of defect.

It is easy to withdraw the stock while it is still in the retail pharmacy, or with the wholesaler, but it is difficult to recall the dispensed medicines. Good pharmacy practice cannot expect and accept 'INABILITY" to respond to recall orders. Detailed information about the patient, his address, phone number, e-mail and good habit of keeping his PMR is the best solution to reach the patient. The collected medicines should be kept separate and appropriately labeled as "Recalled Medicines Not For Sale". The record should be maintained as follows :

- Date of Recall.
- Name of the product.
- Instructing authority.
- Details of the product: Mfg. Dt., Batch No., Exp. Dt. and manufacturer.
- Stock details: Name of distributor, No. of units purchased, sold and in balance.
- Medicines collected from: Name and phone number of patient, No. of units collected.
- Receivers record: Name of authority to whom products are returned, date, quantity and signature of receiver.
- Reason for recall.
- Name and signature of the pharmacist.

In addition to above documents, the pharmacies should develop and maintain the following documents:

i) Standard operating procedures (SOP) for purchase of medicines, storage, rejection and disposal.
ii) SOP for dispensing or distribution of drugs in hospitals.
iii) Hygiene documents, cleaning and disinfectant procedures.
iv) Records of complaints, side effects, adverse drug reactions.

APPLICATION FORMS

a) Drug information forms: Pharmacists are a best source for drug related information and both patients and doctors could benefit from it. For that, pharmacists can take help of drug information centers (DIC) nearby and provide authentic information with references if needed. Pharmacies should provide blank forms to the needy persons for filling in information about the drugs and they and the Pharmacists should act liaison between the needy person and DIC. He can send the query to DIC and provide the information received by DIC to the needy. Formats for inquirer and provider of information may be as follows (Fig. 5.7 and 5.8):

Drug Information Center

State Pharmacy Council

DRUG INFORMATION REQUEST FORM

Date of enquiry   : .... Time: Received by:

Mode of request: ☐ Direct access   ☐ During ward rounds   ☐ Telephone

Name of enquirer: ....   Profession: . ...

Address   : ....   Phone   : ....

Query: ....

Purpose of enquiry: ☐ Better patient care   ☐ Update knowledge

Reply needed   ☐ Immediate   ☐ Within 1Hr.   ☐ Within a day

Patient Details:

Age: ....   Weight: .... Sex: M   ☐   F   ☐

Current disease: ....

Current drug therapy: ....

Pathological status   : Liver ....   Kidney ....   Other ....

If Pregnant woman: ☐ First Trimester   ☐ Second Trimester   ☐ Third Trimester

Additional information: ....

....

Signature of Enquirer   Signature of Pharmacist

Figure 5.7: Drug Information Request Form

Drug Information Center

State Pharmacy Council

DRUG INFORMATION DOCUMENT

Receiving Enquiry

Date of enquiry   : ....   Time :   Received by:

Name of enquirer : ....   Profession: . ...

Address   : ....   Phone : ....

Query: ....

Patient Details:

Age: ....   Weight: ....   Sex: M ☐   F ☐

Current disease: ....

Current drug therapy: ....

Pathological status   : Liver ....   Kidney ....   Other ....

If Pregnant woman: ☐ First Trimester   ☐ Second Trimester   ☐ Third trimester

Mode of Enquiry:

Mode of request:	☐ Direct access	☐ During ward rounds	☐ Telephone
Purpose of enquiry:	☐ Better patient care	☐ Update knowledge	
Question category:	☐ Indication	☐ Pharmacology	☐ ADR
	☐ Administration	☐ Efficacy	☐ Poisoning
	☐ Availability	☐ Interactions	☐ Pregnancy/ Lactation
Urgency to reply	☐ Immediate	☐ Within 1Hr.	☐ > A day

Mode of Reply

Date of reply   :   ....   Time of Reply: ....

Time taken to reply :	☐ < 10 Min	☐ 15-30min	☐ 1 Hr	☐ > A day
Form of reply :	☐ Written	☐ Verbal	☐ Printed material	☐ Email
References :	☐ Micromedex	☐ Medline	☐ IDIS	☐ Other

Reason for delayed Reply: ....

Name & sign of Clinical Pharmacist   Name & Sign of H.O.D.

Figure 5.8: Drug Information Document

2) Adverse Drug Reactions (ADR) : Identification and reporting of adverse drug reaction is one of the duties of clinical pharmacist. It can be used to evaluate safety of drugs during marketing phase. Central Drugs Standard Control Organisation (CDSCO), a government body analyses the ADR and can even recommend to ban unsafe drugs. For voluntary reporting of ADR an online form is available on www.cdsconic.in. Medical professional or pharmacist should play proactive role in collecting and reporting ADR. Typical format for reporting ADR and advice about reporting is given in Figure 5.9

3) Displays: Every pharmacy should display the common instruction, as shown in fig.5.10.

Jeevan Pharmacy, Pune

Mr. U. R. Sathi, B.Pharm.

Reg. No. 753712

Ph. No. 020-25285436

E-mail : jeevansathi@pdca.com

Dear Customers

- The medicines should be stored at room temperature, away from heat, moisture and direct sun light.
- Keep medicines out of the reach of children.
- Take the missed dose as soon as possible, but skip missed dose if it is almost time for the next regular dose. Do not take two doses at a time.
- Do not change prescribed drug or brand without permission of physician or pharmacist.
- Do not keep outdated medicine or medicine no longer needed.
- Be sure that any discarded medicine is out of the reach of children.
- Preferentially take medical advice from family physician and family pharmacist.
- Adopt good habits of life style.

Figure 5.10 Typical Display in Pharmacy

ACCREDITATION

It is well proven that organisations with set norms, procedures and standards function better than those without. However, except the rules mentioned under Schedule N of Drugs and Cosmetics Act, no other norms or standard procedures have been set to run medical stores. With emergent retail chains, there is a need to develop professionalism by pharmacists in the functioning of pharmacies, to compete with each other and emerge successful. With changing socio-economic scenario, Indian population is expecting and will accept services from audited pharmacies.

Accreditation is a process of quality assurance whereby the routine activities, services, systems and supporting processes within the pharmacy are critically appraised to ensure that

CDSCO

Central Drugs Standard Control Organisation
Directorate General of Health Services,
Ministry of Health & Family Welfare, Government of India.
Nirman Bhawan, New Delhi 110011
www.cdsco.nic.in

Adverse Drug Event Reporting Form

For VOLUNTARY reporting of
Adverse Drug Events
by health care professionals

Report #	
To filled in by Pharmacovigillance centres receiving the form	

A. Patient information

1. Patient identifier initials (First, last)	2. Age at time of event:	3. Sex ☐ F ☐ M
	or	
Date of birth:	(dd/mm/yy)	4. Weight _____ kgs.

B. Suspected Adverse Event

5. Outcomers attributed to adverse event (check all that apply)

☐ death _____
   (dd/mm/yy)
   permanent impairment/damage
☐ life-threatening
☐ hospitalization - initial or prolonged

☐ disability
☐ congenital anomaly
☐ required intervention to prevent
☐ other: _____

6. Dates of event starting (dd/mm/yy)	7. Dates of event stopping (dd/mm/yy)

8. Describe event or problem

9. Relevant tests/laboratory data, including dates

10. Other relevant history, including pre-existing medical conditions (e.g., allergies, race, pregnancy, smoking and alcohol use, hepatic/renal dysfunction, etc.)

Confidentiality: The patient's identity is held in strict confidence and protected to the fullest extent. Programme staff is not expected to & will not disclose the reporter's identity in response to a request from the public. Submission of a report does not constitute an admission that medical personnel or contributed to the event.

C. Suspect Medication (s)

11. Name (Brand and/or generic name)	(Labeled Strength)	(Manufacture)
# 1		
# 2		

12. Dose	Frequency	Route used	13. Therapy dates (if unknown, give duration)	
			# 1 From	To
			dd/mm/yy	dd/mm/yy
# 2			# 2	

14. Diagnosis for use (separare indications with commas)
1
2

15. Event abated after use stopped or dose reduced
1 ☐ yes ☐ no ☐ Not Applicable
2 ☐ yes ☐ no ☐ Not Applicable

16. Lot # (if known)	Exp. date (if known)
# 1	# 1
# 2	# 2

17. Event reappeared after reintroduction
1 ☐ yes ☐ no ☐ Not Applicable
2 ☐ yes ☐ no ☐ Not Applicable

18. Concomitant medical products and therapy dates including self medication & herbal remedies (exclude those used to treat event)

D. Clinician (if not the reporter)

19. Name and Professional Address : _____

_____ Pin code: _____

Tel No.: _____ Speciality : _____
with STD code

E. Reporter (see confidentiality section below)

20. Name & address	Phone

21. Date of this report (dd/mm/yy)

22. Health professional? ☐ yes ☐ no	23. Occupation	24. Also reported to ☐ no one else ☐ manufacturer ☐ user facility ☐ distributor
25. If you do not want your identity disclosed to the manufacturer, place an "x" in this box ☐		

Figure 5.9 Advice about reporting ADR to CDSCO

pharmacies develop performance standards in accordance with good pharmacy practices (GPP) guidelines. Thus, the concept of accreditation of pharmacies is based on the need to have quality system in place that would help to upgrade the existing system with the aim of continuous improvements.

Indian Pharmaceutical Association (IPA) has undertaken a project on "Accreditation of Pharmacies in India" in collaboration with WHO India Country Office. In the near future, a manual on accreditation will be prepared explaining different standards according to GPP including layout, design of pharmacy, housekeeping, personnel, cleanliness, documents, etc. The objectives are to develop a rating system for pharmacies based on quality of systems and supporting processes within the pharmacy.

Concept Clear : **Stock Related Records**

Purchase record: Inventory record.
Cash memo: Billing of sold items, cosmetics, OTC and prescription drugs.
Expired Medicine Record: Expired medicines and its disposal.
Returned Medicine Records: For medicines, unused/expired, returned by patient.
Recalled Medicine Record: For medicines that are recalled in emergency.
Application record: Drug information, ADR reporting.
Accreditation: Developing a rating system for pharmacies.

6 Storage and Stability of Medicine

WHO Expert Committee on specifications for pharmaceutical preparations states that "Inadequate storage and distribution of pharmaceutical products can lead to their physical deterioration and chemical decomposition, resulting in reduced activity and, occasionally, in the formation of toxic degradation products". Storage conditions address the required environmental conditions in terms of temperature, relative humidity and exposure to light at various stages of manufacturing, storage and distribution. Product expiration date is based on these storage conditions; and protecting the quality of the product until expiration date, is an important professional function of the pharmacist.

Degradation of Drugs

Degradation of drugs occurs under tropical conditions of high ambient temperature and humidity. In general, each 10°C change in temperature doubles the rate of chemical reaction, which is the main factor governing expiry of the product. The amount of moisture adsorbed by drugs or excipients influences dissolution rate of drugs, or hardness and disintegration time of tablets and thus affects physicochemical properties of dosage forms. These changes may alter bioavailability and therapeutic efficacy of the product. Selection of containers and storage of products at suitable storage condition, minimise drug degradation. A primary pack enhances product stability, whereas secondary pack further provides protection in transportation and handling.

Degradation of pharmaceutical substance is of following types:

1) **Physical:** Loss of ingredient, loss of volatile additives (flavours), precipitation, creaming,

---

phase separation, change in viscosity, colour, etc. Microbial growth and contamination are also included under physical stability. It causes cloudiness or precipitation in solutions, breaking of emulsions, caking of suspensions, discolouration, gas generation, etc.

2) Chemical: Chemical degradation of drugs such as oxidation, hydrolysis, photolysis, polymerisation, etc., or chemical interactions as between drugs, drug-additive or product-container.

3) Biological: Changes in bioavailability, toxicity, irritation, etc.

Signs of Physical Instability: At the time of dispensing (compounded, as well as manufactured product) pharmacists should check the product for signs of instability. The USP-24 provides some general guidelines to detect physical stability. Physical changes may be the result of chemical instability and such formulations should not be dispensed; eg. deposition of salicylic acid crystals on surface of solid dosage form or on the wall of the container in which aspirin is packed.

Liquid dosage forms:

- Solutions: Cloudiness, turbidity or precipitation of dissolved drug; changes in colour, flavour and taste. Discolouration of liquid extracts, precipitation, etc.
- Suspensions: Non-dispersible cake, increase or decrease in viscosity, large particles, change in colour, flavour and taste.
- Emulsions: Cracking, development of rancid odour, bigger droplets.

Solid dosage forms:

- Powders: Caking of powder or discolouration. The dry powders for reconstitution are sensitive to moisture, therefore these should be observed for presence of fog or liquid droplets inside the container, and for objectionable odour, etc. Effervescent powders and tablets are moisture sensitive; swelling of tablet/powder mass, caking and development of gas in the container are signs of generation of carbon dioxide.
- Capsules: Change in physical dimensions, hardening or softening, sticking of two or more units, adherence of units to walls of container.
- Uncoated tablets: Excessive powder or pieces of tablets, cracked, chipped tablets, discoloration, softening or moist appearance.
- Coated tablets: Cracked, moist or discoloured coat, mottling, twinning.

Semisolid dosage forms:

- Creams: Cracking, bleeding, lumps or grittiness, crystal growth, contraction due to loss of water.

- Ointments: Lumps or grittiness, crystal growth, bleeding, change in consistency.
- Suppositories: Hardening, softening, crystal growth. Change in colour, development of rancid odour.

Sterile dosage forms: Any sign of colour change, haziness, surface film or gas formation may be due to microbial contamination. Check for presence of particulate matter and leakage of container at the time of dispensing. For eye and eardrops, check for broken/damaged dropper.

Expiration period

Expiry date or shelf life is the period of storage up to which a given product remains stable and stability of medicinal product is the capability of it to remain in its original quality. This is calculated on the basis of chemical stability of active molecules and it is the time period up to which a drug retains 90 per cent of its original concentration. It is also called as t_{90}.

The Schedule P of Drugs and Cosmetics Act, 1940, gives the information on expiry date and storage conditions. Under usual circumstances, most of proprietary medicines dispensed in an original pack have a shelf life of one to five years. Manufactured pharmaceuticals are labeled with date of manufacturing and expiry date in terms of 'Month-Year.' Some examples of medicines with their shelf life are as follows:

i)   12 months: Bacitracin lozenges, Liquid serum, Typhus vaccine,
ii) 18 months: Penicillin tablets, Amoxycillin trihydrate dry syrup.
iii) 24 months: Ampicillin dry syrup, Chloramphenicol eye drops, Vitamin B_2 injection, Vitamin C injection.
iv) 36 months: Calcium pantothinate tablet, Rifampicin capsule, Vitamin B_{12} injection.
v)   48 months: Chloramphenicol capsule, Thiamine monohydrate.
vi) 60 months: Riboflavin, Tuberculin PPD, Gentamycin sulphate.

The compounded products have expiry date of one month from the date of manufacturing. Transfer from original pack to dispensing container, or dilution of product, will reduce shelf life, which is usually two weeks; when any product is to be used within 24 hours, it is called as freshly prepared preparation. Compounded products have actual DD-MM-YY.

Concept Clear :	Stability of Pharmaceutical product

Degradation : Physical, Chemical and Biological.
Shelf Life: Period of storage upto which a product retains its 90 per cent concentration.
Instability: Chemical, Physical and Biological changes.
Exp. Date: Manufactured products: 1-5 years. Label: 'Mfg. DT.' and 'Exp. DT.' in term of 'Month -Year.'

STORAGE CONDITIONS

Storage conditions are usually defined with respect to temperature, humidity and exposure to light. If official monographs are considered, then nearly 7 per cent medicines should be stored between 2 and 8 °C, 79 per cent require 8-30 °C. Stability, container, storage condition and labeling are interlinked and therefore proper labeling is important for maintaining the stability of the product. *Monograph of Indian Pharmacopoeia* mentions storage conditions as summarised in Table 6.1

Table 6.1: Pharmacopoeial storage condition

Sr. No.	Storage Condition	Interpretation
1	Cold	Any temperature not exceeding 8 °C and usually between 2 and 8 °C.
2	Cool	Any temperature between 8 and 25 °C.
3	Room Temperature	Temperature prevailing in working area
4	Warm	Any temperature between 30 and 40 °C.
5	Excessive heat	Any temperature above 40 °C.

A survey conducted by IPA Delhi branch in 2002, reveals some important facts about storage of medicines in India. Proprietary medicines bear different terminologies for label storage conditions, meaning of which neither remains the same in different parts of a country, nor simple to be understood by consumers. For example, storage conditions for about 70 per cent drugs official in *Indian Pharmacopoeia* is 'room temperature'; but, in India room temperature ranges from below freezing point to upto 45-50 °C. Secondly, only 10 per cent of the retail pharmacies are air-conditioned to provide temperatures less than 30°C.

Practicing the storage of medication : In addition to proper storage during manufacturing, transport and in retail pharmacies, patients should know the meaning and importance of storage conditions. However, the storage conditions mentioned in pharmacopoeia, or on proprietary medicines, are difficult to be interpreted by the common man and hence the community pharmacists should interpret and simplify them.Table 6.2 gives general method for storage.

Table 6.2: Simplified Storage Conditions For Medicines

S.N.	Storage Condition	Temp °C	Meaning	General Method for Storage
1	Cold place	2 - 8	Do not store above 8°C, but do not freeze	Store in refrigerator but not in freezer.
2	Cool place	8 - 25	Do not store above 25-30°C.	Store at room temperature. When temperature is above 30°C, area should have AC
3	Protect from moisture	Room Temp. RH < 60%	Keep in dry place. Temperature up to 30°C.	Should not be stored in humid areas like bathrooms and should be provided by manufacturer in a moisture-resistant container.
4	Protect from light	No direct sunlight	Keep in dark place/ away from direct sunlight. Temperature should be below 30°C.	Store in cupboard or drawer, and should be provided by the manufacturer in a light-resistant container.

Except in the regions having extreme environmental conditions, normal shelves, drawers and refrigerators are enough to store average medicines. However, India is a tropical country and several places are very hot and/or humid, some places are ice-cold, whereas some have intense light. Therefore, pharmacies must be designed in such a way that there is minimum direct sunlight falling on the medicines. The pharmacies in hot climatic areas (temperature above 30°C) should be air-conditioned. In the cold climatic regions, the pharmacies will require heaters, especially in winters. It is better to make provision of temperature and humidity indicators in the pharmacies. Some general guidelines for storage of medicines are given below:

i)   If the product has no special instructions regarding storage, then it should be stored in dry, clean shelves at room temperature (up to 30°C).

ii) Light and temperature sensitive medicines should not be stored in counters.

iii) The vaccines and sera must be kept in freezers and ice-packs must be used for transporting them.

iv) Medicines such as insulin, adrenaline injections, contraceptives and vaccines like DPT, DT, TT and Hepatitis should be stored in refrigerators, but not be kept in the freezer.

v)   Do not keep insulin vials and vaccines on the fridge or television, because the surface may be hot.

vi) When room temperature is above 30°C, the pharmacy should be air-conditioned or have air-circulating fans.

Storage and Stability of Medicine

vii) Patients should not put the medicines in a luggage bag that could be kept near the engine of a motor-vehicle or airplane. Coolant bags should be used in summer to carry medicines like insulin.

viii) Patients should be instructed to "Store the medicines in closed shelves/drawers away from direct sunlight. Insulin-like medicines should be stored in refrigerators or in earthenware pots".

ix) Earthenware pots half-filled with water can be used to simulate conditions of a cool place. The medicines are placed in a plastic bag or any other waterproof bag and suspended at the mouth of the pot. It can be called as 'Freezer of the Poor'.

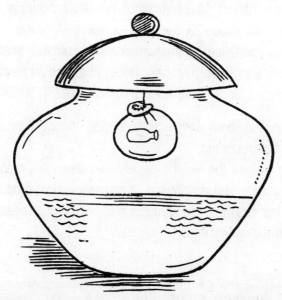

Figure 6.1: Earthenware Pots to store medicines

Ensuring proper storage of medicines: Pharmacies should be so designed as to protect medicines from direct sunlight and they should have air conditioning provisions to monitor temperature and humidity. Shelves should protect medicines from air borne dust. The design of furniture and fixtures should not allow growth of rodents and insects. A document should be maintained for design qualification of premises, interiors, routine inspections and repairs. The premises should be inspected every quarterly for floor and roof leakage if any, to ensure that shelves are well marked and to ensure the working of refrigerators. A complete stock verification should be conducted every month and documented in stock records. The expired products should be segregated, so they can be disposed off every month or every quarter, depending on the policy of the pharmacy. Computer billing provides an easier means to maintain daily stock. It also helps to put emergency orders and to identify expired products. The fire extinguishers and electricity generators should be checked every half year, to assure their working. As part of good dispensing practices, chief pharmacists and drug inspectors should sign the design qualification, records and general storage policy of the pharmacy.

GOOD DISTRIBUTION PRACTICES

Maintenance of temperature is necessary not only during manufacturing and storage in retail pharmacies, but also when the product has to be transported or shipped; and later when it is in the patients' custody. Almost 40 per cent of the pharmaceutical products are highly sensitive to temperature and about 25 per cent of vaccines reach their destination in a degraded state. During transportation, by truck, train, ship or aircraft, pharmaceutical products can get subjected to varied temperature ranges. Taking into account these practical problems, W.H.O. (2004) recommended Good Distribution Practices (GDP), which states that:

- Where special storage conditions are required during transit, they should be provided, checked, monitored and recorded.
- Temperature mapping across the vehicle should be done and recorded.
- Containers used for storage and distribution of pharmaceutical products should not have an adverse effect on the quality of the products and should offer adequate protection from external influences, including bacterial contamination.

Concept Clear: Storage conditions

- Cold place 2-8 °C, Cool place 8-25 °C, Dry place: Upto 30°C & RH < 60per cent, Protect from light: Away from direct sunlight and upto 30 °C.
- Facilities: Air conditioning, refrigerators, ice-packs, coolant bags, fire extinguishers and electricity generators.
- Ensuring storage: Design of pharmacy, facilities, furniture, documentation, periodic inspections, design qualifications.
- Good distribution practices: Provide, monitor and record interior temperature of vehicle.

7 Posology

Posology (Greek *Posos* - how much; *logos* - science) is the science of doses. Since the exact dose of any given drug, to produce the desired therapeutic effect varies from person to person, the doses of drug are usually expressed in the form of the range. The prescribed dose is that which exerts a therapeutic effect in the majority of subjects. It should be of minimum amount for eliciting the desired therapeutic response and maximum amount that can be tolerated by average subjects.

Factors Affecting the Dose

1) Age: Children do not react to all drugs in the same way as the adults do and with a few exceptions, drugs are more active and more toxic to children than to adults. This is due to many reasons; eg. newborn infants have relatively high total body water content, low body fat content, immature renal and hepatic functions, different protein binding capacities and gastric acidity. But in some cases, activity of certain metabolic pathways such as, conjugation and oxidation is more in children, than the adults and necessitate the administration of high doses on mg/kg basis than those required in adults; eg. theophylline. In geriatric patients, since the metabolism of drugs may be diminished; and many metabolic functions decline with age, they require different doses than the younger patients. Thus, with some exceptions, drugs tend to produce greater and more prolonged effect at the extremes of life. For example, renal function is low at birth, particularly in premature neonates and increases dramatically over the first two weeks of life. Due to aging, renal function progressively declines and may be significantly reduced in elderly patients. It means the dose requirements of drugs excreted renally are highly variable. Higher the rate of renal clearance, more will be the dose of drug required.

---

2) Body weight: The relative proportion of muscular and adipose tissue in the individuals governs the distribution and clearance of a drug from the body. Therefore, a dose for children is usually calculated on body weight basis, in terms of mg/kg/day. Because of higher metabolic rate, children generally require higher dose per kilogram than adults. But this method poses problems while calculating dose for obese children. Due to more weight, they are liable to be given higher doses than required. Since, obesity produces a corresponding increase in renal and hepatic function, it is better to calculate a dose based on ideal body weight of the child of that particular age.

3) Surface area: Many physiological factors such as plasma volume, oxygen consumption, and requirement of body fluid electrolytes, calories and glomerular filtration are proportional to the surface area. The surface area is also used to calculate dose; for example, anticancer drug methotrexate is administered on mg per sq.m. of body surface. The average body-surface area of a 70 kg adult is about 1.7 to 1.8 square meters.

4) Sex: On the basis of weight, female adults generally require smaller doses than males. Gender-based response to a drug may be due to unequal ratio of lean body mass to fat mass. On the basis of total body weight, the percentage of adipose tissue is greater and percentage of water is lower in adult females as compared to adult males.

5) Pathological conditions: Because of pathological conditions like renal function impairment or liver disease, many drugs remain in the body for longer periods of time.

6) Route of administration: Whether the drug is administered orally, topically or by injection determines effectiveness of its action. Drug administration by injections produces rapid drug action as a maximum amount of drug is available to elicit pharmacological effect. The intravenous dose of a drug is often smaller than the subcutaneous dose and this in turn is smaller than the oral dose. Drugs that are extensively metabolised in the liver (first pass metabolism) may need to be administered in higher doses. After oral administration, isosorbide dinitrate (antianginal drug) undergoes first pass metabolism. To avoid this first pass metabolism, it is also administered as a sublingual tablet. When the drug is given orally, then the dose is almost double than that of the sublingual dose.

7) Time of administration: Since, most of the drugs have better absorption from small intestine, they reach the site of absorption faster if taken on an empty stomach. Thus, any change in gastro intestinal emptying rate is likely to affect the dose. A number of drugs require to be given in higher doses, if given after a meal, eg. ferrous sulphate if administered in between meals is more effective than when administered immediately after meals.

Several physiological functions are altered during bed rest as compared to when the patient is active, including reduction in gastric emptying rate, increase in cardiac output and renal flow. It changes absorption, distribution and elimination of a drug.

8) Frequency of administration: Drugs having short plasma life get rapidly excreted from the body. In such cases, to maintain steady state plasma concentration, it requires frequent dosing. Controlled drug delivery systems are developed to reduce the frequency of administration.

9) Tolerance: Tolerance is a diminution in responsiveness, as use of the drug continues. If tolerance occurs, large doses of a drug are required to elicit an effect that is ordinarily produced by the normal therapeutic dose of drug. Examples of drugs which may produce tolerance after chronic administration are narcotic drugs like morphine, pethidine, heroin, alcohol, barbiturates, amphetamine, caffeine and nicotine, etc.

10) Elimination rate of drug: The body considers drugs as foreign substances (xenobiotics) and continuously works at eliminating them. Hydrophilic drugs are easily eliminated from the body via urine, whereas hydrophobic drugs stay in the body by partitioning into fat tissue and lipoidal membranes. Therefore, doses of the former type of drugs may be higher than those of the latter type.

11) Genetic polymorphism: Human body counters xenobiotics by enzymatically converting water-insoluble form into appreciably more hydrophilic form, which is then excreted in the urine. The enzyme system that probably plays the most crucial role in elimination of about 60 per cent of the drugs is the family of cytochrome P450 (CYP450) enzymes. The genetic mutations of these enzymes are reported, which produces altered enzymes with low or no activity or also hyperactivity, it is called as genetic polymorphism. Thus, certain individuals may show no or low metabolism of certain drugs and some may show hypermetabolism. Secondly, CYP450 enzymes are also induced or inhibited by many drugs, thereby altering the capacity of an individual to metabolise a drug. The inducers of CYP450 are smoking, alcohol, omeprazole, isoniazide, rifampin, phenytoin, carbamazepines, etc. These can accelerate rate of metabolism of co-administered drugs, needing more doses. The inhibitors include amodarone, cimetidine, ciprofloxacin, grapefruit juice, ketoconazole, lansoprazole, ciprofibrate, disulfiram, furafylline, etc. They may increase toxicity of co-administered drug. For example, grape juice increases toxicity of sildenafil, drug used to treat erectile dysfunction.

12) Idiosyncrasy and hypersensitivity: Idiosyncrasy is defined as a 'genetically determined abnormal or unusual response to a drug'. It occurs in a small proportion of individuals. For example 'salicylism' produced by chronic dosing of aspirin.

Hypersensitivity or drug allergy is an adverse reaction to particular chemical resulting from a previous exposure to the substance, occurring in only a small fraction of all people receiving the particular drug. Most common allergic effects are skin rashes, edema, anaphylactic shock, bronchospasm, serum sickness syndrome, etc.; and examples of drug which may produce it are penicillin, sulfonamide, phenacetin, etc.

13) Drug interactions: When different drugs interact amongst themselves or with food in the body, it is called drug interactions. Acute administration of alcohol has been shown to reduce the clearance of drugs like diazepam, paracetamol and tolbutamide. The intake of coffee has been shown to increase the bioavailability of paracetamol. Thus, in such cases, amount of drug required will be less. On the other hand, smokers may require an increased dose of theophylline to maintain therapeutic plasma level.

Synergism: When two or more drugs given together results in a total effect greater than the sum of their independent affect, it is called as synergism; eg. codeine and aspirin.

Addition: When the effect of two or more drugs given together is equal to the sum of their individual effect, it is called as addition; eg. ephedrine and aminophylline.

Antagonism: When two or more drugs given together produce effects opposite to each other, on the same physiological system, it is called as antagonism; eg. acetyl choline and atropine, ephedrine and phenobarbital.

Calculation of Doses:

A) According to Age:

1) Young's formula-

$$\text{Children dose} = \frac{\text{Age (years)}}{\text{Age} + 12} \times \text{Adult dose}$$

This formula is used to calculate dose of children below 12 years of age.

Exercise 7.1 : If the adult dose of paracetamol is 500 mg, what will be the dose for a child of 4 years?

$$\frac{4}{4+12} \times 500 = 125 \text{ mg}$$

Proprietary preparations: The proprietary paracetamol liquid preparation for paediatric use are syrup or suspension: 125 mg/5ml; Kid tablets: 125 mg. Adult tablet: 500 mg.

2) Dilling's formula-

$$\text{Children dose} = \text{Age (Year)} \times \frac{\text{Adult dose}}{20}$$

This formula is used to calculate dose for children between ages 4 and 20 years.

Exercise 7.2 : If the adult dose of ampicillin is 250-500 mg 3-4 times/day. What will the dose of a child of age 10 years be?

a) $\dfrac{10}{20} \times 250 = 125$ mg b) $\dfrac{10}{20} \times 500 = 250$ mg

Proprietary Preparations of ampicillin: Dispersible table for kid: Ampicillin 125 mg and 250 mg. Capsule: 250 mg and 500 mg.

Young's and Dillings' formula are generally used for calculation of children's dose. The other formulas include.

3) Cowling's formula: $\dfrac{\text{Age (years)} + 1}{24} \times$ Adult dose

4) Fried's formula: Child dose $= \dfrac{\text{Age (Months)}}{150} \times$ Adult dose

5) Bastedo's formula: Child dose $= \dfrac{\text{Age (years)} + 3}{30} \times$ Adult dose

6) Gaubin's formula: Dose for children of various ages is fraction of adult dose.

Age (years)	Parts of Adult dose	Age (years)	Parts of Adult dose
Under 1	1/12	14 - 20	2/3
from 1 - 2	1/8	21 - 60	Full adult dose
2 - 3	1/6	60 - 70	4/5
3 - 4	1/4	70 - 80	2/4
4 - 7	1/3	Over 90	1/2
7 - 14	1/2		

B) According to Body Weight:

1) Clark's formula:

Child dose $= \dfrac{\text{weight (pounds)}}{150} \times$ Adult dose or $\dfrac{\text{weight (kg)}}{70} \times$ Adult dose

Here, the average weight of an adult is taken as 150 lb or 70 kg.

Exercise 7.3 : The adult dose of Nimesulide is 100 mg b.i.d. What should be the dose for a child of 30 kg?

$\dfrac{30}{70} \times 100 = 43$ mg b.i.d

Proprietary Preparations: Nimesulide Tab: 100 mg and suspension 50 mg/5 ml.

C) According to Surface Area:

Recently, the calculation of doses according to surface area, has gained wide acceptance. Number of body functions and requirements are proportional to the surface area of the body. If we know weight (W in Kg) and height (H in cm) of a child, surface area (S in m²) can be calculated using formula-

$$Log\ S = 0.425\ log W + 0.725\ log\ H + 1.85$$

Formula to calculate child dose using surface area is,

Surface area of child in (m²)

$$Child\ dose = \frac{Surface\ area\ of\ child\ \left(m^2\right)}{1.8} \times Adult\ dose$$

The average body weight and surface area of children is given under percentage method.

Exercise 7.4 : If adult dose of mefenamic acid is 500 mg t.i.d., what will the dose for a 3 month old child, who suffering from juvenile idiopathic arthritis? Calculate it in percent of an adult dose.

$$Child\ dose = \frac{0.32}{1.8} \times 500$$

$$= 88\ g$$

Adult dose is 500mg

Therefore, 88 mg is 18 per cent of adult dose.

(D) Percentage Method

Age	Body weight (kg)	Height (cm)	Body surface area (m²)	Percentage of adult dose
> 1 month	3.4	50	0.23	12.5
1 month	4.2	55	0.26	14.5
3 month	5.6	59	0.32	18
6 month	7.7	67	0.40	22
1 year	10	76	0.47	25
2 years	14	94	0.62	33
3 years	18	108	0.73	40
7 years	23	120	0.88	50
12 years	37	148	1.25	75

E) Veterinary dose: In general, the dose of an adult (70 kg) and a dog of weight 18 kg is the same. If dose of an adult dog is assigned 1 g, then the comparative dose for others is, Dog: 1 g; cat 0.5 g; swine 2 g; sheep/goat 3 g; horse 16 g; cattle 24 g.

Exercise 7.5 : Haloperidol, an antipsychotic drug, can be given to adults in doses of 5 mg, 2 or 3 times a day. What will be the dose for a six month old infant, a child of 5 years and a boy of 16 years?

a) Dose for an infant of: six months

According to Fried's formula $= \dfrac{6}{150} \times 5 \, mg = 0.2 \, mg$

b) Dose for a child of 5 years: According to Young's formula-

$= \dfrac{5}{5 + 12} \times 5 \, mg = 1.47 \, mg \, (1.5 \, mg)$

c) Dose for a boy of 16 years: According to Dilling's formula $= \dfrac{16}{20} \times 5 = 4 \, mg$

Haloperidol for oral use is available in the form of tablets of various strengths, viz., 0.25 mg, 1.5 mg, 2 mg, 5 mg, 10 mg and 20 mg and drops contains 2 mg/ml, and 10 mg/ml of drug. A dropper bearing calibrations of 0.25 ml, 0.5 ml, 0.75 ml and 1 ml is provided. From these, the convenient dosage forms can be given to patients.

Exercise 7.6 : How many theophylline tablets, each containing 200 mg are needed to provide 13 mg/kg/day in divided doses for a week for patients weighing 50 kg ?

The dose of theophylline is 13 mg/kg/day

∴ For 50 kg patient, 13 mg x 50 kg = 650 mg.

Since each tablet is of 200 mg. One tablet three time a day is suitable dose.

∴ For 7 days, 21 tablets are required.

Proprietary theophylline tablets contain 200 and 300 mg of drug.

Exercise 7.7 : How many milliliters of Amoxicillin syrup containing 125 mg/5ml of drug is required to provide dose of 20 mg/kg/day in divided doses for four days to a child weighing 45 lbs.?

1 lb = 458.5 g   ∴ 45 lbs = 20.632 kg.

Dose of Amoxicillin for children under 20 kg is 20-40 mg/kg/day for 3 to 10 days.

∴ 20 kg x 20 mg = 400 mg/day.

The composition of Amoxicillin syrup is 125 mg/5 ml.

∴ 5 ml of syrup t.i.d. for 4 days will be required.

∴ 15 ml per day x 4 day = 60 ml.

The proprietary amoxicillin syrup contains 125 mg/5 ml in 30 ml and 60 ml volumes, and 250 mg/5 ml in 30 ml capacity. Kid tablets are of 125 mg and 250 mg.

The dose, caution and advice to the patients regarding the commonly used drugs, is summarised in Table 7.1.

Modern Dispensing Pharmacy

Table 7.1 : Posology and Patient Counselling For Some Drugs*

No.	Drug	Dose	Caution	Patient Counselling
1)	**Acetazolamide** Diuretic	Oral : Initial 250 mg. o.d., up to 1.0 g/day in divided doses.	• Lactation, pregnancy; • Do not take more than a dose of aspirin (if prescribed);	• Take in morning.
2)	**Acyclovir** Antiviral	Oral : 200 mg 5 times for 10 days, IV : 10 mg/kg over 1 hr, 8 hrly. Topical : 5% ointment q.i.d. for 7 days.	• Contraindicated in lactation, Allergy; • Pregnancy, renal impairment.	• Use rubber gloves to apply ointment.
3)	**Albendazole** Anthelmintic	Oral : Hook worm, roundworm, threadworm : 400 mg single dose. Tapeworm : 400 mg o.d. for 3 day.	• Contraindicaded in pregnancy, lactation and neonates;	• Take with food. • Take iron suppliment.
4)	**Allyloestrenol** Progestogen to prevent abortion	Oral : 5-10 mg daily in divided doses.	• Pregnancy first 4 months, Liver dysfunction; • Genital carcinoma, diabetic; • Do not take with aspirin and antacids.	• Do not discontinue dosing abruptly; • Do not change dose.
5)	**Alprazolam** Anxiolytic	Oral : 0.25 - 0.5 mg t.i.d., Max : 4 mg/day	• Lactation pregnancy, children; • Renal and liver impairment.	• Avoid alcohol; • Do not drive; • Do not discontinue dosing abruptly;
6)	**Amitriptyline** Antidepressant	Oral : Initially 25 mg t.i.d., up to 150 mg daily.	• Lactation, pregnancy, epilepsy; • Liver impairment;	• Avoid alcohol; • May cause dizziness when standing up quickly; • Do not drive.

* For further reading refer CIMS.

No.	Drug	Dose	Caution	Patient Counselling
7)	**Amlodipine** Calcium chan-nel blocker.	Oral : Initial 5 mg o.d., increase up to 10 mg over in 7-14 days.	• Lactation, pregnancy, children; • Renal and liver impairment.	• Do not discontinue dosing abruptly; • Do not drive; • Do not change the brand; • May cause dizziness while standing up quickly.
8)	**Amoxycillin** Bactericidal	Oral : 250-500 mg t.i.d., IM : 50-100 mg/kg/day in 3 divided doses, IV : 1.0 g t.i.d. in meningitis.	• Lactation; • Allergy to penicillins; • Renal and liver impairment.	• Do not discontinue the dosing; • Complete the course of medication.
9)	**Ampicillin** Bactericidal	Oral : 250-500 mg. 3-4 times daily, IV : 2.0 g q.i.d.	• Lactation, allergy to penicillins; • Renal impairment; • Interfere in urine sugar test.	• Take 30 min before food or on empty stomach. • Complete the course of medication.
10)	**Aspirin** Platelet inhibitor	Oral : 75-100 mg to 150 to 325 mg.	• Allergy, last 3 months of pregnancy; • Pre-operation period; • Lactation, pregnancy; • Ulcer, asthma; • Renal and liver impairment.	• Take with food; • Do not crunch/chew SR tablet.
11)	**Atenolol** Beta-blocker	Oral : 25-50 mg o.d. up to 100 mg. o.d. IV : 5 mg IV over 5 min.	• Lactation, pregnancy, diabetes, asthma; • Renal and liver impairment;	• Do not discontinue the dosing abruptly; • Do not drive. • Take 30 min before food;
12)	**Azithromycin** Bactericidal	Oral : 500 mg o.d. for 3 days.	• Lactation, pregnancy, children, allergy to penicillin; • Renal and liver impairment.	• Complete the course of medication; • Do not take with antacids.

No.	Drug	Dose	Caution	Patient Counselling
13)	**Beclomethasone** Corticosteroid	Topical : 0.025% w/w cream, 1-2 times daily. Inhalation : 400-800 mcg/day. Nasal : 50 mcg/spray, 2 spray b.i.d. in each nostril.	• Allergy, asthma; • Lactation, pregnancy.	• Rinse mouth after each inhalation; • Refer chapter 13 for direction to use of inhalers.
14)	**Betamethasone** Glucocorticoid	Oral : 0.6 - 7.2 mg/day. IM/IV : 4-20 mg q.i.d.	• Lactation, pregnancy, children; • Diabetes, hypertension; • Ulcer, psychosis.	• Take with food; • Do not discontinue dosing abruptly.
15)	**Bisacodyl** Laxative	Oral : 5 to 10 mg at bed time. Rectal : Suppository, 10 mg in morning.	• Pregnancy; • Avoid in intestinal obstruction, signs of appendicitis.	• Take on an empty stomach. • Do not take milk or antacid within 1 hr; • Take after food.
16)	**Bisoprolol** Beta-blocker	Oral : 2.5 or 5 mg o.d. up to 20 mg/day.	• Lactation, pregnancy.	• Do not discontinue the dosing abruptly;
17)	**Bromocriptine** To treat hypoglycaemia	SC/IM/IV : 0.5 to 1 mg.	• Lactation, pregnancy, children; • High blood pressure.	• Take with food; • Avoid driving.
18)	**Captopril** ACE-inhibitor	Oral : 6.25 to 50 mg t.i.d. Max : 150 mg/daily.	• Lactation, pregnancy; • Renal impairment.	• Take on empty stomach. • Do not take potassium suppliments.
19)	**Cefadroxil** Bactericidal	Oral : 1-2 g as single dose or in 2 divided doses.	• Lactation, pregnancy, allergy to cephalosporins; • GI diseases, renal impairment.	• Take with food. • Complete the course of medication.

88

No.	Drug	Dose	Caution	Patient Counselling
20)	**Celecoxib** NSAID, Cox-2 inhibitor	Oral : 200 mg o.d. or 100 mg b.i.d.	• Lactation, pregnancy; • Asthma, allergy.	—
21)	**Cephalexin** Bactericidal	Oral : 1-2 g daily in 3-4 divided doses.	• Lactation, pregnancy, allergy to cephalosporins and penicillins. • GI diseases, renal impairment	• Take with food • Complete the course of medication.
22)	**C h l o r a m - p h e n i c o l** Bactericidal	Oral : 2-3.5 g daily in 4 divided doses.	• Contraindicated in pregnancy and lactation; • Sensitivity; • Renal and liver impairment; • Avoid all other medicines;	• Take after food • Complete the course of medication.
23)	**Chlordiazep- oxide** Anxiolytic	Oral : 20-40 mg daily, upto 50-100 mg/day in divided doses.	• Lactation, pregnancy.	• Avoid alcohol; • Do not drive; • Do not discontinue abruptly;
24)	**Chloroquine** Antimalarial	Oral : initial 600 mg, followed by 300 mg 6-8 hrly, on 2nd and 3rd day 300 mg o. d. IV : 10 mg/kg over 8 hrly. IM : 3.5 mg/kg over 6 hrly.	• Pregnancy, lactation, allergy, retinal damage, children. • Renal and liver impairment; • Epilepsy.	• Take with food. • Consult eye specialist, if required.
25)	**Chlorprom- azine** Antipsychotic	Oral : 25 mg - 1 g daily in divided doses. Max : 2.0/day. IM : 25-50 mg, 3-4 times day.	• Lactation, pregnancy; • Do not take with antihistaminics	• Avoid alcohol; • May cause dry mouth and constipation.

No.	Drug	Dose	Caution	Patient Counselling
26)	**Chlorpropam-ide** Antidiabetic	Oral : Initially 100 or 125 mg daily, then up to 500 mg daily.	• Contraindicated in pregnancy and in lactation.	• Avoid alcohol; • Do not discontinue the dosing abruptly; • Do not change the brand; • Avoid excessive exposure to direct sunlight.
27)	**Cimetidine** Histamine H_2 receptor antagonist	Oral : 200 mg - 400 mg bid or q.i.d. for 4 to 8 weeks. Max : 2.4 g daily. IM & IV : 300 mg 6-8 hrly.	• Renal, liver and thyroid impairment • Not to take more than a single dose aspirin (if prescribed). • Lactation, pregnancy, • Renal impairment.	• Do not take antacids within 1 hr. • Avoid taking with antidepressant. • Avoid alcohol and smoking.
28)	**Ciprofloxacin** Bactericidal	Oral : 250-500 mg b.i.d. IV : 100-400 mg b.i.d.	• Contraindicated in pregnancy, lactation, children, allergy; • Renal impairment;	• Take 30 mins before food • Avoid driving • Complete the course of medication. • Do not take antacids, milk, calcium or iron suppliment.
29)	**Cisapride** In constipation	Oral : 10 mg t.i.d.	• Lactation, pregnacy; • Hepatic impairment; • Avoid erythromycin, ketoconazole.	• Take 15 minutes before food, • In case of irregular heart beat, or pulse, contact the physician.
30)	**Clarithromycin** Bactericidal	Oral : 250 - 500 mg b.i.d. up to 1.5 g daily.	• Lactation, pregnancy, allergy; • Renal impairment;	• Take with food. • Complete the course of dosing.
31)	**Cloxacilin** Bactericidal	Oral : 500 mg q.i.d., up to 18 g daily. IM : 250-250 mg q.i.d. IV : 1-4 g q.i.d.	• Lactation pregnancy allergy; • Liver diseases.	• Take 30 min before food. • Complete the medication course.

No.	Drug	Dose	Caution	Patient Counselling
32)	**Danazol** Attenuated androgen	Oral : 200 mg - 800 mg in divided doses b.i.d. for 6 months.	• Lactation, pregnancy. • Renal and cardiac dysfunction.	• Avoid excessive exposure to direct sunlight; • Do not change dose; • Do not discontinue dosing abruptly.
33)	**Dexamethasone** Glucocorticoid	Oral : 3-6 mg/day. IM/IV : 0.5-20 mg. Topical : 0.01% cream, 4-6 times daily.	• Lactation, pregnancy, children; • GI ulcer, diabetes, hypertension.	• Take with food; • Do not discontinue the dosing abruptly.
34)	**Diazepam** Anxiolytic	Oral : 2.5 to 10 mg 2-4 times daily. Max : 10 mg/day. IM/IV : 2-20 mg, 3-4 hrly.	• Lactation, pregnancy; • Renal and liver impairment.	• Avoid alcohol; • Avoid driving; • Do not discontinue the dosing abruptly.
35)	**Diclofenac** NSAID	Oral : 50 mg b.i.d./t.i.d. SR Tab : 100 mg o.d. IM : 75 mg 1-2 times daily. Topical : Diclofenac diethyl-ammonium ~ diclofenac 1% w/w, 3-4 times daily.	• Lactation, pregnancy, GI Ulceration • Impaired renal, cardiac and liver function. • Do not take aspirin during this therapy.	• Take with food; • Do not crush / chew SR tablet. • Avoid driving.
36)	**Diltiazem** Calcium chan- nel blocker	Oral : 180 mg/day in 3-4 divided doses. Max : 240 mg/day. SR Tablets or capsule : 90-120 mg b.i.d. to 180 mg b.i.d.	• Lactation, pregnancy, diabetes • Renal and liver impairment	• Take on an empty stomach with glass of water. • Do not discontinue dosing abruptly. • Do not crush/chew SR tablet/ capsule.

No.	Drug	Dose	Caution	Patient Counselling
37)	**Diphen-hydramine** Antihistamine	Oral : 25-50 mg, 1-4 times daily	• Contraindicated in pregnancy, hypersens. • Epilepsy.	• Take with food. • Avoid driving. • Avoid alcohol.
38)	**Docusates** Fecal softner	Oral : 100 mg, 4-5 times a day. Rectal : Enema, 50-120 mg.	• Pregnancy • Avoid with liquid paraffin. • Avoid rectally in fissures.	–
39)	**Domperidone** Antiemetic	Oral : 10-20 mg, 4-8 hrly.	• Pregnancy	• Take 15 min before food.
40)	**Enalapril** ACE-inhibitor	Oral : 2.5 mg to 10-20 mg o.d.	• Lactation, pregnancy; • Renal impairment.	• Do not take potassium suppliments. • Avoid alcohol.
41)	**Erythromycin** Bactericidal	Oral : 1.0 g daily b.i.d. or q.i.d.	• Lactation, pregnancy. Allergy. • Liver diseases.	• Take 30 mins before food; • Complete the course of medication.
42)	**Ethinyl oestradiol** Oestrogen oral contraceptive	Oral : 0.05 mg daily from 5th day of menstrual cycle for 21 days.	• Contraindicated in pregnancy and lactation., • Jaundice, vaginal bleeding.	• Take with food or milk.
43)	**Famotidine** H₂ receptor antagonist	Oral : 20 mg-40 mg b.i.d. for 4-8 weeks. IV : 20 mg b.i.d.	• Lactation, pregnancy. • Renal impairment children.	• Take with food. • Avoid alcohol.
44)	**Felodipine** Calcium channel blocker	Oral : 5-10 mg/day in divided doses.	• Lactation, pregnancy; • Liver dysfunction.	• Do not discontinue dosing abruptly. • Take with food; • Do not crush or chew tablet. • Avoid alcohol. • May cause dizziness while standing up quickly.

No.	Drug	Dose	Caution	Patient Counselling
45)	**Flurazepam** Hypnotic	Oral : 15-30 mg at bed time	• Lactation, pregnancy • Liver and respiratory impairment. • Do not take with antihistaminics	• Avoid alcohol. • Do not take antacids within 1 hr. • Do not drive.
46)	**Frusemide** Diuretic	Oral : 40-80 mg once or twice daily. IM : 20-80 mg/day. IV : 20-80 mg slow IV (1-2 min).	• Lactation, pregnancy • It should be taken with potassium suppliment.	• Do not take if tablets show colour change. • Avoid excessive exposure to direct sunlight. • May cause dizziness while standing up quickly.
47)	**Furazolidone** Antidiarrhoeal	Oral : 100 mg q.i.d.	• Lactation, pregnancy. • Avoid decongestants.	• Avoid alcohol. • Take with food. • Urine turns brown coloured. • Take at regular time intervals as directed by physician.
48)	**Glibenclamide** Antidiabetic	Oral : Initially 2.5 mg daily, then upto 20 mg/ day, 30 min before breakfast.	• Contraindicated in pregnancy, lactation. • Renal and liver impairment. • Not to take more than a single dose of aspirin (if prescribed)	• Take immediatly before breakfast or first meal. • Do not discontinue the dosing abruptly.
49)	**Glimepiride** Antidiabetic	Oral : 1-2 mg o.d. with first meals. Max : 8 mg o.d.	• Contraindicated in pregnancy, lactation. • Renal and liver impairment.	• Do not change the brand. • Take immediately before breakfast or first meal. • Do not discontinue the dosing abruptly. • Do not change the brand.

No.	Drug	Dose	Caution	Patient Counselling
50)	**Glyceryl trinitrate** Antianginal	Sublingual : 0.5 mg every 3 min, up to 0.8 to 2.4 mg every 5-10 min. Oral : 2.5-6.5 mg 8-2 hrly. Transdermal and IV infusion.	• Lactation and pregnancy.	• Do not crush/chew/swallow the sublingual tablet. • May cause dizziness while standing up quickly. • Do not discontinue dosing abruptly.
51)	**Haloperidol** Antipsychotic	Oral : 0.5 to 5 mg, 2-3 times daily. IM : 2-5 mg every 4-6 hrly.	• Lactation, pregnancy, epilepsy	• Take with food; • Take with caution in very cold or very hot weather; • Avoid alcohol; • May cause dizziness while standing up quickly. • Do not drive. • Avoid excessive exposure to direct sunlight.
52)	**Ibuprofen** NSAID	Oral : 1.2-1.8 g daily in divided doses. S.R. : 300-600 mg b.i.d.	• Lactation and pregnancy; • G.I ulceration, asthma; • Do not take aspirin during this therapy.	• Take with food • Do not crush/chew SR tablet • Avoid driving.
53)	**Indomethacin** NSAID	Oral : 25 mg, 2-3 times daily; S. R. Tab/Cap : 75 mg o.d.	• Avoid in lactation, pregnancy, and children • G.I. ulcer, hypertension, asthma. • Do not take aspirn during this therapy.	• Take with food. • Do not crush/chew SR tablet/ capsule. • Avoid driving.

Posology

No.	Drug	Dose	Caution	Patient Counselling
54)	**Mefenamic, acid** NSAID	Oral : 500 mg t.i.d.	• Avoid in lactation. • Pregnancy, children. • Renal and liver impairment. • G.I. ulcer, asthma • Do not take aspirin during this therapy.	• Take with food. • Avoid driving.
55)	**Isosorbid dinitrate** Antianginal.	Sublingual : 5-10 mg Oral : 5 to 10 mg q.i.d. S. R. tablet : 20 to 40 mg b.i.d.	• Lactation, pregnancy.	• Take on empty stomach with glass of water. • Do not crush/chew/swallow sublingual tablet and S. R. tablet. • Do not discontinue dosing abruptly. • Do not drive.
56)	**Ketoprofen** NSAID	Oral : 50 mg, 2-3 times daily. S.R. tab : 100/200 mg o.d. IM : 200 mg in divided doses. Topical : 2.5% gel, 2-3 times daily.	• Avoid in lactation, pregnancy and children; • Renal impairment; • G.I. ulcer, asthma. • Do not take aspirin during this therapy.	• Take with food. • Do not crush/chew S.R. tablet • Avoid driving.
57)	**Lansoprazole** Proton pump in-hibitor	Oral : 15-30 mg daily in morning.	• Lactation, pregnancy; • Liver disease.	• Take before food, • Avoid alcohol and smoking.
58)	**Lisinopril** ACE-inhibitor	Oral : 2.5 mg o.d. upto 40 mg/day	• Lactation and pregnancy; • Renal impairement;	• Do not drive. • Avoid alcohol.
59)	**Loperamice** Antidiarrhoeal	Oral : 2 mg after each loose motion. Max : 16 mg/day	• Lactation, pregnancy; • Liver dysfunction, severe colitis, • Allergic to loperamide.	• Do not use for children under 2 years.

No.	Drug	Dose	Caution	Patient Counselling
60)	**Mebendazole** Anthelmintic	Oral : Round, whip and hookworm : 100 mg b.i.d. for 3 days. Threadworm : 200 mg b.i.d. for 30 days. Pinworms : 100 mg o.d.	• Contraindicated in pregnancy, lactation, allergy and in infants. • Liver impairment.	• Take with food. • Liver disease.
61)	**Mesalazine** Antiinflamma-tory	Oral : 2.4 g daily in divided doses. Rectal : Enema, : 1 g daily.	• Lactation, pregnancy; • Liver dysfunction; • Avoid with lactulose.	—
62)	**Metformin** Antidiabetic	Oral : 500 mg t.i.d. with meals, upto 3 g/day.	• Contraindicated in pregnancy and lactation. • Renal, liver, thyroid and cardiac impairment. • Not to take more than a single dose of aspirin (if prescribed).	• Take with food. • Avoid alcohol. • Do not discontinue the dosing abruptly. • Do not change the brand.
63)	**Metoclopramide** Antiemetic.	Oral : 5 to 10 mg at bed time. Rectal : suppository 10 mg in morning.	• Avoid in intestinal obstruction, signs of appendicitis.	• Do not take milk or antacid within 1 hr; • Take on an empty stomach.
64)	**Metronidazole** Antibacterial	Oral : 2.0 g as single dose or 500 mg b.i.d. for 7 days. IV : 15 mg/kg over 1 hr followed by 7.5 mg 1 kg over 1 hr, 6 hrly.	• Lactation, pregnancy, allergy; • Renal and liver impairment.	• Take with food; • Avoid alcohol; • Avoid driving; • Urine may show reddish-brown colour, it is normal.

No.	Drug	Dose	Caution	Patient Counselling
65)	**Nalidixic acid** Bactericidal	Oral : 1.0 g q.i.d. for 1-2 weeks	• Lactation, pregnancy, allergy and infants below 3 months. • Renal and liver impairment. • Convulsions.	• Take with a glass of water; • Avoid excessive exposure to direct sunlight. • Complete the course of medication. • Avoid driving.
66)	**N a p r o x e n** NSAID	Oral : 250 mg b.i.d. Topical : 10% gel, 2-3 times daily.	• Avoid in pregnancy, lactation, and in children; • GI ulcer, asthma; • Renal and liver impairment; • Do not take aspirin during this therapy.	• Take with food. • Avoid alcohol. • Avoid driving.
67)	**Nifedipine** Calcium chan-nel blocker	Oral : 10-20 mg every 6-8 hrly. Max : 80 mg. S.R. tab : 30-60 mg o.d.	• Lactation, pregnancy, diabetes, • Liver and renal impairment.	• Take with food or milk. • Do not crush or chew S. R. tablet. • Do not discontinue the dosing abruptly.
68)	**N i m e s u l i d e** NSAID	Oral : 100 mg b.i.d. Topical : 1% gel, 3-4 times day.	• Avoid in pregnancy, lactation, • GI ulcer, • Renal and liver impairment.	• Take with food.
69)	**N i t r a z e p a m** Hypnotic	Oral : 5-10 mg at bed time	• Lactation, pregnancy, • Do not take with antihistaminics.	• Avoid alcohol. • Do not take antacids within 1 hr. • Do not drive.
70)	**Norfloxacin** Bactericida	Oral : 400 mg b.i.d. for 3-10 days, up to 800 mg b.i.d.	• Lactation, pregnancy, children. • Convulsions. • Renal impairment.	• Take 30 min before food. • Avoid antacids, milk within 2 hrs. • Avoid driving; • Complete the course of medication.

No.	Drug	Dose	Caution	Patient Counselling
71)	**Omeprazole** Proton pump Inhibitor	Oral : 10-20 mg daily for 4-8 weeks Max : 40 mg	• Lactation, pregnancy, • Liver disease.	• Take before food. • Avoid alcohol and smoking. • Do not open or chew capsule.
72)	**Oxytetracyline** Bactericidal	Oral : 1-2 g day in 4 divided doses 6 hrly. Topical : 30 mg/g ointment 2-3 times daily.	• Contraindicated in pregnancy, lactation, allergy and in neonates. • Renal and liver impairment.	• Take on empty stomach. • Avoid milk, antacids or iron suppliment. • Complete the course of medication.
73)	**Paracetomol** Antipyretic, analgesic	Oral : 0.5-1.0 g 4-6 hrly. Max : 4 g/day. IM : 150 mg.	• Renal and liver impairment. • It may change the results of blood sugar level.	• Take with a glass of water. • Do not use continuously for more than 10 day.
74)	**Pheniramine maleate.** Antihistamine	Oral : 25 mg, 2-3 times daily, 50 mg b.i.d. Slow IV, IM : 22.75. mg/ ml, 1-2 times daily.	• Contraindicated in lactation, hyper-sensitivity children • Hypertension, epilepsy.	• Avoid driving. • Avoid alcohol.
75)	**Piperazine** Anthelmintic	Oral : Roundworm : 4 g o.d. morning for 7 days. Threadworm : 2 g o.d for 7 days.	• Contraindicated in lactation, allergy, epilepsy; • Renal and liver impairment. • Pregnancy.	• Complete the course of medication.
76)	**Piroxicam** NSAID	Oral : 10-30 mg daily, IM : 20 mg.	• Avoid in pregnancy and lactation. • Children, hypertension. • GI ulcer, asthma. • Do not take aspirin during this therapy.	• Take with food; • Avoid alcohol; • Avoid driving.

No.	Drug	Dose	Caution	Patient Counselling
77)	**Prednisolone** Glucocorticoid	Oral : 5 to 60 mg daily IM : 40-120 mg weekly. IV Slow : 10-40 mg over 20 min.	• Lactation, pregnancy • GI ulcer, diabetes, hypertension.	• Take with food • Do not discontinue the dosing abruptly.
78)	**Primaquine** Antimalarial	Oral : 7.5 mg b.i.d. for 14 days.	• Contraindicated in pregnancy, allergy, and infants.	• Take with food. • Do not change dose or brand. • Complete the course of medication.
79)	**Propranolol** Beta-blocker	Oral : 10-40 mg, 3-4 times daily. S.R. tab : 60-240 mg o.d.	• Lactation, pregnancy, asthma. • Renal and liver impairment.	• Do not discontinue the dosing abruptly. • Take with food. • Do not crush or chew S.R. tablet. • Avoid alcohol.
80)	**Ranitidine** H$_2$-receptor antagonist	Oral : 150 mg b.i.d. or 300 mg o.d. IV., IM. 50-100 mg.	• Lactation, pregnancy • Renal impairment.	• May cause drowsiness. • Do not take antacid within 1 hr. • Avoid alcohol and smoking. • When once daily dose is prescribed take it at bed time.
81)	**Roxithromycin** Bactericidal	Oral : 150-300 mg b.i.d. for 7 days.	• Pregnancy, allergy. • Liver impairment • Avoid other medication if possible.	• Take 30 min before food. • Complete the course of medication.
82)	**Rifampicin** Anti T.B.	450 or 600 mg / day for first 2 months and then 10-15 mg / kg three times a week for 4-6 months.	• Pregnancy, lactation • Renal and hepatic disorders • Check list of drug interactions	• Take co-therapy under advice of physician

No.	Drug	Dose	Caution	Patient Counselling
83)	**Salbutamol** Antiasthmatic	Oral : 2-4 mg, 3-4 times daily. S.R. tab : 4-8 mg b.i.d. Inhalation : 100-200 mcg aerosol 3-4 time daily	• Hypersensitivity, pregnancy; • Renal impairment. • Cardiac drug should be taken with care.	• Do not crush/chew S.R. formulation. • Do not change the brand. • Take with a full glass of water.
84)	**Sparfloxacin** Bactericidal	Oral : 400 mg on first day, followed by 200 mg o.d. for 7 to 14 days.	• Contraindicated in pregnancy and lactation, allergy and children. • Renal impairment. • Epilepsy.	• Avoid antacids, minerals / within 2-4 hrs. • Complete the course of medication. • Avoid driving. • Avoid exposure to sunlight.
85)	**Spironolac-tone** Diuretic	Oral : 50-100 mg/day Max : 400 mg / day.	• Contraindicated in pregnancy and in lactation. • Renal and liver impairment. • Take potassium supplement.	• Avoid alcohol. • Take in morning.
86)	**Streptokinase** Thrombolytic	IV : 1.5 million units over 30-60 min. Intracoronary : 2.5 to 3.0 lac units over 30-60 min.	• Pregnancy, diabetic; • Peptic ulcer.	• Take on empty stomach with a glass of water.
87)	**Terbutaline** Antiasthmatic	Oral : 2.5-5 mg, 2-3 times daily. Inhalation : 250-500 mcg 3-4 times daily. SC, IM, IV : 0.25 mg up to 4 times daily.	• Hypersensitivity, pregnancy, lacta-tion, hypertension.	• Do not change the brand.

Posology

No.	Drug	Dose	Caution	Patient Counselling
88)	**Theophylline** Antiasthmatic	Oral : 80-240 mg t.i.d. Max : 900 mg/day. S.R. : 200 mg b.i.d. 400 mg o.d. or b.i.d.	• Contraindicated in lactation, hyper-sensitivity, neonates. • GI ulcer, liver dysfunction.	• Take with food. • Do not crush/chew S.R. tablets capsules. • Avoid smoking. • Do not change the brand.
89)	**Thyroxine** Thyroid hormone	Oral : 0.05-0.2 mg/day.	• Lactation, pregnancy. • Cardiac failure.	• Do not discontinue dosing; • Change the brand.
90)	**Tinidazole** Antiprotozoal	Oral : 2 g o.d. 3-5 days.	• Contraindicated in pregnancy, lactation and allergy.	• Take with food. • Avoid alcohol.
91)	**Tolbutamide** Antidiabetic	Oral : Initially after the 1 g/day, first meal, up to 3 g/day.	• Contraindicated in pregnancy and lactation. • Renal, liver and thyroid impairment. • Not to take more than a single dose of aspirin (if prescribed).	• Avoid alcohol. • Avoid excessive exposure to direct sunlight.
92)	**Trazodone** Antidepressant	Oral : Initial, 50 mg/day at bed time for 3 days, increase up to 100 mg.	• Allergy, • Epilepsy and cardiac diseases, • Renal and liver impairment.	• Take with food; • It may cause dizziness while standing quickly.
93)	**Tromadol** Analgesic	Oral : 50-100 mg, 3-4 times daily. SC, IM, IV : 100 mg.	• Respiratory and cardiac problems. • Pregnancy, lactation, infants • Avoid sleeping pills, anti-histaminics.	• Avoid driving. • Avoid alcohol; • Take with food, avoid driving. • Give instruction for proper injection.

No.	Drug	Dose	Caution	Patient Counselling
94)	**Insulin** Diabetes	SC : Initial 0.2-03 units / kg / day, up to 0.5-1 unit/ kg/day. IV : 6 units/hr.	• Hypoglycaemia, allergic reaction.	• Do not use insulin if it looks grainy, lumpy. • Do not discontinue the dosing and • Do not change the brand. • Discard the vial 30 days after opening it for injection.
95)	**Vasopressin** D i a b e t e s insipidus.	SC/IM : 5-20 units every 4 hrs.	• Lactation, pregnancy. • Hypersensitivity, asthma. • Renal impairment.	—
96)	**V e r a p a m i l** C a l c i u m c h a n n e l blocker	Oral : 40-80 mg t.i.d. Max : 480 mg/day. IV : 5-10 mg over 2-3 min.	• Lactation, pregnancy. • Liver impairment.	• Do not discontinue dosing abruptly. • Do not crush/chew SR tablet. • Avoid alcohol.
97)	**Vinblastine** Antineoplastic	Inj. 10 mg	• Contraindicated in pregnancy, bacterial infection. • Avoid aspirin/ibuprofen-like drugs. • Liver impairment.	• Avoid contact with eyes; • Avoid alcohol; • Keep in refrigerator, but do not freeze. • Avoid exposure to direct sunlight. • May cause constipation.
98)	**Vincristine** Antineoplastic	IV : 25-75 mcg/kg weekly.	• Contraindicated in pregnancy • Avoid aspirin-like drugs. • Liver impairment	• Keep in refrigerator, but do not freeze.
99)	**Xylometazoline** Nasal decongestant	Nasal drops : 0.1%, 2-3 drops into each nostril 8-12 hrly, up to 7 days.	• Hypersensitivity ocular infection. • Pregnancy, lactation hypertension.	• Do not exceed dosing more than 7 days.
100)	**Zidovudine** Anti-AIDS	Oral : 100 mg 4 hrly or 200 mg 8 hrly.	• Contraindicated in lactation, anaemia. • Renal and liver impairment.	• Take on an empty stomach. • Avoid driving. • Advice on prevention of AIDS.

8 Physicochemical Incompatibility

Incompatibility studies are considered to be the first step in the rational compounding of a dosage form. Once an active ingredient is identified, it has to be compounded into an effective dosage form. The design of a stable, efficacious, safe, attractive and easy-to-administer dosage form requires careful study of the physical and chemical properties of the drug and the additives to be used in fabricating the dosage form.

Incompatibility is an undesirable result of mixing, prescribing and/or administering together two or more antagonistic substances, which may affect the safety, purpose or appearance of the product. Such undesirable results may be the consequences of interaction between formulation ingredients, or of the product formed due to these interactions; or may be the pharmacological consequences aroused from drug-drug or drug-food interactions. The former types of incompatibilities are a result of physicochemical interactions; whereas, latter are called as therapeutic interactions or incompatibilities.

Up-to-date knowledge of physicochemical properties of drugs and therapeutics is vital. The pharmacists should be able to detect any possible physicochemical or therapeutic incompatibilities, even if two or more different prescriptions are issued for a patient at a time. Incompatibilities are easier to prevent than to correct. The ability of the pharmacists to interpret the prescriber's intention is the key to correct an incompatibility. Most of the prescription drugs now carry a product insert, which lists the composition, indications, contraindications, side effects, recommended storage, and other valuable information. The current indices of medicinal products, such as CIMS/ MIMS, give all such information and also reviews on current topics and drug profiles of new drugs. USP-DI is the official drug information index. Many of the manufacturers publish trade journals, brochures and catalogues for physicians. In developed countries such publications are simultaneously directed to the pharmacists. Though none of these publications contain any significant amount of physicochemical compatibility data, these are very helpful in describing contraindications, toxicity, and other therapeutic incompatibilities. Due to undeveloped dispensing practices in India, the manufacturers underestimate the role of the pharmacists in prescription writing, which accounts for poor identification of therapeutic incompatibilities.

Concept Clear: Incompatibility

Incompatibility is an undesirable result of prescribing, compounding and administering two or more antagonistic substances, which may affect the safety, purpose or appearance of the product.
- Therapeutic incompatibility
- Physicochemical incompatibility.

DRUG AND DOSAGE FORM

Drugs may be defined as agents intended for use in the diagnosis, mitigation, treatment, cure or prevention of diseases in human beings or animals. When administered orally, applied topically, inserted in body cavities or injected in body, these agents either repair a body organ or restore its function to normal conditions, hemostasis. Drugs are obtained from the following sources:

i) Natural Sources:
   a) Plants   :   Atropine, Reserpine, Morphine, etc.
   b) Animal   :   Insulin, Vaccines, Enzymes, etc.
   c) Mineral   :   Kaolin, Liquid paraffin, etc.
   d) Microorganisms :   Antibiotics, etc.
ii) Semi-synthetic drugs :   Antibiotics, Morphine derivatives, etc.
iii) Synthetic drugs   :   Aspirin, Paracetamol, Pro-drugs such as Omeprazole, etc.

Drugs can be further classified as follows:

i)   Source   :   Natural, semi-synthetic, synthetic.
ii)   Chemical nature   :   Inorganic, aliphatic, aromatic, heterocyclic, etc.
iii) Category   :   Analgesic, Antipyretic, Hypnotic, etc.
iv)   Therapeutic activity :   Active ingredient, Lead Compound, Pro-drug, Inactive drug, etc.
v)   Federal regulation :   Over-the-counter (OTC) drugs, Prescription/Legend drugs.

Dosage Form: Drugs cannot be used for administration in their native forms, and in order to obtain the maximum therapeutic effect, they are formulated into dosage forms, such as, tablets, capsules, solutions, suspensions, ointments, etc. Dosage form is a blend of a drug component with a non-drug component produced in a definite physical form, shape and size, intended to be administered by a particular route of administration. The non-drug components, known as 'additives', are used to maintain overall stability of the dosage form.

Reasons for designing dosage form

i) Very small quantity of a pure drug is difficult to weigh and measure.

ii) Dosage form, owing to its definite size, shape and mechanical strength, is easy to administer by a selected route.

iii) A unit dosage form provides greater accuracy in dose.

iv) Quality dosage forms show predicted and reproducible therapeutic response.

v) As compared to drugs in powder or liquid forms, solid dosage form is easy to handle, transport and store.

vi) Improvement in physicochemical stability is possible by admixing suitable stabiliser in a dosage form.

vii) With the addition of organoleptic additives, dosage forms acquire improved palatability and acceptance.

Types of dosage forms:

i) Sterile dosage forms: Sterile indicates total absence of living microorganisms. It should not be confused with the term pyrogen-free. Pyrogens are metabolic by-products of microorganisms. Chemically, pyrogens are lipopolysaccharide in nature. When injected, they produce fever and such preparations are called as pyrogenic. Ophthalmic products must be sterile, and injections must be sterile and apyrogenic.

ii) Non-sterile dosage forms: The conventional dosage forms, such as tablets, capsules, liquid orals and topical semisolids, are the non-sterile products. These contain pyrogens, but are free from pathogenic microorganisms. The route of administration determines the number and type of microorganisms that are allowed in non-sterile products. By virtue of normal defense mechanism, the human body can tolerate a comparatively high level of microbes when contaminated topical dosage form is applied on an intact skin, as compared to oral ingestion of a contaminated dose.

Drug Delivery Systems

Recently, one of the most exciting developments in modern pharmaceutical formulation is the design of organ targeted and controlled drug release dosage form, which are termed as Novel Drug Delivery System, Targeted Drug Delivery, Controlled Drug Delivery, Therapeutic Systems, etc. They are intended to optimise the value of the medication delivered, either by delivery of the drug to the appropriate target area or by controlling drug concentration in the body over a convenient dosing interval. Such preparations offer the convenience of once- or twice-a-day dosing, based on constant drug delivery for a prolonged period of 8 to 24 hours. After absorption of drug, the system achieves a concentration in blood that is high enough to be therapeutically effective, but low enough not to cause toxicity. These systems also result in reduced dosing frequency, reduced dose and improved patient compliance. Examples of these are sustained release tablets, transdermal drug delivery systems, occular drug delivery systems, intrauterine devices, magnetically controlled devices, etc.

At the compounding level, the aim of the formulation pharmacist is to design a patient-acceptable and reasonably stable dosage form to fulfill the intention of the prescribing physician. The dosage form is compounded on the basis of physicochemical incompatibilities between drug-drug, drug-additive, product-container and expected therapeutic efficiency of the product. The Pharmacists, on the basis of their knowledge of incompatibility, select additive to build physical, chemical stability and biological activity in the product. The Pharmacists, in addition to scientific knowledge, use their artistic sense for selection of colour, flavour and sweetening agent to impart palatability, so as to increase patient acceptance of the product. Formulations should be less complicated and contain minimum required ingredients. The compounded products should maintain their stability for a month.

In short, compound development is a creative work of designing and developing a new product and encompasses various activities, such as development of a new drug, or improvement of existing products.

Concept Clear : Drug and Dosage Form

- Drug is an agent which, when administered, repairs a body organ, or its functioning to normal condition. Drug is a pure synthetic chemical, part of which is derived from plant or animal, microorganisms or mineral compounds.
- Dosage form is a blend of drug component with non-drug component produced in definite physical form, shape and size, intended to be administered by a particular route of administration. These include tablets, capsules, solutions suspensions, creams, etc.

PHYSICOCHEMICAL INCOMPATIBILITY

If mixing of two or more drugs or a drug and excipients, by a particular method, results in a physicochemical change in the properties of a drug or dosage form, or production of a new chemical substance having different pharmacological action, it is called as physicochemical incompatibility. When incompatibility is prevented by addition, substitution or elimination of one or more ingredient, it is called an adjusted incompatibility. Some interactions are a little difficult to correct. Such interactions can be tolerated if they do not affect therapeutic value of the formulation; otherwise, the prescription is referred back to the prescriber for advice.

The physical and chemical incompatibilities are either visible or invisible and rapid or delayed. The rapid and visible incompatibilities include colour change, effervescence and precipitation. When the incompatibility is slow, the physicochemical changes are visible after dispensing the product. Though such a change in product may not affect the therapeutic value of the product, it may undermine the patient's confidence in the pharmacist or the physician. Pharmacists must use their knowledge and skill 'Secundum artem' to prevent incompatibility, for which they can follow certain rules. These are given below:

i) Modify the order of mixing.
ii) Dispense with 'Shake well before use' label.
iii) Recommend storage condition.
iv) Allow ingredients to react before packing.
v) Add physical stabiliser (suspending/ emulsifying agent).
vi) Add chemical stabiliser (antioxidant/ buffer).
vii) Add preservative.
viii) Modify the consistency by adding softening/stiffening agent.
ix) Select soluble, compatible or stable form of drug.

1) Physical Incompatibility

Physical changes such as insolubility, precipitation, immiscibility or liquefaction occur by mixing two or more substances. The resultant product may have undesirable colour, appearance or heterogenic drug distribution. Physical properties such as particle size, shape, crystalline properties, melting point, hygroscopicity, solubility, partition coefficient, ionisation constant, optical activity, etc., should be studied to avoid incompatibility. To identify compatibility, on the basis of literature, information on some binary mixtures of a drug and excipient should be prepared and evaluated. The number of ingredients should be kept to a minimum. More the ingredients In a formulation, greater is the possibility of interactions. A common method of reducing the number of ingredients is to use an excipient that performs more than one function. The product developed should be stable in the container in which it is packed. In some cases, product-container interactions are possible, such as adsorption or absorption of some ingredients of the product by the plastic or rubber and precipitation, or degradation of drug by the alkaline nature of glass containers.

Types of physical incompatibilities are as given below.

i) Insolubility

a) Insoluble drug: When a drug is insoluble in a solvent, it may create problems in proper administration of the dose. For example:

i) Insolubility ↔ Solubility enhancers: Dose accuracy and bioavailability of a liquid containing insoluble drug is poor. Compounding a solution of chemically equivalent soluble salt of an insoluble drug can correct such a problem, eg. salts of alkaloids. Solubility enhancers such as co-solvent, solubilising agents, complexing agent can be used to facilitate solution, eg. Paracetamol elixir.

ii) Insolubility ↔ Alteration in volume: Instead of use of co-solvents, if possible, the amount of original solvent can be doubled to get a complete solution of a given drug. But the increased dose of a resulting solution should be convenient to administer.

iii) Settling ↔ Suspending agent: The drug in mixtures containing insoluble solids (suspensions), during storage, settles to the bottom at times. For uniform dose, the sediment should be easy to re-disperse and dispersed phase should remain uniformly suspended for enough time so that the dose can be received. Insoluble drugs are of two types, diffusible and indiffusible. Lighter and diffusible drugs such as light kaolin and light magnesium carbonate, remain evenly distributed in a vehicle for a long time, which is enough to ensure uniformity of the dose. These prescriptions are labelled as 'Shake well before use'. In addition to this, an increase in the viscosity of the vehicle by adding a thickening agent, delays settling of indiffusible drugs such as chalk or calamine.

iv) Poor wettability ↔ Levigating agent: Some drugs have poor wettability with a given vehicle and these either float on the surface, or sink at the bottom of the vehicle. Levigation of such solids with wetting agents, such as glycerin, propylene glycol or hydrophilic surfactants, help in the uniform distribution of the hydrophobic drug in water, eg. sulphur lotion.

b) Precipitation of drug: The precipitation of a drug may occur during compounding or storage. A drug in dissolved state and precipitated state shows different pharmaceutical and therapeutic properties. For example:

i) Poor solvent ↔ Order of mixing: Precipitation of dissolved drug may occur when the solution of drug is added in a poor solvent. It is advisable to dissolve a drug in a good solvent. A well diluted solution is then added in a poor solvent in small amounts with stirring after each addition; eg. addition of alcoholic solution of a drug in water, addition of resin tincture in water or addition of gum mucilage in alcohol.

Prescription No. 8.1

℞

Benzoin tincture	— 4 ml
Glycerin	— 10 ml
Rose water, to make	— 100 ml

Prepare lotion. Apply locally.

Benzoin is resin. It is an astringent and a protective agent. It should be slowly added in water with stirring after each addition. The resultant colloidal dispersion will not require addition of suspending agent. However, rapid mixing may result in the formation of a gummy mass. Which is difficult to disperse. Label the container as 'Shake well before use.'

ii) Precipitation ↔ Suspension: Though solution of an insoluble potent drug is possible by replacing the chemical equivalent of soluble salt, crystallisation of the drug during storage sometimes makes it a complicated dosage form. In such cases, it is advisable to prepare suspension of an insoluble form instead of solution, eg. suspension of insoluble barbiturates.

iii) Cap-locking ↔ Co-solvents: Liquid preparations, especially those containing syrups, may show crystallisation of sugar in the closure, resulting in cap-locking. Addition of glycerin, propylene glycol or sorbitol minimises it.

iv) Grainy semisolids ↔ Non-uniform cooling: Partial solidification of higher melting point waxes may occur when cool spatula is used for mixing, or when a hot product is poured in a cool container. Grains also develop during preparation of creams, if the aqueous phase and oil phase do not have same temperatures at the time of mixing. This can be prevented by avoiding localised cooling.

ii) Liquefaction: Eutectic substances such as camphor, menthol or thymol, if mixed together, undergo liquefaction, eg. Eutectic powders, Insufflations. Liquefaction can be corrected in either of the following ways:

i)   Dispensing individual ingredient separately.

ii)   Compounding powder using diluents.

Prescription No. 8.2

℞

Menthol	— 30 mg
Camphor monobromate	— 30 mg
Chloral hydrate	— 130 mg

Compound powder. 1 at bed time.

Diluents such as lactose, magnesium oxide or magnesium hydroxide are separately mixed with eutectic substances and such mixtures are mixed to produce the final product. Diluents prevent physical contacts of liquefiable substances.

iii) Allowing completion of liquefaction and absorbing the liquid using adsorbents such as substances like kaolin.

iii) Immiscibility: Oil phase, in addition to its medicinal value, is component of dosage forms for various reasons such as, vehicle, solvent or source of higher free fatty acid to form soap in emulsions. The poor distribution of immiscible oil with water is pharmaceutical incompatibility. For example:

i) Immiscibility ↔ Emulsifying agent: When oil and water are made miscible by the use of an emulsifying agent; the resulting dosage form is termed as emulsion.

Castor oil is a laxative. To improve its palatability, it should be produced in oil-in-water type of emulsion. The external water phase masks the unpleasant taste of castor oil. Additionally, use of flavouring agent is recommended.

Prescription No. 8.3

℞

Castor oil	—	15 ml
Acacia powder	—	4.0 g
Cinnamon water, to make	—	60 ml

Take once at bed time.

ii) Salting out ↔ Redissolution: Many substances may precipitate from a saturated solution, when some other substance is dissolved in the solution, eg. salting out of volatile oils from aromatic water during preparation of solution of water-soluble drug. To overcome this, a suitable emulsifying or solubilising agent should be included in the formula, or such aromatic water should be allowed to stand for redissolution, or separated oil. Since excess electrolyte causes precipitation of the emulsifying agent, in preparation of emulsions, electrolytes should be used in the optimum quantity.

iii) Flavour oils ↔ Miscible form: Volatile oils which are used as flavouring agents, are water immiscible and are required in small quantities. Therefore, these are incorporated in the form of their water miscible and diluted form, such as aromatic water and flavoured syrups, eg. peppermint oil, is used as aromatic water, or o/w emulsion.

iv) Inhalations ↔ Dispersing agents: Inhalations contain volatile and water immiscible oils such as eucalyptus oil, menthol. For uniform distribution, these oils are adsorbed on an inert adsorbent and it is formulated as a suspension. eg. Eucalyptus oil and menthol inhalation.

v) Common solvent ↔ Monophasic system: Addition of common solvent dissolves immiscible components of formulation producing monophasic liquids, eg. addition of alcohol in soap liniment.

iv) Unpalatability: The taste is more intense when the drug is in its dissolved state. The insoluble drug in the form of suspensions, or solid dosage forms, are more palatable than their solutions, eg. chloramphenicol palmitate suspension.

2) Chemical incompatibility

The chemical interaction between two or more substances forms an undesirable substance. Rapid incompatibilities should be corrected by the pharmacists before dispensing the medicine. Delayed incompatibilities may be dispensed by ensuring slow rate of chemical reaction and the latter is best achieved by storing the product in a refrigerator or in a cool place. Chemical incompatibilities are given below:

i) Precipitation: Precipitation of a drug takes place either due to pH change or due to a chemical reaction between drug-drug or drug-additives. When the precipitated product is therapeutically active, it is formulated as per the procedure used to prepare mixtures containing diffusible solid or indiffusible solid. If the resultant precipitate is inactive or toxic, such a prescription is referred back to the physician.

a) pH change: Modern medicines are often salts of weak acids and weak bases. The unionised forms are insoluble in water and ionisable salts are soluble in water. A pH change, not only changes solubility, but it also changes rate of degradation. If the resultant precipitate has therapeutic value and it is chemically stable, one can tolerate the incompatibility. A suitable co-solvent can be used to increase solubility, otherwise a suspension is formulated. For example, Morphine hydrochloride, above 2.5 per cent concentration, is insoluble and results in the formation of diffusible precipitate under alkaline condition. The solubility of precipitated morphine in alcohol is 1 in 100. Thus, incompatibility can be treated either by (i) preparing suspension of diffusible precipitate or (ii) using alcohol as co-solvent to prepare solution.

Caffeine citrate, above 2.2 per cent concentration, under alkaline condition, produces indiffusible precipitate; but when alcohol is used, it tolerates a higher concentration of caffeine citrate without precipitation.

b) Precipitation by chemical reaction:

i) Drug-drug interactions: Active ingredients react with other drugs or additives, yielding diffusible or indiffusible precipitate. Caffeine citrate is a mixture of equal weight of caffeine and citric acid. The citric acid reacts with sodium salicylate to liberate salicylic acid in the form of precipitate. It causes gastric irritation. However, when only caffeine is used, it forms a soluble complex with sodium salicylate. Therefore, caffeine citrate should be replaced with half the amount of caffeine to get clear solution. Some other examples are given in Table 8.1.

II) Alkali metal soaps, ammonium soaps get precipitated by addition of hard water.

iii) Flavour ↔ pH: Liquorice looses its flavour due to precipitation in presence of acid. Acid reacts with glycyrrhizin, a flavouring constituent of liquorice, forming glycyrrhizinic acid precipitate.

Table 8.1: Precipitation by chemical reaction

No.	Drug	Reacting substance	Method of compounding
1)	Strychnine Alkaloids	Soluble iodides/bromides Tannins	Diffusible suspension Indiffusible suspension
2)	Quinine HCL	Salicylates	Indiffusible suspension
3)	Sodium salicylate and benzoates	Acids (citric acid from lemon syrup)	Indiffusible suspensions. Replace lemon syrup with lemon tincture and simple syrup.
4)	Sodium salicylate	Ferric salts	Indiffusible suspension or precipitate is soluble in presence of sodium bicarbonate.
5)	Barbiturates	Ammonium bromide	Indiffusible suspensions. Replace ammonium bromide with sodium bromide.

ii) Redox reactions: Some drugs, or their dosage forms, undergo oxidation when exposed to air, excessive temperature and due to overdilution of liquids, incorrect pH or presence of catalyst. The common catalyst includes metal ions, enzymes, and bacteria. A drug in the liquid state is more sensitive to oxidation than in insoluble state, and granular substances get less exposed to oxygen than fine powders. The frequently occurring oxidation-reduction type of incompatibility includes:

a)   Auto-oxidation of oils, fats, phenolic substances, aldehydes and vitamins can be controlled by addition of primary antioxidants, such as alpha tocopherol, propyl gallate, BHA, BHT.

b)   Paraldehyde, tannins, epinephrine, procaine HCl, sulphacetamide and related compounds undergo oxidation activated by heat. These require protection against trace metal ions. In addition to proper storage, antioxidants such as ascorbic acid, sodium metabisulphite, sodium sulphite and complexing agents, like EDTA, are used to control oxidation.

c)   Preparations containing riboflavin, folic acid and ascorbic acid show incompatibility. Riboflavin is light sensitive, and the alkaline solution is quite unstable in heat and light, forming biologically inactive fluorescent degradation product. Surfactants accelerate photo-decomposition of riboflavin. Riboflavin is more stable at pH 6 to 6.5 and it should be stored in a dark place. A solution of folic acid is photostable, but the presence of riboflavin causes decomposition of folic acid.

d)   When dry powders contain both oxidising and reducing agents, the mixture may explode. The inter-particulate friction developed during mixing increases chances of redox reaction, eg. explosive powders. Therefore, such reacting substances should be dispensed separately or powders should be mixed lightly by spatulation method. The tablets containing oxidising and reducing agents should be packed separately to avoid friction.

iii) Hydrolysis: Hydrolysis can be controlled by avoiding moisture contact or by changing pH. The cocaine HCl undergoes hydrolysis to a greater extent (up to 30 per cent) at pH 6, as compared to when the pH of cocaine solution is 2 to 5.

Thiamine HCl may be autoclaved without appreciable decomposition below pH 5. At higher pH it undergoes decomposition.

Aspirin is sensitive to water and gets converted to a more irritant acetyl salicylic acid. It should be granulated without using water.

Paracetamol is stable between pH 5 and 7. Ibuprofen shows more solubility above pH 6, therefore to compound suspension of these two drugs in combination, pH of liquid should be 5-6.

Table 8.2: pH Dependent Solubility of Ibuprofen and Stability of Paracetamol

Parameter	pH 1.1	pH 2	pH 4	pH 5	pH 6	pH 7	pH 8
Paracetamol Degradation half life (yrs)	—	0.73	—	19.8	21.8	—	2.28
Ibuprofen Solubility (mg%)	2.1	—	2.9	12	53	244	—

iv) Racemisation: The conversion of an optically active form to an optically inactive form, without changing chemical constitution, usually results in reduced therapeutic activity, eg. adrenaline, norephedrine, etc.

v) Effervescence: Two or more ingredients of formulation react to generate carbon dioxide. To overcome such reactions, either (a) Mix the reacting ingredients in an open container and allow the reaction to complete before filling in final container. The rate of reaction can be increased by using hot water, (b) Change one or more reacting ingredients or (c) Dispense reacting substances separately, e.g. gargles containing borax, sodium bicarbonate and glycerin.

The boric acid formed from borax reacts with glycerin to form monobasic glyceryl boric acid, which liberates carbon dioxide when reacted with sodium bicarbonate. To hasten the reaction, ingredients should be mixed in an open container using hot water as vehicle.

Prescription 8.4

℞

Compound sodium borate solution NF.
Sodium borate — 15 g
Sodium bicarbonate — 15 g
Liquified phenol — 3 ml
Glycerin — 35 ml
Distilled water, to make — 1000 ml

vi) Complexation: A number of additives, such as macrogols or surfactants, form a complex with drug, or additives like preservatives, resulting in reduced effectiveness. The complex formed has poor absorption or penetration in cell membrane, and in turn has poor preservative or poor therapeutic effect. The complex should be reversible. Complex formation may also reduce irritation, eg. povidone-iodine soluble complex. Calcium forms an insoluble complex with tetracycline, reducing its absorption. Complexes formed by sequestering agents with metals are water-soluble. Potassium iodide forms a soluble complex with iodine.

vii) Colour change: The colour change is visible incompatibility. When the colour reaction is rapid it is allowed to complete before dispensing. Delayed colour change after dispensing, may confuse the patient regarding the authenticity of the dosage. The latter type of problem can be corrected by avoiding colour reaction, or by adding a dark colour to mask any colour change during storage. The typical example explaining oxidation and colour change is Sodium Salicylate, mixture BPC.

Prescription No. 8.5

℞

Sodium Salicylate, Mixture BPC

Sodium salicylate	- 5.0 g
Sodium metabisulphite	- 0.1 g
Conc. Orange peel infusion	- 5.0 g
Chloroform water, DS	- 50.0 ml
Water, freshly boiled & cooled, to make	- 100.0 ml

It explains oxidation and colour change. In acidic gastric content, Sodium salicylate converts into salicylic acid. The precipitate of salicylic acid causes irritation to the gastric mucosa. The alkaline microenvironment, due to presence of sodium bicarbonate, minimises the formation of salicylic acid. However, during storage, the alkaline solution undergoes oxidation by atmospheric oxygen and becomes brownish-black. The coloured product is safe and has therapeutic value, but it may confuse the patient regarding the drug's effectiveness. The sodium metabisulphite is added as antioxidant to control the oxidation and, in turn, the colour change. Orange peel infusion is a flavouring agent and chloroform water has preservative and flavouring properties. Since the preservative is volatile, the preparation should be used within two weeks.

Category and dose: Analgesic. 5 ml 3 times a day.

Label: Take with the aid of water after meal.

Patient counselling: To avoid GI irritation, the preparation should be given after meals with plenty of water. Avoid administering it to patients with peptic ulcer and to children under 12 years.

viii) Incompatibility with containers: The product filled in a container may react chemically with the container, or get absorbed by the container, or the closure. Some examples are:

i) Glass containers leach alkali, which may change solubility of a drug, or an additive, or cause chemical degradation.

ii) Rubber closures may adsorb preservatives.

iii) Plastic containers may soften, due to chemicals such as methyl salicylate.

iv) Metal containers catalyse rate of chemical reaction. Metal containers are usually internally coated with epoxy resin to prevent unwanted chemical interactions and to prevent grey marks on tablets due to abrasion.

TECHNICAL PROBLEMS

Formula ingredients, compounding process, equipment used have influence on physicochemical stability of a drug and its dosage form. some examples are mentioned below.

i) Compression ↔ Disintegration: Compression of tablet at low pressure may result in tablets with poor mechanical strength, but it shows fast disintegration; whereas, tablets made at high pressure, or using granules prepared by dry granulation, may show delayed disintegration.

ii) Low dose drug ↔ Triturations: The potent drugs having low dose can be diluted with diluents by preparing triturates. Low dose powders are mixed with diluents by the doubling up method.

iii) Mixing of additive ↔ Change in mixing order: To prevent loss of volatile additives, these should be added in liquids just before filtration/filling. To ensure uniform colouration of insoluble drugs, such as kaolin, instead of dissolving colour in the vehicle, it should be triturated with the drug.

iv) Emulsification ↔ Mixing technique: Emulsification is effective by triturating immiscible mixtures under high shear, but with intermittant pauses.

v) Air entrapment ↔ Mixing technique: In highly viscous liquids, problems may arise due to air entrapment during compounding, which may result in increased volume, filling variation and instability. Avoid vigorous mixing, or mix in a closed vessel, preferably under vacuum.

Improvisation

When any particular dosage form is difficult to handle, administer or apply, two alternatives are possible, (a) Change the dosage form or (b) Compound new dosage form using existing dosage form. The compounding of new dosage form of improved quality using the existing dosage form is termed as improvisation. For example, (i) Tablets are crushed or capsules are opened and resultant powder is used to compound a liquid for easy oral administration. The antibacterial tablets or capsules are crushed and the powder is used to compound a topical product. (ii) Many times the pharmacist prefers to use a prefabricated dosage form as a source of active ingredient, mainly to avoid weighing extremely small quantities of a potent drug. Two or more tablets can be crushed and the powder can be filled in capsules. (iii) Sometimes a physician directs an ingredient to be incorporated in the content of a pre-filled capsule. (iv) Dispersion of dispersible analgesic tablets in water may be used as gargle for treating throat inflammation. (v) In treatment of complex skin infections, the physician prescribes two or more marketed creams or ointments. Such products are prescribed with the direction 'Mix in equal quantity and apply'. The patient may not be able to mix the medicines properly and hence the pharmacist should prepare and dispense such a mixed or diluted product. (vi)The best example of improvisation of modern medicines is reconstituted suspension. Since antibiotics have poor stability in aqueous medium, these are compounded in the form of dry powders. Dry powders are stable for 1 to 2 years. Such dry powders are reconstituted using freshly boiled and cooled water. The resultant liquid should be used within 14 days.

The following reasons should be considered for improvement of dosage form:

i)   Drug combinations or dilutions are required, (a) when such a product is not available in the market, (b) when the patient complains of it being unpalatable, showing side effects, or other such problems, in a commercial product.

ii)   After interpreting the physicians' intention.

iii) The pharmacist had to select a suitable vehicle and a container.

iv)   The improvised product has to be used within seven days after compounding, e.g. compounding of erythromycin ointment using erythromycin soild dosage form.

It is an example of compounding by improvisation:

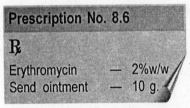

Prescription No. 8.6

℞

Erythromycin   — 2%w/w
Send ointment   — 10 g.

Dosage forms: Erythromycin is a broadspectrum bacteriostatic agent. Topically it is used in acne treatment in concentration of 2 to 4 per cent. Tablets and capsules containing 250 mg of erythromycin are available.

Base selection: The following points should be considered to compound semisolid dosage form by improvisation.

a)   In general, water miscible ointment base is used for wet skin, i.e., cuts and infections. For dry skin and conditions such as allergy and itching, an oily base is used.

b)   Base used for improvisation should be compatible with the original product. Incompatibility is possible due to change in pH, presence of opposite charged surfactant or ions.

c)   Base should not change physicochemical properties of the drug or dosage form, eg. aqueous cream should not be diluted with an oily base.

d)   Dilution with base should not reduce the drug release rate.

e)   If the product is to be applied on a small specific area, the base should produce viscous product; whereas, for application on a larger skin surface, the product should be thin, and non-sticky.

An emulsifying base having moderate properties is more suitable for present prescription. Anhydrous bases have poor cosmetic value, due to their greasy, staining nature and being difficult to wash. Water-soluble bases, due to their solubility in sweat, may not retain the drug in contact with acne for a long period of time. Emulsifying base is water miscible, washable and comparatively less oily. It may improve skin-product contact and consequently the penetration of drug in the acne.

Working formula:

Powdered solid dosage form equivalent to 200 mg (2% w/w) of erythromycin.

Emulsifying ointment — to make 10 g.

Open the capsule and take weight of powder, or weigh the tablet. Suppose the weight of tablet is 300 mg, that is, 250 mg of drug is present in 300 mg of dosage form. Therefore, 200 mg of drug is equivalent to 240 mg of powdered tablet.

3) Compounding: Open the capsule, or crush the tablet. Pass powder through sieve # 85. Compound the product by trituration method. It should be labelled as 'For external use only' and 'Use within one week'.

All these incompatibilities are interlinked and have to be studied as a part of the development of a dosage form in the mutual correlation. Briefly, the designed dosage form should be such that it fulfils the expectation of the physician and the patient. The physician is interested in treatment of his patients effectively, with no side effects. The expectations of patients include an attractive and pleasantly flavoured dosage form that can be conveniently handled and administered. The pharmacist, therefore, is morally, legally and socially responsible for the quality of dosage forms, which can fulfill these requirements.

Concept Clear : Physicochemical Incompatibility

Mixing of two or more drugs, or a drug and excipients, by a particular method, results in physicochemical changes in the properties of the drug or dosage form, or production of a new chemical substance having different pharmacological action.

Types of incompatible interactions are as follows:

i) Physical incompatibility: Insolubility, liquefaction, immiscibility.

ii) Chemical incompatibility: Precipitation by pH change/chemical reaction, redox reactions, hydrolysis, effervescence, complex formation.

Incompatibility with container: Leaching, absorption, hardening/softening of container.

iii) Technical problems: Problems and shortcuts in procedure, mixing techniques, etc.

Improvisation: Improvement/modification in a final product.

9 Therapeutic Incompatibility

THERAPEUTIC INCOMPATABILITY

In the modern era, pharmacists mainly deal with therapeutic incompatibilities; and errors in the dispensing of medicines is one of the main reasons behind it. Two or more drugs can be prescribed with the intention of producing a specific degree of action. When the intensity of drug action, or the nature of action, differs from that intended, the effects are termed as therapeutic incompatibilities.

Today, too many drugs and brands are awaiting prescription from physicians. The physicians have a wide choice to prescribe from and the pharmacists must help, as well as countercheck, the prescribed medicines for ensuring rational prescription. Pharmacists must be able to avoid therapeutic incompatibilities. They must have knowledge of pharmacokinetics and pharmacodynamics of drugs. Pharmacokinetics deals with distribution and elimination of the absorbed drug and determines the effective drug level in body fluids and tissues. Pharmacodynamics deals with induction of pharmacological effect, therapeutic and/or side effects, as a function of concentration of drugs in the body, e.g. solutions show more rapid drug absorption than suspensions or tablets. Surfactants increase rate and extent of absorption of certain drugs by increasing area of contact at the site of absorption and also by increasing the membrane permeability. Metabolic inactivation of a number of drugs, following oral administration, can occur in the liver and therefore administration of such drugs by rectal or sublingual route avoids this first pass inactivation.

The design of dosage form also depends on the nature of the disease or illness for which the drug is intended. Therefore, it is necessary to study factors like-route of administration, by which a drug can be conveniently administered and onset and duration of its action when administered by that route; age of patient, condition of patient, such as ability to swallow, consciousness, etc. Flavoured and sweetened oral liquids are more convenient for children than the solid dosage forms, which are difficult to swallow. Unconscious patients can be treated best by injections or rectal administration of drugs.

The typical examples of therapeutic incompatibilities are as follows:
1)   Medication errors
2)   Drug-interactions

MEDICATION ERRORS

Medication error is any preventable drug event that may cause, or lead to, inappropriate or irrational medication use, which may cause harm to the patients. Medication errors can be made by doctors, pharmacists, nurses and patients.

Medication error is the single largest cause of human suffering and according to an American study, more than 28 per cent patients hospitalised, are admitted due to medication errors. In India this figure may be higher, but due to unavailability of data it cannot be figured out. Such errors usually occur due to overdosing, sub-therapeutic dose, consumption of wrong medicine, or possibility of drug interactions. It not only increases the degree of harm, but also increases the cost of therapy. The factors that contribute to medication errors can be categorised as:

1)   Prescription errors
2)   Dispensing errors
3)   Selection errors
4)   Bagging errors
5)   Administration errors

1. Errors In Prescription Writing

The prescription should be neatly and correctly written by the medical practitioner, otherwise interpreting it is a major hassle for the pharmacists. Most of the today's prescriptions are written in English, but a number of times, spelling mistakes and illegible handwriting are major reasons in misunderstanding the prescription. An improper prescription is one of the main causes of dispensing errors. Some of the reasons of errors in prescription writing are given below.

a) SALA Medicines: The availability of near about lakhs of brands in the market is main reason due to which medical practitioners are unable to reproduce and write correct name and correct spelling of the medicine. There are certain medicines whose names are similar in spelling or pronunciation and hence these are called as Sound Alike Look Alike (SALA) medicines. For example,

is 1 tablet twice a day for three days. It is not wise to cut strips and dispense any odd number of tablets. For kids, suspensions or sachets is preferred.

In some cases, dosing is complicated, in which case a readymade kit can be used. As health professionals, pharmacists should also discuss with doctors about dose calculation, ready to use packs, etc., eg. chloroquine, an antimalarial drug, has variable doses over the period of a course. For adults, the initial dose of 600 mg (chloroquine base) followed by 300 mg after 6 to 8 hours, on day one. On second and third days, a single dose of 300 mg/day is advised. But in practice, a dose of 500 mg tablet once a day for 3 days or 250 mg tablet twice a day for three days is given. To avoid confusion, Chloroquine Compliance Kit is available, i.e., CLO-KIT (Indoco), PARAQUIN KIT (Ethico), Y-VEX KIT (Ethico), which contain tablets of different strengths in different colours, which can be easily identified by a common man, e.g. adult dose of CLO-KIT is one orange coloured tablet for initial dose, followed by one pink tablet after 6, 24 and 48 hours.

e) Dose and Direction: Pharmacists should check the dose, dosage regimen and direction to use. The CIMS, USP DI and other commercially available drug indices should be referred.

In addition, prescription should mention the vehicle to be used, time for taking the medicine, i.e., before or after meals, etc. Aspirin causes GI irritation and should be taken after food.

Prescription No. 9.1	Prescription No. 9.2
℞ Tab. Aspirin 300 mg. 1-1-1 × 3 days.	℞ Granules Ispaghula - 3.5 g Send 3 sachets Take one sachet at bedtime whenever constipation occurs

Ispaghula husk acts as both, laxative and anti-diarrhoeal, depending on amount of water co-administered with granules. Here, the patient is suffering from constipation. To act as laxative, ispaghula granules should be taken with at least 300 ml of water. Therefore, the directions to use should mention amount of water to be taken during dosing.

Concept Clear: Errors in Prescription

- SALA Medicines
- Types of dosage form
- Strength of medicine
- Quantity to be dispensed
- Dose and Directions

Therapeutic Incompatibility

2. Dispensing Errors:

Dispensing errors are the errors in supply of medicines. It may be due to supply of wrong medicament, or wrong dosage form of a particular medicament, or insufficient or excess dose of the drug. The reasons for dispensing errors are as follows:

a) Poor handwriting: One should expect readable prescriptions with clear-cut dosing directions. Even today, some prescriptions are very difficult to read and are intentionally done so, so as to keep the therapy secret. Thus, understanding the written medicine and its dose, becomes a major job for pharmacists. A silly mistake in mentioning the type of dosage form, or spelling it wrongly, may adversely affect the patient.

b) Long prescriptions: Too many medicines written in the prescription not only increase chances of medication errors during dispensing, but also the possibility of drug interactions and complexity in administration. Ideally, a prescription should bear two, or maximum three, medicines at a time. Long prescriptions increase chances of not dispensing, or dispensing twice some of the medicines, by pharmacists. Sometimes medicines may be out of stock and cannot be dispensed and hence the patients avoid purchasing these medicines later, which can lead to incomplete therapy. Endorsing the dispensed medicines by pharmacists can minimise such errors.

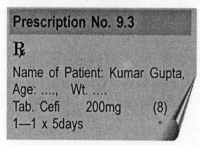

Prescription No. 9.3

℞

Name of Patient: Kumar Gupta,
Age: ...., Wt. ....
Tab. Cefi   200mg   (8)
1—1 x 5days

c) Incomplete patient information: An ideal prescription contains important information such as age, weight and sex of patient; dosage form, generic/brand name of drug, dose and units to be dispensed, e.g. prescription 9.3 is for Cefixime whose dose is 200-400 mg/day for adults and 8 mg/kg/day for children. It is available as tablets and capsules of 100 and 200 mg and dispersible tablets containing 50, 100 and 200 mg of drug. Tab. Cefi (Khandelwal) is available as DT-tab of 100 mg and tablet of 200 mg. In this prescription, the doctor has forgotten to fill in the age and weight of the patient. According to the prescribed dose, the patient is an adult. But it creates confusion and hence the age of the patient should be confirmed.

d) Deviation in attention of pharmacist: Focused attention during dispensing is of prime requirement. Any deviation in attention due to phone calls, watching television and improper mood of pharmacists, may directly or indirectly affect the dispensing of right medicines. Environmental factors such as lighting and heat can distract health professionals from their medical tasks. Excessive workload, fatigue and anxiety can also lead to wrong dispensing.

e) Misunderstanding of verbal orders: Spellings and pronunciation of SALA medicines, incorrect pronunciation of OTC/prescription medicines by patients may be cause of medication errors.

effect is antagonistic. Antagonistic effect between beta-blockers and bronchodilators may cause bronchopasm. Antagonism may be beneficial; e.g. caffeine is intended to overcome the cerebral depressant action of acetophenetidin. Antagonistic drugs can be prescribed with an intention to overcome adverse effects of each other, e.g. antacid contains magnesium hydroxide gel (laxative) with aluminum hydroxide gel (constipative).

b) Addition and Synergism: When interacting drugs having similar action are given in their full individual doses, and they produce effect which is the sum of individual effects, it is termed as addition, e.g. co-administration of sedative and hypnotic drugs. When the action produced by combination is greater than that would be expected from the sum of their individual actions, it is termed as synergism, i.e., morphine with diazepam, alcohol and antihistaminics. Drugs of such combinations should be prescribed in reduced doses. Two sympathomimetic drugs have additive effect. The prescription should be referred back to reduce the doses. .

Addition and synergism are desirable if toxicity or side effects are reduced by the lower dosage used and when a prescription becomes less expensive, e.g. the combination of sulfonamides show less nephrotoxicity, diuretics can be prescribed with antihypertensive drugs to monitor blood pressure. Drugs that act by different mechanisms are combined together for treatment of a particular disease, e.g. penicillin and sulphonamides for infections.

iii) Adverse drug reactions: ADR is any response to a drug, which is unintended, noxious, and which occurs at prescribed standard dose. The ADR is either a side effect or extension effect. Extension effects are excessive pharmacological actions, normally dose related, and are also classified as Type A reactions. Though a patient receives a standard dose, due to some pathological abnormality, such as renal failure or liver damage, it produces high plasma drug levels. The effects due to sudden drug withdrawal are also type A reactions, e.g. NSAID in renal failure, narcotic analgesics in liver diseases may cause adverse reactions. Development of anxiety, dysphoria is due to benzodiazepine withdrawal.

The abnormal side effects, or novel responses, of the drug are classified as type B reactions, e.g. allergic reactions such as anaphylaxis due to penicillins, photosensitivity due to sulpha drugs.

iv) Contraindication: Some drugs are not prescribed, or not taken in specific physiological or pathological condition, e.g. aspirin containing drugs are not given to treat peptic ulceration, and to children below 16 years of age. Salicylates interfere with blood clotting by acting as anti-coagulants; therefore, aspirin therapy should be discontinued a few days before heart surgery. Sodium containing electrolyte powder is contraindicated for hypertensive patients. Sulpha drugs such as sulphadiazine should be contraindicated in patients taking urinary acidifier such as ammonium chloride. Number of drugs are avoided being prescribed to pregnant and lactating mothers.

---

v) Drug-Alcohol / Tobacco interaction: While prescribing to a patient for curing a particular disease, physicians take care of drug interactions. However, most of the time a prescriber is not aware of simultaneous drug therapy, or type of food or drinks the patients are taking during therapy. In day-to-day life, number of common substances, such as caffeine (tea, coffee), nicotine (tobacco, cigarettes), alcohol (beer, wine, ayurvedic Asawa), etc., may cause interactions with drugs. Chronic alcohol ingestion activates enzymes that transform acetaminophen into chemicals that lead to liver damage. Alcohol decreases bioavailability of tolbutamide. Cigarette may reduce plasma concentration of carbamazepine and imipramine and increase bioavailability of glutethimide.

vi) Drug-food interactions: Food changes the gastric pH and gastric emptying time. It can increase gastric pH upto 6 and prolong gastric residence for 2 hours. Most of the drugs have better absorption from small intestine, therefore drugs taken on full stomach usually show delayed action, eg. paracetamol. On the contrary, enteric coated tablets should be taken on an empty stomach, preferably half-an hour before food. It protects the enteric coat from reaction of food-induced pH and helps rapid entry of the dosage form into the small intestine.

vii) Composition of product: Drug-drug interactions are less complicated to avoid than the interactions with unlabeled additives in the medication. The manufacturers are not required to list all additives on the label. Therefore, additives of one formulation may interact with drug or additives of another medicine, if these are simultaneously administered; e.g. absorption of certain antibiotics may gets reduced if co-administered with a tablet containing dicalcium phosphate as diluent. For the same reason, tetracyclin-like antibiotics are not taken with milk or antacids.

Prescription No. 9.4

℞

Cap. Tetracycline hydrochloride   250 mg
1 q.i.d. for 5 days.

viii) Polypharmacy: The therapeutic incompatibilities are most common when a patient is taking medications for acute illness such as pain, fever, infections or diarrhoea, during chronic drug therapy for diseases such as asthma, hypertension, and diabetics. The therapeutic incompatibility usually takes place when more than one physician is prescribing for the same patient, or when the patient simultaneously purchases OTC drugs.

ix) Errors in writing a dose: Errors in prescription writing regarding dose, dosage form, strength or directions to use may lead to undesirable pharmacological effects, e.g. diazepam is prescribed as 0.5 g, which is 500 mg. The actual dose of diazepam is only 5 mg. Pharmacists should follow the procedure of dispensing of incomplete prescription.

ROLE OF COMMUNITY PHARMACISTS

All possible therapeutic incompatibilities can be avoided by taking therapy consultation from a family physician and medication consultation from a family pharmacist.

i) Patient Medication Record (PMR) contains all the current information about patients and their medical therapy. Therefore, assessing the prescription against PMR and updating the information of dispensed medicines, during every dispensing, can definitely minimise chances of errors.

ii) Review the patient's existing drug therapy, including any over-the-counter medications or herbal or dietary supplements and inquire about old and new allergies before giving prescribed medications.

iii) Computer software programs designed to check patient information, drug duplicates, expired drugs or SALA medications, can reduce medication errors.

iv) Pharmacists should read a prescription at least twice and should carry out a double check after each dispensing.

v) Pharmacists can ensure simple steps to minimise errors such as keeping the prescription and medication containers together during dispensing.

vi) Pharmacies should have adequate staff and no or minimum distractions during dispensing.

vii) Introducing bar coding technology can greatly enhance the accuracy of drug dispensing and administration.

viii) Pharmacists should have current knowledge concerning changes in medications and treatments.

ix) Non-pharmacy personnel should not be allowed to dispense.

x) Patients and families should be encouraged to ask questions about all medications ordered.

PRESCRIPTIONS FOR PRACTICE

Prescription No. 9.5

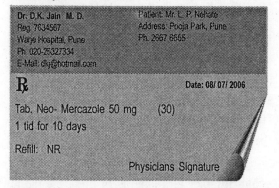

Dr. D.K. Jain M. D.
Reg. 7634567
Warje Hospital, Pune
Ph 020-25327334
E-Mail: dkj@hotmail.com

Patient: Mr. L. P. Nehate
Address: Pooja Park, Pune
Ph. 2667 6655

℞   Date: 08/ 07/ 2006

Tab. Neo- Mercazole 50 mg   (30)
1 tid for 10 days

Refill: NR

Physicians Signature

Reading the Prescription :

- The accompaning prescription for Tab. Neo-Mercazole 50 mg, to be taken 1 tablet three times a day for 10 days.
- Tab. Neo- Mercazole (Nicholas Piramal) contains Carbimazole 5 mg that is an antithyroid drug. The usual dose of drug is 15-45 mg per day.
- It means the prescription is intended for Tab. Neo-Mercazole 5.0 mg, which is misprinted/written as 50 mg.
- The drug being potent, the said tablet is only available in single strength, 5 mg; dispense the prescription by *Secundum artem*. Contact doctor and make a note on the prescription.

Prescription No. 9.6

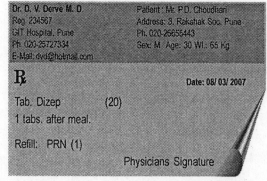

Dr. D. V. Derve M. D.
Reg. 234567
GIT Hospital, Pune
Ph 020-25727334
E-Mail: dvd@hotmail.com

Patient : Mr. P.D. Choudhari
Address: 3, Rakshak Soc. Pune
Ph. 020-26655443
Sex: M Age: 30 Wt.: 65 Kg

℞   Date: 08/ 03/ 2007

Tab. Dizep   (20)
1 tabs. after meal.

Refill: PRN (1)

Physicians Signature

Reading the Prescription:

- The present prescription is for Tablet Dizep, 1 tablet after meals for 20 days. Additionally, it is ordered to refill whenever occasion arises.
- Tab Dizep contains Diazepam 5 and 10 mg; it is brand product of Intas. Based on this information, following questions arise,
- What is the disease condition of the patient? Is the patient suffering from psychological problems such as anxiety, insomnia, etc.? Why has the doctor not written the strength of such a potent drug? Why should the tablet be taken after meals? Why is a refill allowed?
- Pharmacists have to discuss the disease condition while filling PMR.
- Answer to all these questions is here.

Mr. Choudhari has visited a doctor who is a specialist in GIT problems. He is suffering from indigestion. With the Intention of treating him with digestive enzymes, the doctor wrote down Tab. Dizec (GSK), which is mixture of Pancreatin 175 mg, sodium tauroglycocholate 50 mg and Simethicone 2 mg. The patient has to take a tablet after meals for 20 days. Secondly, whenever the patient has any problem, the doctor has directed the pharmacist to review the patient; and if any additional dosing is required, he has authority to refill the prescription. Contact the prescriber for new prescription.

Prescription No. 9.7

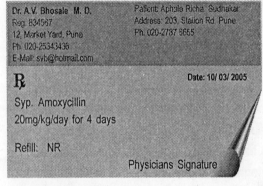

Dr. R. Dies M. D.
Reg. 79834567
Gaurishankar, Satara
Ph. 0231-26327334
E-Mail: rdies@hotmail.com

Patient: Mr. S. P. Kulkarni
Address: 213, Station Rd. Satara
Ph. 2687 6655
Sex: M   Age: 70   Wt: 70 Kg

℞   Date: 08/ 03/ 2007

Tab. Altiazem 60 mg   (10)
½ bid for 10 days

Refill: NR

                    Physicians Signature

Reading the Prescription:

- The present prescription is for Tab. Altiazem 60 mg, ½ b.i.d. for 10 days.
- Tab. Altiazem (Menatini) contains Diltiazem, a calcium channel blocker. This tablet is sustained release formulation available in two strengths, 30 mg and 60 mg.
- The drug is potent. Secondly, SR tablets should not be broken, crushed or chewed.

- The intension of the doctor is not clear. Therefore, the pharmacist should contact him over the telephone and get confirmation about the strength of tablet and timings of administrations.
- Fill the prescription only after doctor corrects it.

Prescription No. 9.8

Dr. A.V. Bhosale M. D.
Reg. 834567
12, Market Yard, Pune
Ph. 020-25343436
E-Mail: svb@hotmail.com

Patient: Aphale Richa Sudhakar
Address: 203, Station Rd. Pune
Ph. 020-2787 6655

℞   Date: 10/ 03/ 2005

Syp. Amoxycillin
20mg/kg/day for 4 days

Refill: NR

                    Physicians Signature

Reading the Prescription:

- The present prescription is for Syp. Amoxycillin for a paediatric patient weighing 18 kg.
- Doctor has mentioned the usual dose of amoxycillin and written generic prescription.
- Pharmacist has to dispense quality product and calculate strength and dose of reconstituted syrup.
- He has to counsell the patient regarding method of reconstitution, way of administration and storage condition.

- Calculation:

Dose of amoxycillin 20 mg/kg/day

For 1 kg = 20 mg; therefore for 18 kg = 360 mg/day

The proprietary amoxycillin dry syrups are available in strength of 125 mg/5 ml and 250 mg/ 5 ml in 30 ml and 60 ml capacity.

It means amount of dry syrup containing 125 mg/5 ml amoxycilin for three times a day will be-

Dose of drug: 125 mg for 3 times = 375 mg/ day

Dose of the reconstituted syrup: 5 ml for 3 times for 4 days = 60 ml.

Thus, the pharmacist has to dispense quality amoxycillin dry syrup that contains amoxycillin 125 mg/ml, reconstituted to 60 ml.

Proprietary preparations: ACMOX (Acme), AMOLIN(Dynamic), ARISTOMOX (Aristo), CARYMOX

(Strides), DAMOXY (Dabur), OLYMOX (Shalaks),WYMOX (Wyeth Lederle).

- **Patient Counselling:**
1. Boil the water for 15 minutes and cool to room temperature. Add this water in the bottle up to the volume mark and shake vigorously for complete dispersion of the powder.
2. Shake the bottle each time just before administering the dose. Dose 5 ml three times a day for 4 days.
3. Use the reconstituted syrup within maximum 4 days.
4. It should not be stored for longer period because, it is stable for only 15 days.

Prescription No. 9.9

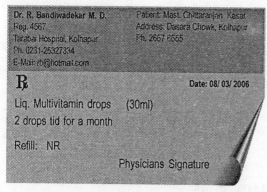

Dr. R. Bandiwadekar M. D.
Reg. 4567
Tarabai Hospital, Kolhapur
Ph. 0231-25327314
E-Mail: rb@hotmail.com

Patient: Mast. Chittaranjan Kasat
Address: Dasara Chowk, Kolhapur
Ph. 2667 6565

℞

Date: 08/ 03/ 2006

Liq. Multivitamin drops   (30ml)
2 drops tid for a month

Refill: NR

Physicians Signature

Principle: Cleanliness and hygiene have high values during paediatric therapy. The tip of droppers should not be touched. Since, the tube type of dropper can be cleaned and dried after each dosing, it requires careful handling. After washing, ensure that no water remains at the opening of the tube. The dry dropper should be well-enveloped, so as to preserve its cleanliness.

Patient Counselling:
1. Open the bottle. Remove the dropper from its envelop without touching the dropper tip.
2. Fit the dropper to bottle.
3. Do not touch the tip of the dropper to any inanimate object. If the dropper has to be washed, no residue of water should remain in the tube, as thus increases chances of contamination.
4. Use the particular dropper provided with the product.
5. Administer appropriate number of drops.

Proprietary preparations: ABDEC DROPS (Parke Davis), ACICON DROPS (Bactolac), ADROVIT (Adley), AROVIT DROP (Roche), BC-VIT DROPS (Bactolac), DROPOVIT (Wyeth Lederle), HOVITE DROPS(Raptakos), VICTOFOL DROPS (FDC).

Prescription No. 9.10: Patient Medication Records

For regular practical work, it would be good practice to select at least 20-25 patients representing different groups, viz., adult males, adult females, infants, children, old patients, patients on chronic therapy, etc. The practical book should contain a list of patients with such special category. For practical purposes, make a PMR of all these patients and use the same names for prescriptions. Below an attempt has been made to show a typical and simple PMR that will give some orientation to the students. Very detailed and easy to operate PMR can be designed with the help of computers. For example, while making the next entry, 'current clinical condition' automatically becomes 'past condition along with date. With one command, pharmacists can have different outputs such as list of patients, total number of asthmatic patients, inventory and daily cash, etc.

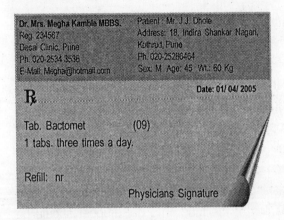

OUTPUT 1:

JEEVAN PHARMACY, PUNE
Patient List

Patient No.	Name of patient	Sex /Age	Chronic disease
1	Dhole Jayant Jijaba	M/45	-
2	Patak Seema Sanjay	F/35	-
3	Rao Monica Ramu	F/05	-
4	Joshi Shrikant Madhukar	M/60	Asthma
"			
1004	Aphale Richa Sudhakar	F/ 3.6 months	-
"			
2005	Shah Shanta Chaturlal	F/58	Hypertension

Therapeutic Incompatibility

OUTPUT 2:

JEEVAN PHARMACY, PUNE
Patient Medication Record

Patient No. : 01

Name : Mr. Dhole Jayant Jijaba

Sex : M   Age : 45

Address: 18 Indira Shankar Nagari, Kothrud, Pune 411 038.

Contacts: Tel: 020 25286464 (R)

Cell. 98220 664455

E-mail.: jaj@hotmail.com

Clinical Condition: Diarrhoea

Past condition: Cold

Allergy: Sulpha

Chronic disease : Nil

Family history : Diabetes to Father

Life style: Business, Traveling, Smoking.

Family Physician: Dr. S.Desai.

Tel.:020-25343536, 9890664422

Date	Rx #	Doctor	Age/Wt	Medicine	Signa	Refill	Charge	Sign.
28/7/4	588	SH Desai	45/60	Cap.ATMOX 250 mg (09)	tid	nr	35.40	SJK
20/2/5	O T C	- - -	45/60	Tab. Crocin 500 mg (10)	sos	-	12.50	SJK
01/4/5	15 09	Megha Kamble	46/62	Tab. Bactomet (09)	tid	nr	28.00	SJK

•••••

10 Pharmaceutical Additives

PHARMACEUTICAL ADDITIVES

Substances which are of little or no therapeutic value, but which are added to the formulation in order to help the production, to maintain physicochemical stability, to improve patient acceptability and to improve the functioning of the dosage form as a drug delivery system, are called pharmaceutical additives. They are also known as pharmaceutical aids, necessities, adjuncts, adjuvants or excipients.

Some substances are not only used as pharmaceutical additives, but they also have some therapeutic value. Therefore, while selecting them, the formulator has to maintain a balance between the desired function and its therapeutic value, eg. agar, castor oil are laxatives; alum, zinc oxide are astringents; chloroform is a general anaesthetic; lactose has nutritive value; lactic acid is a metabolic neutraliser.

Ideal properties of pharmaceutical additives are:

1) Physiologically inert.
2) Physicochemically stable over a wide range of temperature, pH and non-reacting with other ingredients of the formulation.
3) Do not impart any undesired taste, odour or colour to the product.
4) Must be non-toxic, non-irritant and non-sensitising.
5) Should be effective in low concentration.
6) Must be free from microorganisms considered to be pathogenic or otherwise objectionable.
7) Must not interfere with the bioavailability of the drug.
8) Must be commercially available in the form and purity that is commensurate with pharmaceutical standards at a reasonable cost.
9) Must be accepted by regulatory authorities.

Classification

Pharmaceutical additives are classified on the basis of their functions.

1) Diluents, vehicles or bases: lactose, water, white soft paraffin, etc.
2) Physical stabilisers: co-solvents, solubilising agents, supending or emulsifying agents, binders.
3) Chemical stabilisers: antioxidants, buffers.
4) Preservatives: methyl paraben, sodium benzoate.
5) Organoleptic additives: colouring agents, flavouring agents, perfumes and sweetening agents.

Pharmaceutical Additives used in Various Dosage Forms:

Different additives used in the dosage forms are listed below and the common additives are discussed in brief.

I) Liquid Dosage Forms:

1) Vehicles (or solvents and co-solvents): water, aromatic waters, syrups, ethanol, chloroform, propylene glycol, glycerol, polyethylene glycol, vegetable oils, mineral oils, etc.
2) Surfactants:
   a) Solubilising agents : Surfactants with HLB value 15 – 18.
   b) Wetting agents   : Surfactants with HLB value 8 – 10.
   c) Emulsifying agents : o/w emulsifiers, HLB 8 - 18; w/o emulsifiers HLB 3 – 6
   d) Antifoaming agents : Surfactants with HLB 1.5 – 3.
3) Hydrocolloids: viscosity enhancing agents, suspending agents and emulsifying agents such as acacia, tragacanth, clays, cellulose derivative and carbopols.
4) Antioxidants: sodium bisulphate, sodium metabisulphite, butylated hydroxyanisole (BHA), butylated hydroxytoluene (BHT), propyl gallate, citric acid, tartaric acid, ethylenediamine tetraacetic acid (EDTA).
5) Complexing agents: citric acid, tartaric acid, EDTA.
6) Preservative: benzoic acid, sodium benzoate, methyl and propyl paraben, chlorbutanol.
7) Colouring agents: caramel, cochineal, amaranth and other D&C and FD&C colours.
8) Flavouring agents: aromatic waters, flavoured syrups, volatile oils, etc.
9) Sweetening agents: sucrose, syrups, sorbitol, sodium saccharin.
10) Buffers: buffering system based on carbonates, citrates, phosphates or tartarates.
11) Tonicity adjusters: for Injections, ophthalmic and nasal liquids, eg. sodium chloride.

II) Semisolid Dosage Forms:

1) Bases or vehicles

a) Oleaginous bases: petrolatum, beeswax, vegetable oils, stearic acid, acetyl alcohol.

b) Absorption bases: woolfat, wool alcohols, lanolin.

c) Emulsion bases: emulsifying wax, cetrimide emulsifying wax.

d) Water-soluble bases : macrogols.

2) Antioxidants: tocopherols, propyl gallate, BHA, BHT, sodium bisulphate.

3) Buffers: sodium citrate, sodium acetate, etc.

4) Preservatives: methyl paraben, propyl paraben, benzalkonium chloride, phenylmercuric nitrate.

5) Colours: F&D, FD&C and External D&C colours, titanium dioxide, ferric salts.

6) Perfumes: flower oils.

III) Solid Dosage Forms:

1) Diluents (Fillers): lactose, mannitol, dibasic calcium phosphate, etc.

2) Binders: acacia, sodium alginate, starch paste, etc.

3) Disintegrating agents: starch, microcrystalline cellulose.

4) Colouring agents: F&D and FD&C colours.

5) Sweeteners: mannitol, sucrose, saccharin.

6) Flavouring agents: volatile oils.

7) Lubricating agents: magnesium stearate, talc.

8) Anti-adherents: corn starch, colloidal silica.

9) Glidants: corn starch, talc.

Concept Clear : **Pharmaceutical Additives**

Substances, which are of little or no therapeutic value, but which are added to the formulation for a specific function, in order to produce quality dosage form, are called as pharmaceutical additives, aids, necessities, adjuncts, adjuvants or excipients. Their specific functions are:

- Determine physical state of dosage form: base, vehicle.
- Physical stability of formulation: solubilising agent, suspending agent.
- Chemical stability of formulation: antioxidants, buffers.
- Ease in manufacturing of product: lubricants, antifoam agents.
- Organoleptic Additives: colours, flavours, sweeteners.

COMMON ADDITIVES:

According to the type of dosage form, the vehicle and physical stabiliser varies, but other additives such as chemical stabilisers, preservatives and organoleptic additives are more or

---

less same.

i) pH Controlling Agents: Controlling the pH of a pharmaceutical preparation is essential because solubility, stability, physiological compatibility of preparation and the effectiveness of preservative is determined by it. Buffers based on carbonates, citrates, lactates, phosphates and tartarates are included to resist any change in it, eg. monobasic sodium acetate, sodium citrate, potassium phosphate, potassium metaphosphate.

ii) Antioxidants: Antioxidants are effective when used in their soluble form.

i)   True antioxidants act by suppressing the formation of free radicals in the autooxidation, eg. alphatocopherol, butylated hydroxy anisole (BHA), butylated hydroxy toluene (BHT), methyl gallate, ethyl gallate, propyl gallate.

ii) Reducing agents, such as sodium sulfite, sodium bisulfite and sodium metabisulfite are used. These get preferentially oxidised over the drug.

iii) Synergist antioxidants have little inherent antioxidant activity. These are used in combination with the antioxidants mentioned above. These act by regeneration of antioxidant radicals or by chelating metals, e.g. ascorbic acid, tartaric acid, citric acid, hypophosphoric acid and EDTA.

Antioxidants suitable for aqueous preparations include sodium sulphite, sodium bisulphite, hypophosphoric acid, ascorbic acid, and citric acid. For oily liquids, the oil-soluble antioxidants such as alphatocopherol, BHT, BHA and propyl gallate are used. Usual antioxidant concentration is 0.01 to 1 per cent.

iii) Preservatives: Preservatives in non-sterile preparations are intended to stop the multiplication of microbes present and to minimise further contamination during storage. Water is a good medium for microbial growth. In addition to this, presence of syrup and dilute-vegetable extracts provide favourable environment for the growth. Preservatives should have effective solubility in aqueous phase, and should remain in an undissociated state at the pH of the preparation. When a volatile preservative is used as the sole preservative, it can vapourise during the regular opening of the container. Such preparations should be used within two weeks after compounding. Alcoholic flavours and electrolytes make the environment less favourable for microbial growth.

Preservatives are mainly included in liquid preparations for their fungistatic action. For oral solutions, benzoic acid (0.1-0.2 per cent), sodium benzoate (0.1-0.2 per cent), alcohol (15-20 per cent), chloroform (0.25 per cent), glycerin (45 per cent) or preservative system containing 10:1 ratio of methyl paraben and propyl paraben (0.1-0.2 per cent) are used. Dermatological preparations also include preservatives such as phenol (0.5 per cent), cresol (0.3 per cent), chlorocresol (0.1 per cent). Benzalkonium chloride (0.01 per cent) is suitable for ophthalmic, nasal and otic preparations; phenyl mercuric salts (0.001 per cent) for ophthalmic, nasal and topical preparations; thiomersal (0.01 per cent) for ophthalmic preparations.

iv) Organoleptic Additives: The acceptability of a preparation is governed by its sight, touch, smell and taste. In order to mask any objectionable colour, odour and taste, and for psychological benefit of the patients, the below given organoleptic additives are added. They encourage the continuation of the treatment.

Colouring agents are employed for several reasons:

i)   To give aesthetic appeal and impart pleasing appearance to the preparation.

ii) To mask the discoloured, degraded ingredient and thereby to maintain appearance of preparation during its shelf life.

iii) For identification of product.

Colours used in pharmaceutical products are categorised as:

a) Synthetic Colours: Most of these are 'certified'

i)   Colours for Food, Drug and Cosmetics (FD&C)

ii) Colours for Drug and Cosmetics (DC)

iii) Colours for externally applied Drug and Cosmetics (External D&C)
     The commonly used colours from these classes includes, FD&C Blue No.1 (Brilliant blue FCF), FD&C Red No.3 (Erythrosine), FD&C Yellow No.5 (Tartrazine), D&C Blue No.6 (Indigo), D&C Red. No.22 (Eosine), D&C Yellow No.7 (Fluorescein).

b) Natural colours:

i)   Vegetable colours: Chlorophyll (green), carotene (yellow), caramel (black, brown), riboflavin (yellow).

ii) Animal colours: Cochineal (red)

iii) Mineral colours: Titanium dioxide (opaque), ferric oxides (red, yellow). These are insoluble and restricted to external preparations.

Flavouring agents are used to mask the unpleasant smell of the product and to make preparations more palatable. Due to its increased contact with taste buds, taste of the drug is more noticeable in its dissolved state. The liquid dosage forms are critical to flavour and these can be flavoured on the following basis:

i)   Vitamin preparations are coloured deep red with cherry, strawberry or raspberry flavour.

ii) Paediatric drops should have chocolate and fruity flavours and sweet taste. Adults prefer sour taste and citrus and intense flavours.

iii) Viscous flavoured preparation such as flavoured syrup (lemon syrup, orange syrup) or flavour blended with glycerin, sorbitol imparts better mouthfeel effect.

iv) Volatile oils including cinnamon, clove, lemon, orange and peppermint, produce aromatic vapors, which activate olfactory cells. For ease of measurement and to increase miscibility with water, flavouring oils are used in dilute form, such as aromatic waters or emulsions.

Sweetening agents are natural or synthetic agents. Some are given below:

i)   Sugars: sucrose, fructose, glucose, invert sugar, syrup.

ii) Polyhydric alcohols: sorbitol, mannitol, xylitol, glycerin.

iii) Artificial sweeteners: saccharin, cyclamates, aspartame, acesulfam-K.

Sucrose is the choice of sweetener as it masks the taste of salty and bitter drugs. Syrup and liquid glucose imparts body to the liquid. Sorbitol 70 per cent w/w is half as sweet as sucrose. Polyhydric alcohols impart viscosity, a cooling effect and act as humectants, which contributes to the pleasant mouthfeel effect. Saccharin is 500 times sweeter than sucrose and water-soluble sodium and calcium salts are used in liquids. Artificial sweeteners are more suitable for diabetic patients. Non-sugar based sweeteners are non-cariogenic, non-caloric and resist microbial growth.

Concept Clear : **Common Additives**

- pH adjustment ensures solubility, stability and absorption of drug and physiological compatibility of the dosage form.
- Antioxidants are effective in soluble form. These act by preventing auto-oxidation (free radical reactions), preferential oxidation, or by chelate formation.
- Preservatives are effective in their unionised form. The system of using preservative is more effective.
- Organoleptic agents are selected in association with colour, flavour, and category of drug. Viscous-sweet-flavoured liquids impart better mouthfeel effect.

---

11 Monophasic Liquids

Mixtures are liquid preparations intended for oral administration and composed of dissolved or dispersed drug.

Pharmaceutical monophasic liquids (Solutions) are single phase liquid preparations composed of one or more pharmaceutically active ingredients dissolved in a solvent; which are intended to be used internally or externally. Solutions for internal use are either aqueous or hydroalcoholic, whereas, solutions for external use are aqueous or non-aqueous.

According to the route of administration, pharmaceutical solutions are of the following types:

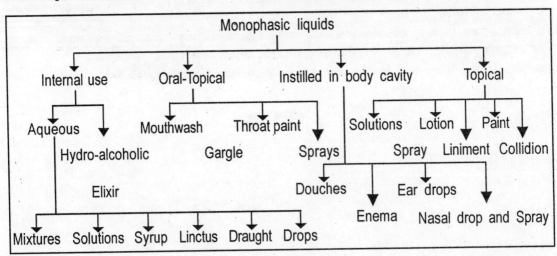

1) Solutions for internal use: mixtures, solutions, syrups, linctuses, elixirs, draughts and paediatric drops.

---

2) Solutions not intended for internal use:
  i) Oral, topical solutions: mouthwash, gargles, throat paints and sprays.
  ii) Solutions to be instilled in body cavities: douches, enemas, eardrops and nasal drops.
3) Solutions for external use: solutions, sprays, liniments, lotions, collodions and paints.

Advantages of Monophasic Liquids

i) Bioavailability of dissolved drug is rapid as compared to its insoluble form. The dosage forms can be ranked in increasing order of bioavailability in the following order.
   Tablets < Capsules < Powders < Suspensions < Solutions.
ii) The drug is more uniformly distributed in liquid vehicle and provides high dosage accuracy than biphasic liquids.
iii) Liquid preparations are easy to swallow and thus more useful for paediatric and geriatric patients.
iv) Clarity of solutions facilitates visual observation.
v) Liquids provide safe means of administering irritant drugs. Unlike solid dosage forms, rapid mixing and dilution of liquids with gastric contents, avoid localised irritation of the alimentary tract. Liquids containing irritant drugs are easily diluted just before administration.
vi) Solution is the only form in which an ingredient can readily be dispensed, eg. hydrogen peroxide solution and strong ammonia solution.

Disadvantages of Monophasic Liquids

i) Number of drugs are poorly soluble in commonly used solvent, water, and require special technique to solubilise them.
ii) Drug in soluble state is chemically less stable than its insoluble state.
iii) Improved contact of soluble drug with the taste buds makes the preparation more unpleasant to taste than the dosage form containing insoluble drug.
iv) Liquids are bulky to handle.
v) Though liquids allow more flexibility in dose, dose accuracy is determined by the accuracy in measuring the dose.

Concept Clear : Monophasic Liquids

Pharmaceutical monophasic liquids are single phase liquids composed of one or more pharmaceutically active ingredients dissolved in solvent; which are intended to be used internally or externally. As per the route of administration, these are :
a) Solutions for internal use.
b) Solutions not for internal use : Oral-Topical solutions and solutions to be instilled in body cavities.
c) Solutions for external use.

FORMULATION OF MONOPHASIC LIQUIDS

Solutions for Internal Use :

1) Drug

Drugs should have sufficient solubility in the commonly used solvent, water. The volume of solvent required to dissolve a dose of drug should be low, so as to restrict the dose of the preparation to 5 ml or in multiples of 5 ml. Milling done to reduce particle size, thus increasing the surface area for enhancement of rate of dissolution, should not affect physicochemical properties of the drug. The amorphous drugs are more soluble than their crystalline form; and the crystalline properties of drugs should not change during processing. The drug should be compatible and remain stable in soluble state and in the presence of solvent and other additives. For instance, solubility profile of paracetamol is: 1 part in 70 parts of water, 8 of ethanol, 9 of propylene glycol, 50 of chloroform and 50 of glycerin. In liquid dosage form, paracetamol is available as syrup and elixir. Due to poor solubility of paracetamol, for preparation of the solution, each 5 ml contains 120 mg paracetamol. water cannot be used as sole solvent. Secondly, due to their toxicity, non-aqueous solvents cannot be used in higher proportions. Therefore, monophasic liquid forms of paracetamol are prepared by co-solvency technique. These contain co-solvents such as propylene glycol, alcohol, and glycerin, to increase solubility of paracetamol To avoid alcohol in paediatric liquids, paracetamol is also available in the form of aqueous suspension. The paracetamol liquid should be maintained at pH 5-6 for better chemical stability. Various approaches are used to enhance solubility of drug in water. They are given below

   i)   Co-solvency using miscible solvents such as, alcohol, propylene glycol and glycerin

   ii) Solubilisation using hydrophilic surfactants

   iii) Complexation using complexing/sequestering agents

   iv) Hydrotropy using salts

   v) pH adjustment

   vi) Chemical modification (salt formation/ chemical complexes).

2) Vehicle

A) Aqueous Vehicles: Water is the choice of vehicle for oral administration due to its physiological compatibility, non-toxicity and availability. Potable water, the water suitable for drinking, is clear, colourless, odourless, and nearly neutral. It is not recommended for compounding because of chemical interactions that may occur between the drug and the dissolved substances present in it. Potable water is recommended for cleaning the equipment. Freshly boiled and cooled water, which is free from vegetative microorganisms is suitable for compounding of liquid orals. Purified water, which is prepared by distillation or deionisation is 100 times free from dissolved solids than potable water. Though water is the most favourable vehicle, most of the modern drugs are insoluble in water, water provides good media for microbial growth and it is not suitable for water sensitive drugs.

Aromatic waters are saturated aqueous solutions of volatile aromatic principles. These are themselves carminative and stomachic and principally used as flavoured vehicle in liquid orals. Syrup is the choice of vehicle for paediatric liquids due to its sweetness and viscosity of flavoured syrups that provides mouth-feel effects. It possesses remarkable taste, masking the bitter and saline taste of drugs. However, it is carcinogenic and not suitable for patients on sugar restricted diets.

B) Non-Aqueous Vehicles: Oral liquids rarely contain more than minor quantities of non-aqueous solvents. Alcohol is a solvent of second choice but it is mainly used as co-solvent. Absolute ethanol contains not less than 99.4 per cent v/v and not more than 100 per cent v/v of C_2H_5OH. Ethanol 95 per cent is a mixture of ethanol and water and contains 94.7-95.2 per cent v/v of C_2H_5OH. Diluted alcohol is 50 per cent v/v of C_2H_5OH in water.

Glycerin, a trihydric alcohol, is a viscous, sweet vehicle, miscible with water and alcohol. In addition to co-solvency, it imparts body to liquid preparations. Propylene glycol is a colourless, viscous and water miscible vehicle. Non-aqueous solvents also have preservative qualities.

Fixed oils obtained from plant and mineral origins are used as solvent for oil-soluble drugs, but due to their unpleasant taste, oils are usually administered in the form of oil-in-water emulsion.

3) Additives

All the additives used in monophasic liquids must be soluble or miscible in vehicle.

a) pH Controlling Agents: Buffers based on carbonates, citrates, lactates, phosphates and tartarates are included to resist any change in pH, eg. monobasic sodium acetate, sodium citrate, potassium phosphate and potassium metaphosphate.

b) Antioxidants: Antioxidants suitable for aqueous preparations include sodium sulfite, sodium bisulfite, hypophosphoric acid, ascorbic acid and citric acid.

c) Preservatives: Preservatives are mainly included in liquid preparations for the fungistatic action. For oral solutions, benzoic acid (0.1 - 0.2 per cent), sodium benzoate (0.1 - 0.2 per cent), alcohol (15 - 20 per cent), chloroform (0.25 per cent), glycerin (45 per cent) or preservative system containing 10:1 ratio of methyl paraben and propyl paraben (0.1 - 0.2 per cent) are used.

d) Organoleptic Additives:

Colour: Monophasic liquid oral preparations are coloured containing soluble FD and C or D and C dyes. Amaranth Solution BPC (red) and Compound Tartrazine Solution BPC (yellow) are commonly used official colour solutions from these classes. Caramel or burnt sugar is used to produce pale yellow to dark brown colours. Other colours include natural colours like riboflavin, saffron, indigo, etc.

Flavours: Due to increased contact of solutions with taste buds, taste of the drug is more noticeable in its dissolved state. Syrup, flavoured syrups; volatile oils such as cinnamon oil, lemon oil, peppermint oil and chloroform are used in the form of aromatic water, emulsion or spirit. Expectorant liquids are usually flavoured with anise water or liquorice extract. Paediatric liquids contain mixed fruit juice and chocolate flavours in sweetened base.

Sweetening agents: Sugar-based sweeteners including sucrose syrup, invert syrup are choice of sweeteners for monophasic liquids. Polyhydric alcohols like sorbitol are useful to improve viscocity and mouthfeel effect. Artificial sweeteners are rearely used and are restricted to their soluble salts only, i.e. Sodium saccharin.

Solutions for External Use :

The basic concept of formulation is the same as that of the monophasic liquid orals. Some of the ingredients used externally are toxic when taken orally.

1) Drug and vehicle

Monophasic liquids for topical use are either aqueous, non-aqueous or mixture of these. Oily preparations are preferred for application on dry skin and aqueous preparations should be applied on wet (broken/cut) skin. Topical route, due to its more physiological tolerance, widens the selection of variety of non-aqueous solvents. High proportion of non-aqueous phase increases spectrum of solubility of drug and additives and improves the overall stability of preparation due to its resistance to microbial growth and reduced hydrolysis of drug.

Alcohol, in external preparations, acts as antiseptic and rubefacient and enhances drug penetration. Rapid evaporation after application produces cooling effect on inflamed area. Industrial methylated spirit, which is exempted from excise duty, contains 5 per cent methyl alcohol and it is an economic solvent for external preparations. Rubefacient rubbing alcohol contains 8 parts of acetone, 1.5 parts of methyl isobutyl ketone and 100 parts of ethanol by volume. The ability of glycerin to retain a drug locally and the soothing effect it produces makes it the vehicle of choice for throat paint. An unhydrous glycerin is used as vehicle in eardrops. Vegetable and mineral oils are used as solvent, carrier and for their lubricating, emollient and occlusive effect.

---

2) Additives

A preservative, which is toxic internally, can be non-toxic when used in external preparations. The site of application also determines selection of preservatives; for example, methyl and propyl parabens cause more Irritation when applied on the nasal mucosa than quaternary ammonium compounds. Dermatological preparations also include preservatives such as phenol (0.5 per cent), cresol (0.3 per cent) and chlorocresol (0.1 per cent). Benzalkonium chloride (0.01 per cent) is suitable for ophthalmic, nasal and otic preparations; phenyl mercuric salts (0.001 per cent) for ophthalmic, nasal and topical preparations; thiomersal (0.01 per cent) for ophthalmic preparations.

External D and C colours are used in external preparations, for example, External D and C Violet No. 2 (Alizurol purple SS), External D and C Yellow No. 7 (Naphthol yellow S). Flower-based perfumes are also preferred in dermatological preparations.

Concept Clear : **Formulation of Monophasic Liquid Orals**

a) **Drug :** Soluble and stable in vehicle.
b) **Vehicle :** Freshly boiled and cooled water, aromatic water, syrup, glycerin, propylene glycol, alcohol.
c) **pH controlling agents :** Acidifying agents, alkaline agents, buffers.
d) **Antioxidants :** Sodium sulfite, sodium bisulfite, hypophosphorous acid, ascorbic acid, citric acid,
e) **Preservatives :** Benzoic acid, sodium benzoate, alcohol, chloroform, methyl paraben and propyl paraben, phenol, cresol, chlorocresol, benzalkonium chloride, thiomersal.
f) **Colouring agents :** FD and C or D and C dyes,
g) **Flavouring agents :** Volatile oils, aromatic water, flavoured syrup, chloroform.
h) **Sweetening agents :** Sucrose syrup, invert syrup, sorbitol, glycerin, sodium saccharin, etc.

COMPOUNDING AND DISPENSING

1) Methods of Formation of Solution

Drug can be formulated in solution form in any one of the following ways:

i) Dissolution: Fine powder of drug is dissolved in the solvent or mixture of solvents. The rate of dissolution is Increased by using heat and agitation.

ii) Chemical reaction: Two or more reactants interact to produce the drug in the solution, eg. strong Ferric chloride solution BPC, Magnesium citrate oral solution USP. The strong Ferric chloride solution involves reaction between iron and hydrochloric acid in the presence of nitric acid, whereas, Magnesium citrate solution is a pleasant laxative based on the reaction between magnesium carbonate and citric acid.

---

iii) Extraction: Crude drugs are often extracted with solvents to produce aromatic water, liquid extracts or tinctures.

The first method is most commonly attempted for compounding of monophasic liquids. Usually ¾th of vehicle is used to dissolve drug and additives. After dissolution of the drug, other soluble and miscible additives are dissolved in drug solution. The resultant solution is subjected to filtration. The remaining amount of solvent is used for rinsing mortar, pastel or beakers and to make up the volume of filtered solution.

2) Filtration : Based on size of solid retained on filtering media, filtration may be termed as fine filtration or coarse filtration. Solutions for internal use and those which are applied on broken skin are made by fine filtration, whereas coarse filtration or straining is used to separate large particles or impurities from biphasic liquids or viscous liquids.

Filter paper is most frequently employed for fine filtration. High quality filter paper such as Whatman filter paper should be used to ensure maximum filtering efficiency. Sintered glass filters are made up of excellent resistance glass. These filters vary in porosity depending on the size of the granules used in the glass filter disc. These are very useful in the filtration of solutions intended for parenteral use, or as alternative to filter paper, where drug reacts with filter paper. A vacuum attachment is necessary to increase rate of filtration.

When possible, the first few millilitres of filtrate should be discarded in order to eliminate possible contamination of filtrate by free fibres associated with most filter papers. It also acts as rinse for the collecting vessel. Alternatively, the filter paper is washed with the vehicle and the filtrate is discarded. The product is filtered before making final volume. The final volume can be adjusted by passing vehicle through the same filter paper. It also gives washing to the residue.

3) Volume Adjustment

For volume adjustment, liquid formulations can be categorised in two types:
i) Amount of vehicle prescribed to make up the volume, and
ii) Amount of vehicle prescribed in exact amount.

In the first case, the filtered solution of drug is transferred in a conical dispensing measure and final volume is adjusted using the remaining amount of solvent. Some formula contains solid and liquid ingredients expressed in mixed units of weight and volume (g and ml) and the amount of vehicle prescribed in exact amount. In such cases, the volume of the liquid produced and the calculated amount may not be the same. Calculation of the formula in same units, based on densities of ingredients, or calculating the original (mixed unit) formula for 20 per cent extra quantities, are usual methods to produce liquid of required volume (Refer exercise 13.8). If preparation is viscous to pour, the volume adjustment is done in tared bottles.

4) Dilution of Liquids

In the case of some liquids, it is recommended that they be diluted during the compounding, or just before administration, for the following reasons:

i)   Dose of liquid oral is less than 5 ml.

ii) Dilution of concentrated form such as mouthwash, gargle.

iii) Minimise gastric irritation, eg. potassium chloride solution and paediatric ferrous sulphate solution.

For the later two reasons, patient is advised to dilute each dose of the liquid with suitable vehicle just before administration. Liquid orals are mostly prescribed in doses of 5 ml or multiples of it. To minimise the error in measurement, the minimum dose of 5 ml is accepted. When the dose of a liquid is fraction of 5 ml, the use of droppers or oral syringes is modern way of dispensing them; otherwise, the pharmacists can dilute and dispense the liquid making the minimum dose 5ml. The vehicle, which is prescribed in the formula, should be used as diluent. However, dilution of a liquid should not affect its overall quality. The diluted preparation should maintain original appearance, palatability, antimicrobial capacity and chemical stability. The dilution may change the stability of the original product; therefore, diluted liquids should be used within two weeks after compounding, e.g. the dilution of liquid containing double strength chloroform water as one of the ingredient with purified water. In this case, Chloroform water, DS, acts as cosolvent, preservative and flavouring agent. The dilution of a liquid using water as vehicle, will reduce its preservative concentration and flavouring property. On the contrary, the dilution of liquid using Chloroform water, DS, will unnecessarily increase the chloroform content. The use of Chloroform water is the correct choice to maintain original qualities in the diluted liquid. (Refer prescription No.11.31 and 12.3). Such problems of dilution are not found in liquids with concentrated aromatic water as one of the ingredients. Dilution of liquid using water will not significantly reduce effective strength of the forty times more concentrated aromatic water. The syrup or non-medicated elixirs is the choice of vehicle for dilution of elixirs, where as, and linctuses are diluted with syrup.

Concept Clear : Compounding of Solutions

- Usually ¾th of the vehicle is used to dissolve drug and additives and the remaining for volume adjustment.
- When the amount of vehicle in the formula of liquid dosage form is prescribed in exact amount (not to make final volume), calculate the original formula for 20 per cent extra quantities.
- If preparation is viscous to pour, volume adjustment is done in tared container.
- Liquids in concentrated form cause irritation to GIT, or when the dose is fraction of 5 ml it has to be diluted. Prescribed vehicle is the choice for dilution.
- Diluted dosage forms should be used within two weeks after the dilution.

---

5) Containers

Plain or amber coloured glass bottles with reclosable child-resistant closure, supplied with 5 ml measuring spoon, are used for liquid orals. When the dose of liquid is less than 5 ml, either it is diluted before dispensing, or a dropper marked with 0.5ml divisions is supplied.

Liquids for oral/topical use are dispensed in plain or amber coloured fluted bottles. Ear drops, nasal drops are supplied in vials with dropper. Throat paint and collodions are supplied with applicator.

6) Storage Conditions

Stability of solutions is affected by the presence of drug in dissolved state. Secondly the aqueous phase contains sugars for microbial growth and loss of volatile components occurs during storage. The compounded liquids should be stored in a cool place and used within one month after compounding otherwise according to the stability of individual liquids, they should be labelled either 'recently prepared' or 'freshly prepared'.

7) Label

The specific instruction for each type of monophasic liquids should explain the direction of use. The orally administered liquids should be labeled as :

'- - -5 ml teaspoonful to be taken in water - - - times a day for - - - days. For other oral-topical and external liquids special instructions should be mentioned.

8) Dispensing of monophasic liquids

The products should not be dispensed if following defects are observed : Cloudiness, turbidity or precipitation of dissolved drug; change in colour, flavour and taste. Discolouration of liquid extracts and precipitation.

Patient counselling : In addition to the general counselling, patients should be educated for methods to use special types of liquids, such as mouthwash, gargle, throat paint, nasal sprays, and ear drops. Importance of dilution should be made clear. Dilution is not a common procedure e.g. linctuses must be taken undiluted and without aid of water; whereas, mouthwash is used after dilution with warm water. Gargles and mouthwashes are not intended for swallowing in large amounts, whereas, linctuses should be sipped and swallowed slowly.

9) Documentation

PMR and CDR are common documents for compounding and dispensing of any type of dosage form. Alongwith general information, the CDR for monophasic liquids specially mention s the name(s) of solvent and order of mixing of ingredients. The slight variation in the mixing order may lead to precipitation of drug.

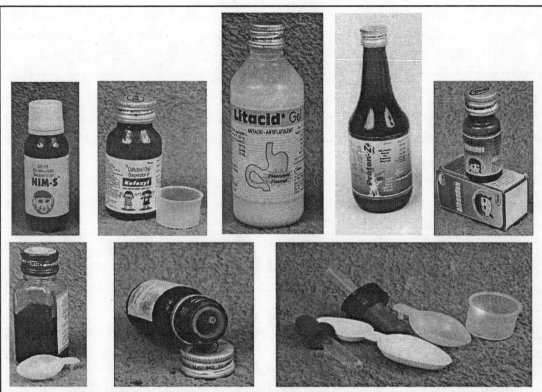

Liquid-orals : Amber bottle 60 ml (Courtesy of Get-Rid Pharma)., Amber bottle 30 ml, White glass bottle 170 ml, Tonic bottle 200 ml, Single dose bottle 10 ml and attached dropper (Courtesy of LiTaka Pharmaceutical). Bottle for viscous liquids and different types of droppers and measures.

Figure 11.1 : Containers for liquid orals

SOLUTION FOR INTERNAL USE

1) Syrups

Definition and Uses: Syrups are sweet, viscous, nearly saturated aqueous solutions of sucrose. Syrups containing medicinal substances are called medicated syrups and those containing flavoring agents are called flavored syrups. Syrup is mainly used as a vehicle, sweetening agent or flavored sweetening base to mask bitter and saline taste in oral liquids.

Formulation : Syrup, IP, contains 66.7 per cent w/w of sucrose, whereas syrup, USP, contains 85 per cent w/v (64.74 w/v) of sucrose. Self-preservative activity of syrup is attributed to its high osmotic pressure and absence of water. The osmotic pressure of syrup is 16 times greater than of an the isotonic solution. The microbial susceptibility of a syrup is inversely proportional to the concentration of sucrose in syrup, but it is not advisable to prepare saturated syrups.

Fluctuations in storage temperature may cause crystallisation of sucrose from the saturated syrups. Secondly, condensate of the vapour may fall into the surface of the syrup, resulting in localised unsaturation, which may provide suitable environment for microbial growth. The crystallisation of sucrose can be minimised by the addition of glycerin, sorbitol or propylene glycol. Presence of a little alcohol in syrups serves as a cosolvent and preservative. Preservatives such as benzoic acid, sorbic acid, sodium benzoate or methyl paraben should be added to syrups in order to preserve them for a long period of time. Syrups have specific gravity of 1.31g.

Flavoured Syrups : Flavoured syrups are almost complete flavouring agents due to their sweet taste and flavour and built in viscous liquid. The viscous-flavoured liquids retain the pleasant taste for prolonged period of time for better mouthfeel effect. Lemon Syrup, BPC (Preparation no. 11.2) and Orange Syrup, BPC (Preparation no. 11.3) are commonly used flavoured syrups. Lemon syrup BPC is prepared by using lemon spirit, citric acid, invert syrup in syrup base. The lemon syrup USP (Citric Acid Syrup) is prepared using lemon tincture (1 ml), citric acid (1 g) in syrup (to make 100 ml).

Orange Syrup, BPC, is 6 per cent v/v solution of orange tincture in syrup. The flavouring property of orange oil is due to the aldehyde content, here calculated as decanal. It also develops terebinthinate odour. The orange tincture is prepared by percolating orange peels with alcohol. The orange tincture is devoid of contents of oil, which undergoes decomposition and thus it is a better way to obtain orange flavour directly from orange peel.

Orange syrup, USP, contains orange peel tincture (5 per cent v/v), citric acid (0.5 per cent w/v), talc, sucrose (82 per cent w/v) in water. Talc is used in the preparation as distributing agent and to remove insoluble matter. The mixture is filtered to get a clear solution. The USP product is acidic in pH.

Artificial Syrups : Sugar-based syrups are caloric and raise the blood sugar level. For on sugar restricted diets, patients sugar-based syrups are not recommended. The polyols, such as sorbitol, glycerin, propylene glycol, or cellulose polymers, such as methylcellulose, hydroxyethylcellulose and artificial sweeteners, are used in place of sugar. Polyols are chemically related to carbohydrates with reducing group of sugar replaced by a primary hydroxyl group. They have low caloric value due to low gastrointestinal absorption. Cellulose is not hydrolysed and absorbed. Artificial sweeteners, such as sodium saccharine and sodium cyclamate, are more than 500 times sweeter than sucrose, non-caloric and they do not elevate blood glucose level. These syrups have excellent consistency and sweetness as that of sugar-syrups. Non-sugar syrups made from polyols and cellulose are recommended cases with reduced glycogenic intake, or zero   glycogenic intake respectively.

- Syrups are sweet, viscous, nearly saturated aqueous solutions of sucrose.
- Syrup IP contains 66.7 per cent w/v of sucrose.
- Syrup USP contains 85 per cent w/v (64.74w/w) of sucrose.
- Self-preservative activity of syrups is attributed to high their osmotic pressure and absence of water.
- It is not advised to prepare saturated syrups.
- Flavoured syrups are sweet and pleasantly flavoured used to impart better mouthfeel effect.
- Terpeneless forms of flavouring substances, such as lemon spirit, and orange peel tincture are choice of sources, of flavour in flavoure syrups.
- Artificial Syrups are sweet, viscous, non-sugars syrups in which the sweet taste is built in to the viscous agent, using artificial sweeteners. Non-sugar syrups, made from polyols and cellulose, are useful in cases with of reduced glycogenic intake and zero glycogenic intake respectively.

Compounding of Syrups

1) Hot process : Weighed quantity of sucrose is added to purified water and the mixture is heated to get clear solution. To prepare syrup, I.P., mixture of sucrose (66.7 g) and water to make 100 g is heated in tared container. If necessary, boiling water is added to adjust the final weight. Volatile flavoring agents or thermolabile drugs are added during cooling. Hot process is quick, but syrups may turn amber to dark brown in colour.

Inversion of Syrup : During heating, sucrose gets hydorlysed to dextrose and fructose, which is indicated by the colour change of the syrup from amber to dark brown. Addition of acids increase the rate of inversion. Reducing sugars formed by inversion of syrup prevent oxidation of drugs and also makes the syrup sweeter. But such syrups are more susceptible to fermentation.

2) Cold process (by agitation) : Agitating of sucrose with water to get a solution is slow process, but it produces colourless and odourless product.

3) Cold process (by percolation) : Syrup, USP, is prepared by percolation. Crystalline, or a coarse granular sucrose (85 g) is placed in percolator. The loosely packed moist cotton is placed in the neck of the percolator and purified water (45 ml) is allowed to pass slowly, till sucrose dissolves. Finally, sufficient amount of water is added in the percolator as washing, and required volume is made (100 ml).

4) Preparation of medicated syrups : Since syrups are nearly saturated and due to strong association between sucrose and water, syrups are not good solvent for water soluble drugs. It is essential first to dissolve the drug in a small quantity of water rather than directly adding it into syrup. Addition of tinctures or fluid extracts to syrups may cause precipitation of alcohol-

soluble resinous and oily substances. Slow addition, with stirring, minimises such separation. When alcohol-soluble matter is not medicinally important, mixture of such substances with water is set aside the insoluble constituents allowed to seperate out. After filtration, sugar is dissolved in filtrate to produce the syrup. Heat-stable drugs can easily be incorporated in hot syrups. Containers and storage : Store in glass bottles / jar. Keep the container well-closed in a cool place. Syrups should be used within two weeks.

Patient counselling : Avoid administering to patients on sugar-restricted diets. Syrups are cariogenic, rinse mouth with water. Do not stores syrup at low or high temperatures.

Proprietary preparations :

- REGLAN SYRUP (CFL) TOMID SYRUP (Gufic) : Metoclopramide 5 mg/ml. In nausea, vomiting.
- LIVOLUK (Panacea) : Lactulose 3.325 mg/ 5ml. In constipation.
- CROCIN (Duphar), FEBREX (Indoco) : Paracetamol 125 mg/5 ml. Analgesic, antipyretic.
- IDIQUIN (Merk), QUINROSS (Merind) : Chloroquine 80 mg/5 ml. Antimalarial.
- WORMIN (Cadila Pharma), EBEN (Gufic) : Mebendazole 100 mg/5 ml. Anthelmintic.
- ASTHALIN (Cipla), SALBU (Pharmacia and Upjohn) : Salbutamol 2 mg/5 ml. Antiasthmatic.
- THEOPED (Protec), T.R.PHYLLIN (Natco) : Theophylline 20mg/ml and 80mg/5ml, respectively. Antiasthmatic.
- ACTIZYME (Synthiko), BECELAC (Dr. Reddy's) : Vitamin B and enzymes. Tonic.

Prescription No. 11.1

℞

Syrup IP

Sucrose   — 66.7 g

Purified water, to make — 100.0 g

Principle :

Syrup, I.P. contains 66.7 per cent w/w of sucrose. The weighed quantity of sucrose is dissolved with the aid of heat. Boiling water is added in a tared container to compensate the water loss by evaporation, and to adjust the weight. The excess of water should not be used initially to dissolve sucrose. Prolonged heating may lead to brown colouration of syrup. Syrups to be stored for long periods should be preserved by adding preservatives methyl paraben. Syrup, IP, has specific gravity of 1.315 - 1.327 g.

Apparatus : Spatula, beaker, glass rod, funnel, measuring cylinder.

Compounding : Use tared container. Add sucrose in water and heat to dissolve it with occasional stirring. Add water to make the final weight.

Container and storage: Pack in glass/plastic bottle. Store in well-closed containers. Use within two weeks.

Category : Sweetening agent

Prescription No. 11.2

R

Lemon Syrup, BPC

Lemon Spirit	— 0.5 ml
Citric acid	— 2.5 g
Invert Syrup	— 10 ml
Syrup, to make	— 100 ml

Principle :

Lemon oil is mainly used as a flavouring agent. The flavour of oil is attributed to the presence of aldehyde, citral. Terpenes present in oil undergo oxidation and acquire terebinthinate odour. Terpeneless lemon oil is 20 times stronger in flavour than natural oil due to higher content of citral. It is also readily soluble in alcohol and it is used in the form of lemon spirit. Lemon spirit is the 10 per cent v/v solution of terpeneless lemon oil in alcohol (90 per cent). Citric acid adds tartness so as to give natural feel and it acts as antioxidant. Invert syrup is sweeter than syrup, but is yellowish-brown in-colour. Reducing sugars present in invert syrup prevent oxidation. Lemon syrup is acidic in pH and not suitable for acid sensitive drugs. e.g. Phenobarbital sodium precipitates at low pH. It has specific gravity of 1.33 g.

Apparatus : Spatula, beaker, glass rod, funnel, measuring cylinder.

Compounding :

i) Dissolve the citric acid in ¾ th volume of syrup.

ii) Add the invert syrup and the lemon spirit. Mix it well.

iii) Make final volume in tared container with syrup.

Container and storage: Pack in glass/plastic bottle. Store in well-closed containers in cool a place. Use within two weeks.

Category and Dose: Flavoured sweetening agent, 2.5 - 5 ml.

Prescription No. 11.3

R

Orange Syrup BPC

Orange tincture	— 6.0 ml
Syrup, to make	— 100.0 ml

Principle :

The orange tincture is devoid of contents that undergo decomposition, but it preserves the flavour of orange. It contains about 4-5 per cent v/v alcohol. Orange syrup has specific gravity of 1.29 to 1.31g.

Apparatus : Spatula, beaker, glass rod, funnel, measuring cylinder.

Compounding : Mix the orange tincture with ¾th volume syrup. Make the final volume in tared container with syrup.

Container and storage: Pack in glass or plastic bottle. Store in well closed containers in a cool place. Use within two weeks.

Category and dose: Flavoured sweetening agent, 2.5 - 5 ml

---

2) Oral Solutions (Mixtures)

The monophasic liquids differ from other classes in respect of the method of administration. These are for internal use; to be swallowed with water. The linctus, drops, draught, though ultimately reach in GI tract, have a specific method of administration.

Proprietary preparations :

- WINTREL (Pfimex) : Salbutamol sulphate 2 mg, bromhexine HCl 4 mg per 5 ml. Bronchitis.
- TOSSEX IMPROVED (Sarabhai) : Codeine phosphate 10 mg, Chlorpheniramine maleate 4 mg, menthol 1.5 mg, sodium citrate 75 mg per 5 ml. Expectorant.
- CYP-L (Albert David), CYLIP (Dolphin) : Cyproheptadine HCl 2mg and lysine monohydrochloride 150mg/5ml. Loss of appetite.
- SOYAMIN 22 (Apex) : Proteins, vitamins, minerals. REVITAL LIQUID (Ranbaxy) : Minerals.

Prescription No. 11.4

℞

Aqueous Iodine Solution I.P.
Iodine — 5.0 g
Potassium Iodide — 10.0 g
Water, freshly boiled & cooled, to make — 100.0 ml

Principle :

Lugol's solution is the synonym for it. Iodine is essential for the formation of thyroid hormones. The human requirement of iodine is 100 to 200 µg daily and the main dietary source of it is drinking water. Potassium iodide, sodium iodide are antithyroid drugs. Oral iodine solution is also used as antidote in alkaloid poisoning. Orally it causes irritation to the GI tract, and should be diluted well with water or milk. It has wider antiseptic action against bacteria, fungi, yeasts, protozoa and viruses. Few drops of iodine solution in drinking water is bactericidal and amoebicidal. Iodine solutions are used as antiseptic in treatment of superficial wounds.

Iodine is very slightly soluble in water (1 g in 3000 ml). Potassium iodide or sodium iodide is used to form water-soluble complexes, KI_3 or NaI_3. Since the dose of iodine is very low, its solution requires 17 times or more, dilution, of solution to make a dose of 5 ml; therefore it is advised to dilute the solution just before use. Sodium iodide-containing solution is less irritant when applied on an open wound.

Each ml contains 50 mg of free iodine and about 130 mg of total iodine. Container used should be resistant to iodine. Antiseptic solutions should be used within a week after compounding.

Apparatus : Spatula, beaker, glass rod, funnel, measuring cylinder.

Compounding :

i) Dissolve potassium iodide and iodine in sufficient amount of water.

ii) Filter the solution. Rinse the beaker with water and filter it in the same solution.

iii) Adjust the final volume with the remaining water.

Container and storage : Store in iodine-resistant container. A cork closure must not be used. Dropper or dosing syringe may be supplied with the container. Store in well closed containers. Use within a week.

Category and dose : Orally as source of iodine, 0.1 - 0.3 ml three times a day daily, well diluted with milk or water. Topical use is as antiseptic.

Label : For external use only (if prescribed for it).

Handling precaution: Iodine is staining, handle with care.

Patient counselling: For oral use, dilute with milk or water. Avoid taking during pregnancy, lactation. It may cause allergic reaction. Avoid administering to hypersensitive patients. Iodine causes staining, handle with care. Iodine solution applied to the skin should not be covered with occlusive dressing. Excessive use may sting and cause tissue damage to open wounds.

Prescription No. 11.5

℞

Ammonium Chloride Mixture BPC

Ammonium Chloride	— 10.0 g
Aromatic Solution of Ammonia	— 5.0 ml
Liquid Extract of Liquorice	— 10.0 ml
Water, to make	— 100.0 ml

Principle :

This preparation is used as expectorant and demulcent. Ammonium chloride and aromatic solution of ammonia are respiratory stimulants. Liquid extract of liquorice is demulcent. Ammonium chloride is freely soluble in water.

Apparatus : Spatula, beaker, glass rod, funnel, measuring cylinder.

Compounding :

i)   Dissolve ammonium chloride in ¾th volume of water. Add aromatic solution of ammonia and Liquid extract of liquorice in it. Filter.

ii)   Rinse the beaker with water and filter it in the same solution.

iii)   Adjust final volume with remaining water.

Container and storage: Store in tightly closed amber coloured glass bottles. a cool place.

Category and dose : Expectorant and Demulcent, 10-20 ml daily in divided doses.

Handling precaution: Inhalation of strong ammonia solution may cause inflammation of respiratory tract. Handle it with care.

Patient counselling : Occasionally may cause dizziness and GI disturbances. Avoid recommending to epileptic patients and patients with impaired renal or hepatic function. Avoid administering to patients who are pregnant. Advice patients to take hot steamy shower, keep warm, take inhalations. Avoid smoking and dusty environment. Advise paracetamol if there is pain and fever. Avoid antihistaminics as these tend to reduce mucous secretion, and hence the expulsion of the resulting viscous mucous is difficult.

Proprietary preparations :

- AVIL EXPECTORANT (Hoechst Marion Roussel) : Each 5 ml contains ammonium chloride

125 mg, pheniramine maleate 15 mg, menthol 1.14 mg in syrup base.

- BENADRYL COUGH FORMULA (Parke-Davis) : Each 5ml contains diphenhydramine HCl 14.08 mg, ammonium chloride 0.138 g, sodium citrate 57.03 mg, menthol 1.14 mg, alcohol 0.262 ml.

Note 1 : Expectorants : There are two types of coughs : productive and unproductive. As the name indicates, productive cough is the body's defence mechanism to expel extraneous material, secretions, and exudates from respiratory tract. It is treated only when it causes discomfort to patient. The patient may experience a feeling of congestion and breathlessness. Unproductive cough should be treated well. The unproductive or dry cough raises no sputum. It may cause hoarseness of voice. The reasons for dry cough include inhalation of foreign particle, irritating fumes, smoke, or as a result of viral infection and flu. The patient suffering from cough should drink 8 to 10 glasses of water per day. The preparations used for cough treatment act by following mechanisms.

1) Liquefy and remove sputum: bromhexine, acetylcysteine are mucolytic. The mechanism involves opening of disulphide bonds in mucus thereby reducing viscosity of mucus.
2) Decongestants: ephedrine, phenylephrine, xylometazole are commonly used nasal and bronchial decongestants.
3) Depress the cough centre: codeine, noscapine.
4) Demulcent and soothing: liquid extract of liquorice, syrup, glycerol. These are useful to relieve cough (irritation or mild inflammation) in larynx. Warm, humid vapours of volatile principles, on inhalation, to relieve cough of lower regions.
5) Expectorants: These are claimed to promote expulsion of bronchial secretions but there is no scientific basis for mechanism. These have stimulatory effect on the respiratory tract, and being inexpensive, are mainly used for placebo function. These include ammonium chloride, ammonium bicarbonate, ammonia solution, ipecacuanha, potassium iodide, squill, volatile oils.

Prescription No. 11.6

℞

Magnesium citrate oral solution USP

Magnesium carbonate	—	15.0 g
Anhydrous citric acid	—	30.0 g
Syrup	—	60.0 ml
Talc	—	5.0 g
Lemon oil	—	0.1 ml
Purified water, to make	—	350 ml

Principle :

The composition, commonly referred to as 'citrates', is a pleasant saline laxative. This is an example of a solution prepared by chemical reaction between magnesium carbonate with citric acid. Magnesium carbonate (15 g) corresponds to 6.0 to 6.47 g of magnesium oxide. Lower is the corresponding magnesium oxide, the lesser is the precipitation in the solution.

Magnesium carbonate + Citric acid = Magnesium citrate + carbon dioxide + water.

Talc acts as adsorbent and filter aid. The pleasant flavour of preparation is attributed to the syrup, lemon oil and carbonation. The carbon dioxide environment is essential for chemical stability, which can be achieved by carbonation using alkali carbonates as follows, or filling carbon dioxide under pressure.

Sodium/Potassium bicarbonate + citric acid = Potassium citrate + carbon dioxide + water.

The tablet of alkali carbonate tablets is placed in a container, which is alternative to avoid possible violent reaction that may occur between powdered alkali carbonate and citric acid. The preparation containing a lower level of citric acid (27.4 g) can be formulated when carbon dioxide environment is created by filling liquid under carbon dioxide pressure. The boiling of the mixture during compounding helps to control microbial contamination. The pasteurisation or sterilisation of solution improves further stability of magnesium citrate solution. Storage in refrigerator adds pleasantness of carbonated beverages to the preparation.

Apparatus : Spatula, beaker, glass rod, funnel, measuring cylinder.

Compounding :

i)   Add magnesium carbonate in 100 ml of water. To this add the solution of citric acid dissolved in 150 ml of water. Mix these to get the solution.

ii) Add syrup and boil the mixture.

iii) Triturate the talc with lemon oil. Add this to hot mixture.

iv) Filter the mixture into a tared bottle. Make the final volume with boiled water.

v)   Cool the solution. Add alkali bicarbonate and shake the airtight bottle to dissolve it.

Container and storage: Store in a cold beverage bottle. Store in an airtight container, and in a refrigerator.

Category and direction to use : Laxative, 200 ml.

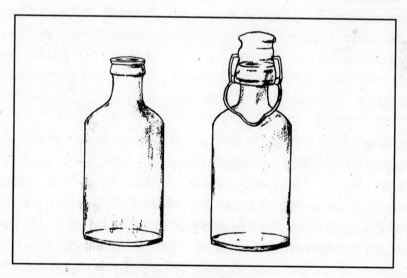

Figure 11.2 : Citrate Bottles

3) Elixirs

Definition and Uses: Elixirs are clear sweetened and flavored hydroalcoholic solutions for oral use. Non-medicated elixirs, such as aromatic elixir Iso-alcoholic elixirs are mainly used as flavored vehicles. Medicated elixirs have their own therapeutic value.

Formulation : Alcohol content in elixirs vary from 3 - 40 per cent. The iso-alcoholic elixir consists of low alcohol, up to 10 per cent and high alcohol up to 70-80 per cent. Instead of using alcohol in high concentration, medicated elixirs can be formulated, using low levels each of alcohol, glycerin or propylene glycol. This keeps the concentration of the non-aqueous solvents low and in turn minimises their adverse physiological effects and burning taste. Since sucrose is slightly soluble in alcohol, elixirs containing high concentration of alcohols are sweetened by using artificial sweeteners.

Table 11.1: Differences Between Elixirs and Syrups

No.	Elixirs	Syrups
1)	Pleasantly flavored hydroalcoholic solution, less sweet than syrup.	Nearly saturated aqueous solution of sucrose. Syrups are sweeter.
2)	Due to co-solvent effect of alcohol, elixirs are suitable to compound poorly water-soluble drug.	Although it is solvent for water-soluble drug, due to saturation it has poor solvent properties.
3)	Although provide palatable means of administration of potent or nauseous drugs, alcohol accentuates salty taste.	Palatable, flavoured syrups provide better mouthfeel effect and syrups are best to mask bitter and saline taste.
4)	Due to high alcohol content, elixirs are not the choice of dosage forms for pediatrics.	Fruit flavored syrups are choice of vehicles for pediatric medications

Compounding : Drug is dissolved in water, or alcohol, as per its solubility. Since sucrose increases viscosity and decreases solubility of drug in water, it must be added after dissolving the drug in a solvent. An aqueous solution is always added to an alcoholic solution with continuous stirring; this helps maintain high alcoholic content and prevent precipitation of alcohol-soluble ingredients. If the mixture becomes turbid, it is allowed to stand to ensure the saturation and coalescence of insoluble oil globules. Talc can be used as dispersing agent and to obtain a clear solution. After filtration, the final volume is made with the vehicle specified in the formula. If required, elixirs are diluted with syrup or non-medicated elixirs.

Containers and storage: Store in tightly closed amber coloured glass bottles away from light.

Patient counselling : Do not dilute with water.

Proprietary preparations :

- BRONCORDIL ELIXIR (USV): Theophylline 80 mg/ml. BRONCORDIL P ELIXIR (USV) : Salbutamol sulphate 1 mg, Theophylline anhydrous 25 mg per 5 ml. Antiasthmatic.
- BROMHEXINE ELIXIR (Ipca) : Bromhexine HCl 4 mg per 5 ml. Mucolytic.
- Rubraplex (Sarabhai) : Elemental iron 114 mg and vitamin B. Anaemia.

Concept Clear : Elixirs

- Elixirs are clear, sweetened and flavoured hydroalcoholic solutions for oral use.
- Mixture of co-solvents is used to minimise adverse physiological effects and burning taste.
- An aqueous solution is always added to an alcoholic solution, with continuous stirring.
- If required, elixirs are diluted with syrup or non-medicated elixirs.

Prescription No. 11.7

℞

Paediatric Paracetamol Elixir BPC

Paracetamol	— 2.4 g
Amaranth Solution	— 0.2 ml
Chloroform Spirit	— 2.0 ml
Concentrated Raspberry Juice	— 2.5 ml
Alcohol (90per cent)	— 10.0 ml
Propylene glycol	— 10.0 ml
Invert Syrup	— 27.5 ml
Glycerol, to make	— 100.0 ml

Principle :

Paracetamol is soluble 1 g in 70 ml of water, 8 ml of ethanol, 9 ml of propylene glycol, 50 ml chloroform and 50 ml glycerin. Due to poor solubility, aqueous preparation only water cannot be sufficient, as sole solvent. The non-aqueous solvents due to toxicity, cannot be used in higher proportion. Therefore, monophasic liquid forms of paracetamol are prepared by the co-solvency technique.

Paracetamol elixir contains alcohol, propylene glycol, chloroform and glycerin as co-solvents. Paracetamol syrup contains alcohol as co-solvent. To avoid alcohol in paediatric liquids, paracetamol is also used in the form of aqueous suspension. Paracetamol is chemically more stable between pH 5 and 6.

Invert syrup and raspberry juice act as sweetening and flavouring agents, respectively. When the dose is less than 5 ml, it should be supplied with a dropper. The preparation should not be diluted; otherwise dissolved paracetamol may get precipitated.

Apparatus : Spatula, beaker, glass rod, funnel, measuring cylinder.

Compounding :

i) Dissolve paracetamol in a mixture of alcohol, propylene glycol and chloroform spirit.

ii) Add mixture of raspberry juice with invert syrup. Mix well. Add amaranth solution. Add ½ amount of glycerin. Filter the solution. Rinse the beaker with glycerin and filter it in the same solution.

iii) Adjust the final volume with the remaining amount of glycerin.

Container and storage: Store in tightly closed amber-coloured glass bottles. away from light.

Category and dose: Antipyretic, Mild analgesic.

Children : 10-15 mg / kg body weight, with Dose frequency of 2 to 3 times a day.

3 months to 1 year : 2.5 to 5 ml;   1 to 3 years   : 5 ml to 7.5 ml

3 to 5 years   : 7.5 ml to 10 ml   5 to 12 years   : 10 – 20 ml.

Patient counselling : Preparation must not be diluted. Avoid administering to patients with impaired renal and hepatic function. Not to be administered for more than 48 hours without physician's advise. Advice patient sto wear light clothing and drink plenty of water. Demonstrate use of thermometer.

4) Linctuses

Definition and Uses : Linctus is a viscous, monophasic liquid containing a high proportion of syrup intended to be sipped and swallowed slowly for treatment of cough. Mostly linctuses contain sedative or expectorant drug and vehicle, that has demulcent or soothing action on the sore mucous membrane of the throat. For prolonged action, linctuses should be given undiluted, but if the dose is less than 5 ml, part of the dose is diluted with syrup or simple linctus.

Formulation : Syrup having expectorant action, such as Tolu Syrup, is most preferable as vehicle. Due to low water content of syrups, dissolution of water-soluble medicament may be difficult. A little water, glycerin or sorbitol is incorporated to increase their solubility. For diabetic patients, syrup is totally replaced by sorbitol solution. Vehicles used in the linctuses have preservative action; in addition chloroform spirit and, benzoic acid are also used as antimicrobial agents.

Container and storage : Store in glass bottle. Store in well-closed container.

Label : Sip and swallow slowly without the aid of water.

Patient counselling : Do not drink water along with or immediately after administration. Avoid administering to patients on sugar-restricted diets.

Proprietary preparations :

- COSCOPIN LINCTUS (Biological E) : Noscapine 7 mg, chlorpheniramine maleate 2 mg, citric acid 28.75 mg, sodium citrate 6.5 mg, ammonium chloride 28 mg, per 5 ml

- DETIGON LINCTUS (Bayer) : Chlophedianol HCl 20 mg, ammonium chloride 50 mg, menthol 0.25 mg, alcohol 0.35 ml.

- SINAREST LINCTUS (Centaur) : Dextromethorphan HBr 10 mg, chlorpheniramine maleate 2 mg, menthol 1.5 mg per 5 ml.

- ZEET LINCTUS (Alembic) : Dextromethorphan HBr 10mg, guaiafenesin 50 mg, phenyl propalamine HCl 25 mg, per 5 ml.

Concept Clear : Linctus

- Linctus is syrup-based, viscous, solution intended to be sipped and swallowed slowly for treatment of cough.
- Vehicles have demulcent or soothing action on the sore mucous membrane of the throat.
- Linctuses should be given undiluted, but if dose is less than 5 ml, part of the dose is diluted with syrup.

Prescription No. 11.8

℞

Simple Linctus BPC

Citric Acid	— 2.5 g
Concentrated Anise Water	— 1.0 ml
Amaranth Solution	— 1.5 ml
Chloroform Spirit	— 6.0 ml
Syrup, to make	— 100.0 ml

Principle :

The demulcent and soothing action of syrup on inflamed mucosa is beneficial to relieve a dry irritating cough. Citric acid, anise water and chloroform are used as flavouring agents. Chloroform acts as preservative also. For paediatric use, 25 ml of simple linctus is diluted to 100 ml with syrup, it is official as Simple linctus,

Paediatric.

Apparatus : Spatula, beaker, glass rod, funnel, measuring cylinder.

Compounding : Dissolve citric acid in ¾ volume of water. Add anise water, amaranth solution and chloroform water. Adjust the volume with syrup in the tared container.

Container and storage: Store in well closed plain bottlea. Use within two weeks.

Category and Dose : Demulcent. 5 ml 3 - 4 times a day.

Label : Sip and swallow slowly without the aid of water. Do not dilute with water.

Patient counselling: Do not drink water along with or immediately after, administration. Contains significant amount of sugar, avoid administering to diabetic patient.

Principle :

Prescription No. 11.9

℞

Codeine Linctus NFI, BNF

Codeine Phosphate Syrup	— 60.0 ml
Tolu Syrup	— 4.0 ml
Vasaka Syrup, to make	— 100.0 ml

Linctus Codeine Co. is the synonym for it. Codeine depresses the cough centre and is useful in relief of sleep-disturbing dry cough. Codeine phosphate syrup is prepared by dissolving 500 mg of codeine phosphate in 1.5 ml of water. It is mixed with 75 ml of syrup. After addition of chloroform spirit (2.5 ml), the volume is adjusted to 100 ml with the remaining syrup. Tolu and vasaka syrups are demulcent and soothing in action, additionally these impart flavour. Codeine linctus, containing codeine phosphate 3 mg/5 ml and 15 mg/ 5 ml is available. Antitussive preparation containing opioid analgesics is not recommended for children below 1 year.

Apparatus : Spatula, beaker, glass rod, measuring cylinder.

Compounding : Mix well and adjust the final volume with vasaka syrup using tared container.

Container and storage : Store in tights closed amber coloured glass bottle. Protect from light. Use within two weeks.

Category and dose : Cough suppressant. 5 to 10 ml 3 to 4 times day. Children : 5 -12 yr, 2.5 to 5 ml. When the dose is less than 5ml, it is dispensed after dilution with syrup or dropper is provided.

Label : Sip and swallow slowly without aid of water.

Patient counselling: Do not drink water along with or immediately after administration. It most occasionally causes constipation. Avoid administreting to children below 1 year, and to patients with impaired renal or hepatic functions. As it contains significant amount of sugar hence, avoid giving to diabetic patients. It may cause drowsiness.

Proprietary preparations :

- CODEINE LINCTUS (Indon), LINCOTUSS OPIOID (Macleods) : Codeine sulphate 15mg/ 5 ml;

- MITS LINCTUS CODEINE CO (AstraZeneca), Syp.CODORIC (Euphoric) : Codeine phosphate 10 mg/5 ml with ephedrin and chlorpheniramine maleate, respectively.

5) Draughts

Draughts are monophasic liquids intended to be taken as a single dose (50 ml) by oral route. The drug is dissolved, or dispersed, in suitable solvent, such as water, syrup and the flavoured preparation is packed as a single dose.

Dilution of liquid is not acceptable because the dilution seriously affects the stability of the preparation, or larger dose or diluted liquid would be inappropriate in the treatment of infants.

Prescription No. 11.10

℞

Paraldehyde Draught, BPC

Paraldehyde	— 4 ml
Liquorice Liquid Extract	— 3 ml
Syrup	— 8 ml
Water, freshly boiled & cooled, to make	— 50 ml

Principle :

Paraldehyde is freely soluble in water. Solubility is higher at low temperature. Liquorice liquid extract is flavoring agent and syrup is sweetening agent. Paraldehyde is quick-acting hypnotic. It has objectionable odour and taste. Paraldehyde should be stored in a dark, cool place and in airtight container. Its contact with cork, rubber and plastic should be avoided. Paraldehyde should not be used if it is brown coloured or has odour of acetic acid. To avoid environmental exposure, mix the ingredients in narrow mouth container and adjust the volume in tared container.

Apparatus : Spatula, beaker, glass rod, funnel, measuring cylinder.

Compounding : Dissolve paraldehyde in ¾ volume of cold water. Add liquorice liquid extract and syrup. Adjust volume with the remaining amount of water.

Container and storage : Store in small amber glass bottle. Store in airtight container in cool and dark place. Avoid contact with cork, plastic or rubber. Use within 24 hours.

Category and dose: Hypnotic. 50ml at once, at bedtime.

Handling precaution: Care should be taken to avoid environmental exposure of paraldehyde or preparation containing it.

Patient counselling: Drink with water. Keep away from children. It may cause drowsiness.

6) Paediatric Drops

These are small dose liquids administered without dilution with the help of dropper. Dilution of liquid is not acceptable because the dilution seriously affects the stability of preparation, or larger dose or diluted liquid would be inappropriate to administer to infants.

Dropper is either graduated in fractions of a millilitre or pre-calibrated. The number of drops delivered by precalibrated dropper are equivalent to the prescribed dose. The former type of dropper is more accurate to measure all types of liquids. Number of drops delivered by dropper may vary in volume depending on the properties of liquid. Though number of drops are the same, the size of drops is different due to the nature of liquid, i.e. surface tension, viscosity, density, temperature of liquid and the rate of dropping.

Proprietary preparations :

- METACIN DROPS (Themis pharma) PARACIN DROPS (Stadmed): Paracetamol, 150mg/ml for analgesic. Antipyretic action.
- PERITOL DROPS (Themis Chemicals), CYPRO DROPS (Geno): Cyproheptadine 1.5mg / ml. Loss of appetite.
- FREND DROPS (Pharmed), TRIFER DROPS (Apex): Iron (III) hydroxide polymaltose complex equivalent to elemental iron 50mg/ml. Haematinic.
- REDPRO PLUS (Pharmasynth), TONOFERRON DROPS (East India): Multivitamin.
- EVION PAEDIATRIC DROPS (Merck) : Vitamin E supplement.
- AROVIT DROP (Roche) : Vitamin A supplement.
- ASTYMIN DROPS (Tablets India) : Amino acid supplements.

Prescription No. 11.11

℞

Paracetamol Syrup, (MEP)

Paracetamol	— 2.40 g
Sucrose	— 50.0 g
Sorbitol syrup	— 20.0 ml
Butterscotch imitation flavour	— 0.075 ml
Vanilline	— 20.0 mg
Peppermint spirit	— 0.165 ml
Methyl paraben	— 120.0 mg
Propyl paraben	— 10.0 ml
Alcohol	— 10.0 ml
Purified Water, to make	— 100.0 ml

Principle :

As discussed in Prescription No. 11.7 liquid forms of paracetamol can be prepared as elixir, syrup and suspension. Elixir contains higher proportion of non-aqueous solvents to affect the solution. The non-aqueous system provides unsuitable environment for microbial growth, but the solvent increases the cost of the preparation. Paracetamol syrup contains the same quantity of alcohol and propylene glycol as the co-solvent, as that of elixir. The co-solvents with water make the system monophasic. The amount of sugars is also not sufficient to provide preservative action, but it provides good media for microbial growth. Therefore, paracetamol syrup contains methyl paraben and propyl paraben as preservative system. By virtue of viscosity, syrups possess better mouthfeel effects than elixirs. Butterscotch imitation flavour, vanillin and peppermint flavour built in sweet syrup, and fortified with cool feeling of sorbitol make the preparation palatable. Sorbitol, also minimise problem of cap-locking. When the dose is less than 5 ml, It should be supplied with dropper.

Apparatus: Spatula, beaker, glass rod, funnel, measuring cylinder.

Compounding :

i)   Dissolve sucrose in $\frac{3}{4}^{th}$ parts of water.

ii) Dissolve paracetamol in mixture of alcohol, propylene glycol and aqueous sugar solution.

iii) Add butterscotch imitation flavour with sorbitol syrup. Mix well. Add mixture of peppermint spirit, vanillin and preservatives.

iv) Filter the solution. Rinse the beaker with water and filter it in the same solution.

v)   Adjust final volume with remaining amount of water.

For other details refer Prescription No. 11.7.

Proprietary preparations :

*   Drops METACIN (Themis); Ultragin (Wyeth) : 125 mg/5 ml.

SOLUTIONS FOR ORAL–TOPICAL USE

1) Gargles

Definition and Uses: Gargles are clear solutions used in the posterior region of the mouth, by agitating the solution with exhaled air, to produce local effect in the throat. These are not to be swallowed in large amounts. Gargles are used to relieve soreness in mild throat infections and most of these have deodorant effect.

Formulation: The commonly used active ingredients in gargle include antiseptics, analgesics, astringents and alkalising agents. Common drugs include, phenol, thymol, menthol, cineole, methyl salicylate, povidone-iodine, potassium chlorate, ferric chloride, borax and sodium bicarbonate. Astringent helps to restore the slack muscles of the , and also relieves dryness by stimulating salivation. Glycerin is the choice of vehicle for gargles, the reasons are as follows:

i)   Due to viscosity, it keeps medicament in contact with membraneous lining of the throat for long periods.

ii) Acts as demulcent.

iii) The sweet taste of glycerin with aromatic substances in gargle gives characteristic flavour.

iv) Acts as co-solvent.

Compounding: Gargles are compounded in tightly closed the same way as the general method described for solutions. Since most gargles are concentrated solutions, prescribed amount of it is diluted with warm water for gargling.

Container and storage: Store in fluted containers. in a scool and dry place.

Label: For external use only. Not to be swallowed in large amounts.

Patient counselling: Dilute with warm water before use. Not to be swallowed in excess.

Proprietary preparations: Gargle and mouthwash

* TANTUM ORAL RINSE (Elder): Benzydamine 0.15 per cent w/v.
* BETADINE GARGLE (Win Medicare), WOKADINE GARGLE (Wockhardt) : PIODIN MOUTHWASH (Biddle Sawyer) : Povidone Iodine 1 per cent w/v.
* KAMILLOSAN LIQUID (German Remedies): Chamomilla oil 15 mg, alcohol 4.16 ml per 10 ml in aqueous base.

Prescription No. 11.12

R

Potassium Permanganate Gargle, NFI 1979

Potassium Permanganate	— 25.0 mg
Water, freshly boiled & cooled,to make	— 100.0 ml

Principle:

Potassium permanganate is soluble in 16 parts of water. Due to its oxidising property, potassium permanganate is used as cleansing agent, deodorant and skin disinfectant. Gargle is the concentrating 1 in 4000 solution, In concentration of 1 in 1000, it is used as mild antiseptic in the treatment of superficial wounds and ulcers. It has been widely used as first-aid in snake bite. For different types of applications, the stronger stock solution can be diluted with freshly boiled and cooled water.

Apparatus: Spatula, beaker, glass rod, sintered glass funnel, measuring cylinder.

Compounding:

i) Triturate the potassium permanganate with 20 parts of water using glass mortar. Decant the solution.

ii) Repeat the procedure by adding 20 ml fresh water and triturating with undissolved potassium permanganate, till it completely.

iii) Filter the solution and Adjust the volume with water.

Container and storage: Store in a fluted container. Cork closure must not be used. Store in tightly closed container, in a cool place. Use within a week.

Category and direction to use: Antibacterial, Antifungal and disinfectant. Dilute with warm water before use.

Label : For external use only. Not to be swallowed in large amounts.

Patient counselling: Dilute with warm water before gargling. Not to be swallowed in excess.

2) Mouthwashes

Mouthwashes are clear solutions intended to be used in the front of the uvula (the tongue-like projection at the middle of posterior edge of soft palate) to clean and refresh the mouth. They are also used in treating diseased state of oral mucous membrane. Although mouthwashes are considered as a separate class, many of these are used as gargles, either as such, or after dilution with warm water. However, mouthwashes have more cosmetic value and are used to maintain oral hygiene. whereas gargles are highly medicated. Mouthwashes contain antiseptic or astringents in pleasantly flavoured vehicle. Like gargles, mouthwashes are used after dilution with warm water and are not to be swallowed in significant amounts.

Concept Clear : Gargle and Mouthwash

- Gargles are clear solutions used in the posterior region of the mouth, by agitating the solution with expired air to produce local effect in throat.
- Gargles are used to relieve soreness in mild throat infections. Most of these have deodorant effect.
- Gargles are highly medicated.
- Mouthwashes are clear solutions intended to be used in the front of the uvula to cleanse and refresh the mouth.
- They are used to clean and refresh the mouth and are pleasantly perfumed.
- Mouthwashes have more cosmetic value.

Prescription No. 11.13

℞

Zinc Sulphate and Zinc Chloride Mouthwash BPC

Zinc Sulphate	—	2.0 g
Zinc Chloride	—	1.0 g
Compound Tartrazine solution	—	1.0 ml
Dilute Hydrochloric Acid	—	1.0 ml
Chloroform Water, DS	—	50.0 ml
Water, freshly boiled & cooled, to make	—	100.0 ml

Principle :

It is used to treat mouth unclears, as astringent and for wound healing. Zinc chloride also desensitises teeth. Zinc sulphate and zinc chloride are very soluble in water. Oxychloride present in the zinc chloride makes the solution turbid. Hydrochloric acid dissolves oxychloride. Tartrazine acts as colour.

Apparatus : Spatula, beaker, glass rod, sintered glass filter, measuring cylinder.

Compounding :

i)   Dissolve zinc sulphate and zinc chloride in 10 ml of water. Add dilute hydrochloric acid to get a clear solution.

ii)   Add chloroform water and tartrazine solution, mix well. Filter.

iii)   Rinse the beaker with water and filter it in the same solution.

iv)   Adjust final volume with remaining water.

Container and storage: Store in tighthtly closed fluted bottles in cool place. Category and direction to use: Astringent, mouthwash. Dilute to 20 times its volume with warm water before use.

Label : For external use only. Not to be swallowed in large amount.

Handling precaution: Zinc chloride is deliquescent and caustic. Zinc sulphate is efflorescent. Therefore should not be exposed zinc salts to environment for prolonged periods.

Patient counselling : Dilute 20 times its volume with warm water before use as mouthwash. Not to be swallowed in excess.

3) Throat Paints

Definition and Uses: Throat paints are viscous preparations of medicaments for local action in the pharynx. Glycerin, because of its viscosity, prevents it being washed away rapidly by saliva and thus a prolonged action is obtained. They are applied to the throat with a brush. Throat paints arc used to treatment of inflammations of various areas of the mouth and throat, including stomatitis, pharyngitis, laryngitis and tonsillitis.

Formulation: The common ingredients used in throat paints are anti-infective agents like phenol, iodine, gentian violet, boric acid and astringents like tannic acid. Iodine is particularly used in treatment of pharyngitis and tonsillitis, gentian violet in treatment of oral candidiasis

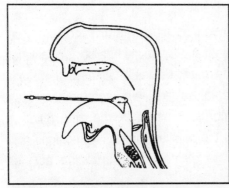

Figure 11.3: Applications of Throat Paint

(thrush), whereas tannic acid is used to relieve a sore throat.

Container and storage: Throat paints should be packed in airtight, coloured, fluted wide mouthed bottles and supplied with brush. These should be kept in a cool place.

Label : For external use only. Not to be swallowed in large amounts.

Patient counselling: Not for swallowing. Apply with brush in throat. Do not drink water immediately after application.

Principle:

Mandl's Paint is the synonym for it. Iodine is anti-infective and potassium iodide has expectorant properties. Potassium iodide and alcohol help to dissolve iodine. Mentha oil gives flavour and glycerin is a viscous vehicle.

Apparatus : Spatula, beaker, glass rod, funnel, measuring cylinder.

Prescription No. 11.14

℞

Compound Iodine Paint INF 1979

Iodine	— 0.31 g
Potassium Iodide	— 0.62 g
Water	— 0.62 ml
Mentha Oil	— 0.10 ml
Alcohol(90per cent)	— 0.94 ml
Glycerin, to make	— 25.00 ml

Compounding :

i) Dissolve potassium iodide and iodine in sufficient amount of water.

ii) Dissolve mentha oil in alcohol. Add it to iodine solution.

iii) Adjust the final volume with glycerin.

Container and storage: Store in iodine-resistant container. Provide brush. Cork closure must not be used. Store in well closed container.

Category and direction for use: Antiseptic. Apply with brush.

Label : For external use only. Shake well before use.

Handling precaution: Iodine causes staining, handle with care.

Patient counselling: Apply with brush (demonstrate way of application). Not to be swallowed in large amounts. Do not drink water immediately after application. May sting if used in excess. Avoid giving to pregnant and lactating mothers. It may cause allergic reaction. Do not dispense to hypersensitive patients.

Tannic Acid Glycerin Paint INF 1979

Tannic Acid	—	20.0 g
Sodium Citrate	—	1.0 g
Dried Sodium Sulphate	—	0.2 g
Glycerin	—	78.8 g

Principle :

It is Tannic acid glycerin, IP. Tannic acid is soluble in water and slowly soluble in glycerin. Aqueous solution of tannic acid oxidises and becomes dark. Sodium citrate liquefies viscous sputum. Sodium citrate and Sodium sulphate prevent darkning of solution. Sodium sulphate is soluble in glycerin. Glycerin acts as soothing agent, and due to its viscosity, keeps the drug in contact with the inflamed throat membrane for prolonged periods of time. Tannic acid glycerin, BPC, is 15 per cent w/w tannic acid solution in glycerin.

Apparatus : Porcelain dish, glass pestle, spatula, beaker, funnel, glass rod.

Compounding :

i)   Mix tannic acid, sodium sulphate, and sodium citrate with ½ volume of glycerin to produce smooth dispersion.

ii)   Add remaining amount of glycerin and heat on sand bath at temperatures not above 120ºC to produce solution.

Container and storage: Store in tightly closed fluted bottle. Provide brush. Store in tightly closed container, in cool place.

Category and direction to use: Astringent, antiseptic. Gum paint. Not to be swallowed in large amount.

Label : For external use only.

Patient counselling : Lightly massage on gum with brush or finger tip. Not to be swallowed in large amounts. Do not drink water immediately after application. Do not administere to patients with impaired hepatic function. Consult a dentist in case of severe pain and bleeding. Rinsing with mouthwash reduces infections. Avoid hot or cold food. Brush teeth 2-3 times a day to prevent formation of plaque.

Proprietary preparations:

• Liq. Limaye's GUM CORRECT (Epic, Satara): Tannic acid 16 per cent, borax 2 per cent, gum acacia 0.5 per cent, glycerin 75 per cent, flavoured base q.s.

• STOLIN GUM ASTRINGENT (Dr. Reddy's): Tannic acid 2 per cent w/v, Zinc chloride 1 per cent w/v, cetrimide 1per cent w/v.

4) Glycerites

Definition and Uses : Glycerites or glycerins are viscous, hygroscopic solutions of medicaments in not less than 50 per cent by weight of glycerin intended to be applied externally. Antiseptic

---

and astringent drugs, like phenol, borax, boric acid and, tannic acid are used for their local action in the form of glycerites. These glycerites are used principally as throat paints. The viscosity is due to glycerin, which helps prolong the contact of medicament with the affected area. Glycerites containing tannic acid, borax, iodine, menthol, acacia have applications in oral hygiene, as they help in prevention and treatment of pyorrhea and minor dental and throat troubles. Such preparations can be applied in various ways, massag on gums, holding a cotton plug soaked with the liquid between the teeth, gargling or using as mouthwash. Glycerites have also found wide use in otic products, where moisture should be excluded, e.g. phenol glycerin, containing 5 per cent of phenol is used as counter-irritant in ear. Non-medicated glycerites such as starch glycerite are used for their emollient action, whereas, tragacanth glycerite is used as a distributing agent. Glycerin solutions are convenient because they possess good physicochemical stability, preservative action and therefore they can be stored until needed.

Containers and storage: Store in fluted bottles. Since glycerites are hygroscopic, they should be stored in tightly closed container.

Proprietary preparations :

- Liq. GUMEX (Pharmadent, Valsad) : Potassium iodide 0.8 per cent, iodine 0.6 per cent, tannic acid 2 per cent, menthol, thymol, camphor each 0.5 per cent, mentha oil and clove oil   each 0.3 per cent, zinc phenol sulphonate 0.8 per cent, phenol 0.2 per cent, glycerin

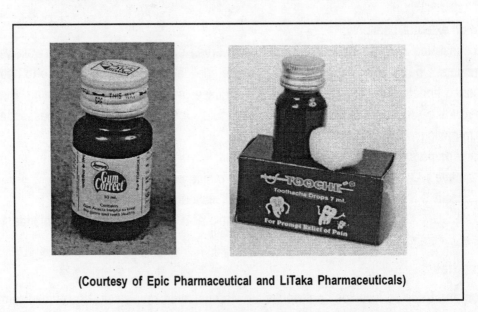

(Courtesy of Epic Pharmaceutical and LiTaka Pharmaceuticals)

Figure 11.4 : Glycerites and Tooth Paints

Monophasic Liquids

Prescription No. 11.16

℞

Borax Glycerin IP
Borax   — 12.0 g
Glycerin — 88.0 g

q.s.

Principle :

Borax is soluble in 16 parts of water and in 1 part of boiling water and 1 part of glycerin. In the dry state, it is efflorescent. Its aqueous solution is alkaline and precipitates metals as insoluble borates. But with glycerin it produces glyceroboric acid. Borax is toxic if taken internally. Glycerin is a soothing agents and, due to its viscosity, keeps the drug in contact with affected area for prolonged periods of time. If required, it is diluted with glycerin.

Apparatus : Porcelain dish, glass pestle, spatula, beaker, funnel, glass rod.

Compounding :

i) Triturate the powdered borax with glycerin to produce smooth dispersion.

ii) Warm the mixture using water bath with constant stirring to get solution. Filter if necessary.

Container and storage: Store in well-closed, thited bottlls, in a dry place Provide application brush.

Category and direction to use : Bacteriostatic.

Label : For external use only. To be used sparingly.

Patient counselling: Do not swallow.

Prescription No. 11.17

℞

Starch Glycerin
Starch   — 10.0 g
Benzoic acid   — 0.2 g
Purified water   — 20.0 ml
Glycerin, to make —100.0 g

Principle :

Starch has absorbent and demulcent properties. When jelled with glycerin, it provides a non-fatty emollient base. Starch is insoluble in water and glycerin. When heated, it produces translucent jelly. Benzoic acid is preservative.

Apparatus : Porcelain dish, glass pestle, spatula, beaker, funnel, glass rod, sand bath.

Compounding :

i) Triturate the starch and benzoic acid with water in the porcelain dish, to produce a smooth dispersion.

ii) Add glycerin and heat the mixture in the sand bath with constant stirring, to get a transparent jelly.

iii) Strain through a muslin cloth.

Container and storage: Store in well-closed, finted bottles, in a dry place. Use within 24 hours. Provide application brush.

Category and direction to use : Emollient. Pill excipient.

Label : For external use only.

5) Sprays

Sprays are aqueous or non-aqueous monophasic liquids, intended for spraying in the throat, nose or on the skin, and also to medicate the upper and lower respiratory tract.

Throat sprays containing antiseptics and deodorants in an aqueous phase, alcohol or glycerin are effectively used to treat laryngitis, pharyngitis and tonsillitis.

Both, nasal and throat spray are used to medicate the respiratory tract. Fine droplets of spray reach the lower respiratory tract. Such devices are called as inhalers. Very small droplets may get exhaled out. Non-volatile solvents, such as glycerin or propylene glycol, are added to control droplet size.

Skin protective and antipruritic drugs are applied on the skin with the help of topical sprays. Medication is applied in a uniform thin layer on to the skin without touching the affected area. This may reduce the irritation that sometimes accompanies on application with the fingertips.

Proprietary preparations :

- WOKADINE SPRAY (Wockhardt), VIODINE SPRAY (Bombay tablets): Povidone iodine 10 per cent w/v and 5 per cent w/v respectively.

SOLUTIONS FOR BODY CAVITIES

1) Nasal Solutions

Definition and Uses : Nasal solutions are aqueous or oily monophasic liquids, rendered isotonic and slightly buffered to maintain the pH at 5.5 to 6.5. Most of them are administered as nasal drops or sprays. Nasal solutions are used intra-nasally to relieve nasal congestion, inflammation and to combat infection. It contains drugs like antihistaminic, sympathomimetic agents (vasoconstrictors) and antibiotics. The shrinking effect of the vasoconstrictor on the swollen nasal membranes affords impressive and immediate relief from congestion.

Formulation: Oily solutions are not preferred, especially mineral oil has been proved to cause lipoid or oil inspiration pneumonia. Oils also interfere with normal ciliary action. A vehicle for nasal solution should be isotonic with mild buffer capacity. It should not modify mucus viscosity and normal ciliary motion. A suitable preservative should be added to suppress growth of microorganisms that may get introduced via the attached dropper.

Containers and storage: Nasal drops are dispensed in 10 to 25 ml capacity amber glass bottles fitted with a screw-caps and droppers. Plastic spray packages are available for dispensing nasal spray. Atomizers produce a coarse spray, which are preferred, rather than a fine mist for nasal application. Nebulisers that produce a fine mist are used to treat respiratory tract.

Label : For external use only.

Patient counselling : Directions to use nasal drops and nasal spray :

i)   Before using nasal drops, wipe mucous away from the nose.

ii) Advice the patient to lie down on a flat surface with the head over the edge of bed to keep the head lower than the shoulders. Insert dropper pipette a little way into each nostril and apply prescribed number of drops.

iii) The patient should remain in this position for few minutes.

iv) Nasal spray : It should always be administered to the patient after making him sit in an upright. Spraying the solution with the head over the edge of a bed could result in the systemic absorption of drug. The excessive and/or repeated use of these preparations can result in a rebound hyperemia or congestion rebound. This secondary effect is worse than the original congestion. Therefore, pharmacists should advice the patients to use the nasal drops or spray sparingly, preferably only 2 or 3 times a day. In of rebound effect, the patient is advised to withdraw application of solution in only one nostril. The complete withdrawl of dosing may cause total nasal obstruction because of bilateral vasodilatation. Once the rebound congestion subsides in the drug-free nostril, within about 1 to 2 weeks, a total withdrawal is then instituted.

Proprietary preparations:

• OTRIVIN Nasal Drops (Novartis), DECON (Cadila Pharma): Xylometazoline HCl 0.05 per cent (paediatric) and 0.1 per cent in an aqueous isotonic solution.

• EFCORLIN NASAL Drops (Glaxo): Hydrocortisone 0.02 per cent, naphazoline nitrate 0.025 percent.

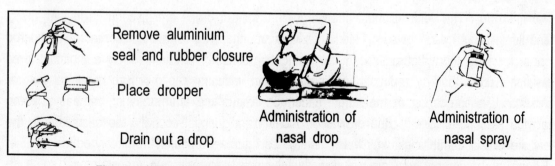

Remove aluminium seal and rubber closure

Place dropper

Drain out a drop

Administration of nasal drop

Administration of nasal spray

Figure 11.5 : Administration of Nasal Drops and Nasal Spray

Prescription No. 11.18

℞

Ephedrine Nasal Drops, BPC

Ephedrine Hydrochloride	— 0.5 g
Chlorbutol	— 0.5 g
Sodium Chloride	— 0.5 g
Water, freshly boiled &	
Cooled, to make	— 100.0 ml

Principle : Ephedrine is a sympathomimetic amine. It is useful in allergic conditions, especially in reversible airways obstruction. Ephedrine type of drugs are likely to cause arrhythmias. It is soluble in 4 parts of water. Chlorbutol is preservative. Sodium chloride is tonicity adjusting agent.

Apparatus : Spatula, beaker, funnel, glass rod, measuring cylinder.

Compounding : Dissolve ephedrine HCl in $\frac{3}{4}^{th}$ volume of water. Add chlorbutol and sodium chloride and make final volume with water.

Container and storage: Store in coloured, fluted bottle, fitted with a dropper or in a plastic squeeze bottle with attached dropper. Store in well closed container in cool place.

Category and direction to use: Nasal blockade in common cold, allergic rhinitis, sinusitis, hay fever. 2-3 drops in each nostril, repeat 2-3 times in a day if required.

Label : For external use only.

Patient counselling: Avoid administering to heart patients. It may cause idiosyncrasy. Explain method of administration.

Proprietary preparations:

- ENDRINE Drops (Wyeth Lederle) : Ephedrine 0.75 per cent, menthol 0.5 per cent, camphor 0.5 per cent, eucalyptol 0.5 per cent, castor oil 0.5 per cent, light liquid paraffin base.

2) Ear Drops

Definition and Uses : Ear drops are solutions, suspensions or emulsions of drugs in water, glycerin or propylene glycol intended for instillation into the ear. These are used for removal of excessive cerumen (ear wax), to treat infection, inflammation or pain and for cleaning and drying the ear.

Formulation : The vehicles most often employed for ear drops are glycerin, propylene glycol and liquid polyethylene glycols. Due to it's viscosity, the drug remains in contact with the ear canal for long. Anhydrous glycerin the being hygroscopic, tends to remove moisture from swollen tissue, thereby reducing inflammation and reducing the moisture available for ear infection. The presence of moisture, macerated tissue and warmness of ear cavity, being provide ideal conditions for the growth of bacteria and fungi. Secondly, the secretions in the ear are fatty and immiscible with water, aqueous solutions are usually not preferred for otic use. Ethanol and isopropyl alcohols are also useful solvents for irrigating the ear canal.

Mineral oil, vegetable oil and hydrogen peroxide have been the commonly used agents for removal of earwax. Drugs used topically in the ear include analgesics, antibiotics, and anti-inflammatory agents. Liquid otic preparations require preservatives such as chlorobutanol (0.5 per cent), thiomerosal (0.01 per cent), or combination of methyl and propyl paraben.

Compounding: Same as that of general method described for solutions, suspensions or emulsions.

Container and storage : Otic solutions are dispensed in dropper bottles.

Patient counselling : The patient is instructed to tilt the head to the side and specified number of drops are placed into the ear. Cotton plug is placed to retain the medication in ear for 15 to 30 minutes. Also advise the patient to remain in this position for a few minutes so the drops do not run out of the ear. It is also advisable to warm ear solutions by rolling the bottle with palms in hand before administration.

Proprietary preparations:

- BETNESOL EAR DROPS (Glaxo Pharma) : Betamethasone 0.1 per cent w/v.
- CHLOROMYCETIN EAR DROPS (Parke-Davis): Chloramphenicol 5 per cent w/v, benzocaine 1per cent w/v.
- CIPROBID E/E Drops (Cadila Healthcare): Ciprofloxacin 0.3 per cent w/v.
- DESOL Ear Drops (Geno): Docusate Sodium 5per cent in aqueous glycerin base.
- GARAMYCIN E/E Drops (Fulford): Gentamycin 3mg/ml.

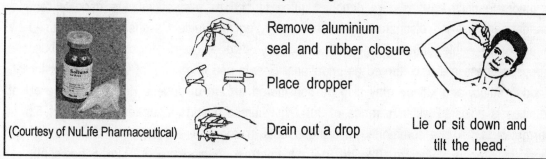

(Courtesy of NuLife Pharmaceutical)

Remove aluminium seal and rubber closure

Place dropper

Drain out a drop

Lie or sit down and tilt the head.

Figure 11.6 : Administration of Ear Drops

Concept Clear : Nasal and Ear solutions

Nasal solutions are aqueous or oily monophasic liquids, rendered isotonic and slightly buffered to maintain pH of 5.5 to 6.5.

Ear drops are solutions, suspensions or emulsions of drugs intended for instillation into the ear for removal of excessive cerumen, to treat infection, inflammation and for cleaning and drying the ear. Anhydrous glycerin is the most beneficial vehicle for ear drops and aqueous vehicles are not recommended.

℞

Sodium Bicarbonate Ear Drops, BPC
Sodium bicarbonate — 5.0 g
Glycerin — 30.0 ml
Water, freshly boiled &
cooled to make — 100.0 ml

Principle :
Sodium bicarbonate is soluble in 11 parts of water. Glycerin serves as viscous vehicle and soothing agent in the inflamed ear. It minimises the harsh effect of alkali. To avoid loss of glycerin during measurement, it is directly added 70 ml solution of drug in water, and volume is adjusted.

Apparatus : Glass pestle, spatula, beaker, funnel, glass rod.

Compounding : Dissolve sodium bicarbonate in ¾ th volume of water. Adjust volume to 70ml. Add glycerin and make the final volume.

Container and storage: Store in well - closed coloured fluted bottles fitted with dropper or in plastic squeeze bottle. Store in a cool and dry place. Use within two weeks.

Category and direction to use: Wax softener. 2-3 drops in each ear, repeat 1-2 times in a day if required.

Label : For external use only.

Patient counselling : As described under ear drops.

3) Douches

Definition and Uses : Douches are aqueous solutions intended to clean, deodorise, soothe or medicate body cavities. Eye douches, often termed as eyewashes, are used to remove foreign particles and discharges from the eyes. Vaginal sterile douches are introduced by means of a suitable rubber syringe, with a specially designed nozzle, for cleansing or antiseptic purposes; these are also termed as irrigations. Enema and irrigations of the ear, nose, throat, bladder, colon, and kidney may also be considered a form of douche. In general, the pH of douches is adjusted within a range of 3.8-4.4; whereas, vaginal douches have pH of 5.5.

Formulation : A The commonly used ingredients in douches are :

Cleansing Agents : Sodium Chloride (0.9 per cent), saponated cresol (0.2-0.5 per cent).

Antiseptics : Mercuric Chloride (1:3000 to 1:10,000), potassium permanganate (0.1-1per cent), lactic acid (0.5-3 per cent).

Astringents : Tannic acid, zinc sulphate, alum, acetic acid.

Deodorants and refreshing agents : Peroxides, perborates, methyl salicylate, thymol, menthol, and eucalyptol.

Douches are often dispensed in concentrated form, which are diluted to volumes of a litre or two, with warm water, before use.

4) Enema

Definition and Uses: Enemas are aqueous or oily solutions, suspensions or emulsions of medicaments intended for rectal administration, to cause bowel evacuation, to bring about local or systemic therapeutic action, or to instill x-ray contrast medium for examination of the lower bowel. Enemas can be broadly of two types :

1) Evacuant enemas (cleansing enemas) and

2) Retention enemas.

Evacuant enemas : Evacuant enemas are employed to cleanse the bowel either to allow better visualisation, or for administration of radiocontrast material during diagnosis, or to decrease the chance of contamination when bowel surgery is indicated. For diagnosis of lower bowel, barium sulphate enema is given as radiocontrast media. The volume of evacuant enema may be as much as one litre. Such large volume enema should be warmed to body temperature before administration. If the enemas is too cold, intestinal cramping may occur, and if is too hot, it may damage the intestinal mucosa.

The mechanism of action of evacuant enema depends upon the ingredients present in it. If tap water is used for evacuation of bowel, it acts by stimulating peristalsis due to their large volume. Enemas containing substances like sodium phosphate, sodium biphosphate, magnesium phosphate and sodium bicarbonate, act by causing osmotic retention of water in the bowel. The evacuation effect of soft soap and turpentine oil is due to their local irritant action on intestinal mucosa. Ingredients like mineral oil, olive oil, glycerin and soft soap are used to lubricate the bowel. Starch mucilage is used for emollient effect and also as suspending agent for insoluble solids in enemas.

Retention enemas : Retention enemas are used for local or systemic effects and their volume does not normally exceed 100 ml. These are very much suitable for patients in whom the oral route must be avoided because of age restictions, mental status or physiological condition. They are especially helpful for administration to in infants and geriatric patients who have difficulty in swallowing. Retention enemas are used to administer anthelmentics (quassia), anti-inflammatory agents (hydrocortisone), sedative (paraldehyde), anti-asthmatics (aminophyllin), basal anesthetics (thiopentone sodium) or nutrients (dextrose).

Containers and storage : Enemas should be packed in coloured, fluted, screw-capped glass bottles. Recently, several plastic squeeze bags with rectal nozzle have been introduced for administration of enema. For the unit dose disposable, polythene or PVC bags, sealed to a rectal nozzle, are more convenient to administer enema. They are stored in a cool place.

Label : For rectal use only.

Patient Counselling : The patient should be guided for administration of enema. The patient should lie on one side with knees bent. Lift buttock during administration of enema and he should remain there for 20-30 minutes.

Proprietary preparations :

- LAXICON ENEMA (Stadmed) : Docusates 0.25 per cent. In constipation.
- NEOTOMIC ENEMA (USV) : Glycerin 15 per cent w/v, sodium chloride 15 per cent w/v : In cas of constipation.
- MESACOL (sun pharma) : Masalazine 4 g 160 ml bottle. Anti-inflammatory.
- ENTOFORAM (Cipla) : Hydrocortisone 10 per cent w/v aerosol form ulcerative colitis.

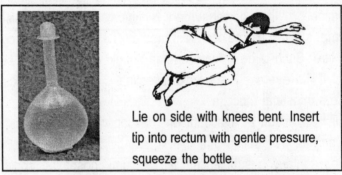

Lie on side with knees bent. Insert tip into rectum with gentle pressure, squeeze the bottle.

Figure 11.7 : Administration of Enema

Concept Clear : Enema

- Enemas are aqueous or oily solutions, suspensions or emulsions of medicaments intended for rectal administration, to cause bowel evacuation, for local or systemic effect or for diagnosis.
- Evacuant enemas are employed to cleanse the bowel and it may be as much as one litre. It is warmed up to body temperature before administration.
- Retention enemas : Retention enemas are used for local or systemic effects and their volume do not normally exceed 100 ml.

Prescription No. 11.20

℞

Soap Enema, INF 1979
Soft Soap — 5.0 g
Purified water,
warm, to make — 100.0 ml

Principle :
Soft soap is formed by saponification of higher free fatty acid with sodium or potassium hydroxides. It acts as evacuant enema due to its local irritation and lubricating properties.

Apparatus : Spatula, beaker, funnel, glass rod, measuring cylinder.

Compounding: Dissolve soft soap in warm purified water.

Container and storage: stored in well-closed, coloured flutted bottles, with syringe or the plastic squeeze bottles/bag with attached long rectal nozzle. Store in well closed container in cool place.

Category and direction to use : Bowel Cleaning. 500 ml by rectal injection. To be warmed up to body temperature before use.

Label : For rectal use only.

Prescription No. 11.21

R

Paraldehyde Enema, INF 1979
Paraldehyde   — 8.0 ml
Sodium Chloride   — 9.0 g
Purified water, to make — 100.0 ml

Patient counselling : As described under enema.

Principle :

Paraldehyde is freely soluble in water. It is hypnotic. The 10 per cent v/v paraldehyde enema is official in BPC.

Apparatus : Spatula, beaker, funnel, glass rod, measuring cylinder.

Compounding : Dissolve paraldehyde and Sodium chloride in water.

Category and Direction to use: Sedative, 30 to 40 ml/kg of body weight to maximum 340 ml by rectal injection. Other information is same as that described in Prescription No. 11.20.

SOLUTIONS FOR TOPICAL APPLICATIONS

1) Topical Solutions

Topical solutions are aqueous or non-aqueous preparations applied externally on skin as general antiseptic solutions, for disinfection of skin lesions including abrasions, cuts, bites, pre-operative and post operative cleansing of wounds, and for surgical hand disinfection.

Proprietary preparations :

- BETADINE (Win-Medicare), PV-DINE (BDH) : Povidone Iodine 5per cent w/v.
- IOPREP ANTISEPTIC SOLN (Johnson and Johnson) : Sodium iodide surfactant base available iodine 1per cent w/v.
- ACEPTIK LIQ ANTISEPTIC (ICI) : Cetrimide 3 per cent w/v, Chlorhexidine gluconate 1.5 per cent v/v.
- DETTOL ANTISEPTIC LIQUID (Reckitt & Colman) : Chloroxylenol 4.8 per cent w/v, terpineol 9.0 per cent v/v, alcohol 13.1 per cent v/v.
- DETTOL-H HOSPITAL CONCENTRATE (Reckitt & Colman), FAIRGENOL H (FDC) : Benzalkonium chloride 40 per cent w/v, Disodium edetate 1.5 per cent w/v.

℞

Cresol with Soap Solution IP

Cresol	— 50.0 ml
Vegetable oil	— 18.0 ml
Potassium Hydroxide	— 10.0 ml
Orange Oil	— 4.2 ml
Water, to make	— 100.0 ml

Principle :

Lysol is the synonym for it. Cresol is bath bactericide and germicide. It is caustic, but less than phenol. The presence of vegetable oil or glycerin reduces. The harsh effects of cresol. Cresol is soluble in 50 parts of water forming a turbid solution. Fixed oils, alkali hydroxides or soap and glycerin are good solvents. Soaps make the preparation clear, but of reduced antimicrobial activity.

Lysol has been the choice of disinfectant for hospital use.

Apparatus: Spatula, beaker, glass rod, funnel, measuring cylinder.

Compounding :

i) Dissolve potassium hydroxide in $\frac{1}{4}^{th}$ volume of water.

ii) Add vegetable oil and heat on water bath till oil droplets disappear. Add cresol and filter the solution. Rinse the beaker with water and filter it in the same solution.

iii) Adjust the final volume in a tared container with the remaining amount of water.

Container and storage : Store in well-closed, amber coloured fluted glass bottles. protect from light. Closure made of cork must not be used. Use within a week.

Category and direction to use: After dilution, it can be used as disinfectant for utensils, floors, etc.

Label : For external use only.

Handling precaution : Cresol is caustic, handle it with care.

2) Collodions

Definition and Uses : Collodions are non-aqueous solutions of pyroxylin in ether-alcohol, with or without medicament intended to be applied to the skin. It leave a film on drying. Non-medicated collodion containing 5 per cent pyroxylin is used as mechanical protective to provide water-repellent seal for minor cuts and scratches.

Formulation : Pyroxylin is nitrated cellulose obtained by the action of a mixture of nitric and sulphuric acids on cotton. The non-aqueous solution of pyroxylin in ether-alcohol is collodion. Collodion, when made pliable and flexible by the addition of castor oil and camphor, is termed as flexible collodion. Colophony is added to improve adhesion. Flexible collodion has the advantage that it can be used on the joints and movable parts of the body without the danger of cracking. Medicated collodions, in addition to its occlusive film, keeps medicament in contact with skin for an extended period of time. Salicylic acid collodion contains 12 per cent of salicylic acid in flexible collodion. It is used as keratolytic agent in removal of corns and warts.

Compounding : The solutions are prepared by shaking. The ingredients with a solvent in a closed container. If any impurity is present, it is removed by decantation.

Container and storage : Air tight, fluted bottles. Keep the container in a cool place. Keep away from open flame.

Label : For external use only, Inflammable. Collodions are applied with brush.

Handling precaution: The principle constituent of pyroxylin is cellulose tetranitrate; it is highly inflammable and harsh to touch.

Proprietary preparation :

- SALACTIN PAINT (NuLife) : Salicylic acid 16.7 per cent, Lactic acid 16.7 per cent in Flexible collodion. Warts, plantars, corns and calluses.

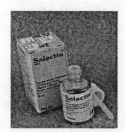 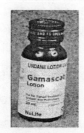 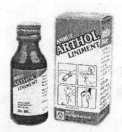

Collodion bottle and applicator, Lotion container (Courtesy of NuLife Pharmaceuticals). Liniment bottle (Courtesy of Amrut Pharmaceuticals).

Figure 11.8: Containers for Topical Liquids

Prescription No. 11.23

℞

Salicylic Acid Collodion BPC

Salicylic Acid	— 12.0 g
Flexible Collodion, to make	— 100.0 ml
Flexible Collodion IP	
Pyroxylin	— 1.6 g
Colophony	— 3.0 g
Castor Oil	— 2.0 g
Alcohol (90per cent)	— 24.0 ml
Solvent Ether, to make	— 100.0 ml

Principle :

Collodions are non-aqueous solutions of pyroxylin intended to form polymer film on the affected area after the solvent is evaporated. Collodions are useful for protection of small cuts and , abrasions. Salicylic acid in higher concentration is caustic and in the form of collodion it is mainly used to heal warts and corns. Pyroxylin is cellulose nitrate. It is soluble in 1 part of alcohol (90 per cent) and 3 parts of ether and it is highly inflammable. Colophony is adhesive resin soluble in alcohol and ether. Castor oil is emollient and plasticiser. Industrial methylated spirit can be used instead of alcohol.

Apparatus : Spatula, beaker, glass rod, funnel, measuring cylinder.

Compounding :

i) Add pyroxylin, colophony and, castor oil in alcohol. Add ether and shake in a closed container, to produce solution.

ii) Keep the solution aside and decant it to get clear filtrate.

iii) Adjust the volume with ether in a tared container.

Container and storage : Store in small air-tight, amber-colored, fluted, bottles or jars. Provide application brush. Keep in a cool place. Keep away from naked flame.

Category and direction to use : Keratolytic. Apply with brush and allow it to dry.

Label : Inflammable. For external use only. Apply with brush on the affected area.

Patient counselling : Prolonged use may be caustic. Keep away from naked flame.

3) Liniments

Definition and Uses : Liniments are solutions or emulsions in aqueous or oily vehicle, intended for massage into the unbroken skin. They are used as counter irritants, rubefacient and soothing.

Formulation : The liniments are either alcoholic, saponaceous, or oily, in nature; aconite liniment, turpentine liniment and methyl salicylate liniment are typical examples of such types, respectively. Alcohol produces rubefacient, counter irritant and mild astringent action, and also facilitates the absorption of the medicament. The oily liniments are milder in action than alcoholic liniments, but are more useful when massage is required. The spreading attribute of alcoholic liniments can be improved by including soap.

Compounding : These are prepared by method for compounding of solutions or emulsions.

Container and storage : Liniments should be dispensed in coloured fluted bottles. Liniments should be stored in well-closed containers in a cool place, because they contain volatile ingredients.

Label : For external use only. Not to be applied on broken skin. Apply with friction. If applicable, shake well before use.

Proprietary preparations :

● LINIMENT MYOSTAL (Solumiks Piramal) : Mahanarayan tel 4 ml, nirgudi tel 4 ml, Gandapuro tel 1 ml, deodar tel 0.5 ml, gandhabiroja 0.2 g, per 10 ml. Counter irritant, topical analgesic.

Prescription No. 11. 24

℞

Soap Liniment, I.P.
Soft Soap	— 8.0 g
Camphor	— 4.0 g
Lemongrass Oil	— 1.5 ml
Purified Water	— 17.0 ml
Alcohol (90per cent), to make	— 100.0 ml

Principle :

Soap liniment, BPC, contains rosemary oil in place of lemongrass oil and *in situ* formation of soap due to reaction between Potassium hydroxide and oleic acid. Soap liniment is used as cleansing agent in seborrhea and acne vulgaris and as antiseptic in treatment of superficial wounds. Camphor is rubefacient, antipruritic, counter irritant. Lemongrass oil has odour as that of lemon oil. It is insect repellant.

Soft soap is made by saponification of vegetable oils, or higher free fatty acids using potassium or sodium hydroxide. It is soluble in water and alcohol. Camphor is soluble in 800 parts of water, 1 part of alcohol and freely soluble in volatile oils. Lemongrass oil is freely soluble in alcohol (70 per cent) and solubility decreases with time. Addition of water in solution of lemongrass oil makes it turbid. Such solution is kept aside for separation of maximum possible undissolved lemongrass oil and filtered to obtain a clear solution. Methylated spirit can be used instead of alcohol.

Apparatus: Spatula, beaker, glass rod, funnel, measuring cylinder.

Compounding:

i) Dissolve soft soap, camphor, and lemongrass oil in ¾th volume of alcohol.

ii) Add water in it and keep aside for few minutes and filter. Rinse the beaker with alcohol and filter it in the same solution.

iii) Adjust the final volume with the remaining alcohol.

Container and storage: Store in tightly closed , amber coloured fluted, glass bottles, in a cool place. Protect from light.

Category and Direction for use: Detergent and mild antiseptic, rubefacient. Apply with friction on unbroken skin.

Label: Alcohol content, 61-65 per cent v/v; For external use only, Inflammable.

Patient counselling: Do not dilute with water. Apply with friction on unbroken skin. Keep away from naked flame.

Prescription No. 11. 25

℞

Camphor Liniment IP, BP
Camphor	— 20.0 g
Arachis oil	— 80.0 g

Principle :

Camphorated oil is the synonym for it. Camphor Is rubefacient, antipruritic, counter irritant. Arachis oil is used as solvent for camphor and to provide lubrication during massage.

Apparatus: Spatula, beaker, glass rod, funnel, measuring cylinder.

Compounding: Dissolve camphor in arachis oil in a closed

container.

Container and storage: Store in tightly closed amber coloured fluted glass bottles. in a cool place.

Category and direction for use: Rubefacient, counter irritant. Apply with friction on unbroken skin.

Label: For external use only.

Patient counselling : Do not dilute with water. Apply with friction on unbroken skin.

4) Lotions

Definition and Uses: Lotions are suspensions, emulsions, combination of emulsion-suspension or aqueous or non-aqueous solutions, designed to be applied to the unbroken skin without friction. Since they are used for their epidermic effect, such as local cooling, soothing, protective, drying or moisturising properties, depending upon the ingredients used, they need not be applied with massage.

Formulation: The therapeutic agents included in lotions are antifungal, anti-inflammatory, anti-infective, anti-pruritic, scabicidal agents, parasiticide and local anaesthetics. Many times they are simple solutions, while others contain insoluble solids such as calamine, sulphur or zinc oxide. Suspension type of lotions are referred to as shake lotions. Bentonite and sodium carboxymethyl cellulose are widely used as suspending agents in such lotions. Natural gums such as acacia or tragacanth, are not suitable as suspending agents for lotions, because of their sticky and irritant nature. Lotions may also be dilute o/w emulsions stabilised by emulsifying agents like emulsifying wax, which also impart body to the lotion, eg. benzoyl benzoate lotion. In white lotion, the insoluble solid is formed by chemical reaction between zinc sulphate and sulfurated potash in liquid state and are not filtered. Since the precipitate produced is nearly colloidal in size range, no suspending agent is required.

Lotion may contain substances such as glycerin or alcohol. Glycerin retains the moist film on the skin for prolonged period of time and it also promotes adherence of the powder layer on the skin surface. The evaporation of the alcohol after application produces a cooling effect in inflammatory conditions, leaving a protective coat of fine powder on the skin surface.

Container and storage: Lotions should be dispensed in coloured, fluted bottles and if they are viscous, wide-mouthed jars may be used.

Label: For external use only. Apply without friction on intact skin. If applicable, shake well before use.

Proprietary preparations :

● STATUM-B LOTION (Crossland): Clotrimazole 1 per cent w/w, betamethasone 0.05 per cent w/v.

- TRIBE-NB LOTION (Jenburkt): Clotrimazole 1 per cent w/v, beclomethasone 0.025 per cent w/v. Antifungal.
- GAMASCAB (Nulife), GAMARIC (Euphoric), Gamma benzene hexachloride 1.1, Scabicide.
- BETNOVATE SCALP (Glaxo pharma): Betamethasone 0.1 per cent. Dermatoses, psoriasis.
- ZOFLUT (Cipla) : Fluticasone 0.005 per cent w/v corticosteroid, Anti-inflammatory.

Concept Clear : Topical Applications

- Collodions are non-aqueous solutions of pyroxylin intended for topical application. These form protective film on the evaporation of the solvent.
- Liniments are solutions or emulsions intended for massage into unbroken skin. These allow drug penetration in skin layers to produce counter irritant or rubefacient effects.
- Lotions are suspension, emulsion or solutions. After application, they deposit the drug on the skin is surface, for superfecial effects.

Prescription No. 11. 26

℞

Salicylic Acid Lotion, BPC

Salicylic Acid	— 2.0 g
Castor Oil	— 1.0 ml
Alcohol (95 per cent),	
to make	— 100.0 ml

Principle :

Salicylic acid is keratolytic, bacteriostatic and fungistatic in nature. Keratolytic agents are often recommended in chronic scaling or thickened lesions. Salicylic acid and sulphur have applications in seborrheic scaling and follicular infections. Salicylic acid is soluble in 550 parts of water and in 4 parts of alcohol. Castor oil acts as emollient to minimise harsh effect of salicylic acid. Alcohol may be replaced by industrial methylated spirit.

Apparatus: Spatula, beaker, glass rod, funnel, measuring cylinder.

Compounding:

i) Dissolve salicylic acid in $\frac{1}{4}^{th}$ volume of alcohol.

ii) Add castor oil and rinse the beaker with alcohol. Adjust the final volume with the remaining amount of alcohol.

Container and storage: Store in well-closed amber coloured fluted glass bottles. Store in well closed containers in a cool place. Protect from light.

Category and direction to use : Keratolytic. Being antidandruff, lotion has to be applied on wet hair and , washed 5 to 10 minutes after application.

Label: For external use only. Inflammable. Keep away from open flame.

Patient counselling: If irritation of eye persists, wash eyes with water. Prolonged use may be caustic. Do not dry the hair near an open flame. Regular washing of hair with antidandruff

---

shampoo is the best alternative for dendruff free hair. Change in shampoo brands is more beneficial. Regular hair cleaning and moistening the scalp with non-sticky hair oil is advisable.

ADDITIONAL EXERCISES

Prescription No. 11.27

℞

Vasaka Syrup IP

Vasaka Liquid Extract	—	50 ml
Glycerin	—	10 ml
Syrup, to make	—	100 ml

Principle :

Vasaka is crude drug consisting of fresh or dried leaves of Adhatoda Vasaka (eg. Adulsa).Vasaka liquid extract is alcoholic extract.

Apparatus: Spatula, beaker, glass rod, funnel, measuring cylinder.

Compounding: Use tared container. Mix vasaka liquid extract with glycerin. Add syrup to make the final volume.

Container and storage: Pack in well-closed glass, or plastic, bottles. up to the mark. Use within two weeks.

Category and dose: Expectorant, 2 - 4 ml

Label: Alcohol 15-18 per cent v/v.

Patient counselling: Avoid recommending it to diabetic patients. It is caloric and cariogenic. Avoid recommending it to children. I am it contains 15-18 per cent v/v of alcohol.

Proprietary preparations:

- TULSIYUKT ADULSA COMPOUND SYRUP (Amrut Pharma): Each 100 ml contains extract of adulsa 4 g, jestamadha 1 g, tulsi 1 g, badishep 500 mg, sunta caried garuct 500 mg, balharda 500 mg, kantakari 500 mg, lemon grass 500 mg, dhayati 250 mg, pudina phool 20 mg, karpoora 20 mg, in syrup.

- DANGIDULSA COUGH MIXTURE (Dangi Labs) : Each 10 ml contains aqueous extract of calamus 30mg, extract of *Glycyrrhiza glabra* 100 mg, extract of *Zingiber officinale* 66.60 mg, extract of *Terminalia bellarica* 33.33 mg, extract of *Pepper longum* 33.33 mg, extract of *Vornonia anthelmintica* 8.33 mg, jawkhar 58.33 mg in syrup base.

Prescription No. 11.28

℞

Tolu Syrup, IP

Tolu Balsam	—	1.25 g
Sucrose	—	66.00 g
Water, to make	—	100.00 ml

Principle:

Tolu balsam is unorganised crude drug obtained from plant. Due to its volatile constituents, it acts as stimulating expectorant. It is insoluble in water. The aromatic constituents dissolve in water to produce saturated aromatic water, which is sweetened with sucrose.

The USP formulation contains tolu balsam tincture and light magnesium carbonate as distributing agent. The tincture is triturated with light magnesium carbonate then water is added and filtered.

Apparatus: Spatula, beaker, glass rod, funnel, measuring cylinder, water bath.

Compounding:

i) Coarse particles of Tolu balsam and 40 ml of water are placed in tared glass vessel. In closed vessel, the mixture is heated gently for half an hour and with frequent stirring. The mixture should weigh 36 g, If it is less, sufficient water is added to adjust the weight.

ii) Cool and filter the solution. Add sucrose and warm to dissolve it.

iii) Adjust the final weight with the remaining water.

Container and storage: Store in well-closed containers. Use within two weeks.

Category and dose: Flavouring agent. Expectorant, 2 to 8 ml.

Patient Counselling : Avoid administering to diabetic patient. It is caloric and cariogenic.

Prescription No. 11.29

℞

Ephedrine Syrup NFI

Ephedrin Hydrochloride — 400 mg

Syrup, to make — 100 ml

Principle :

Refer prescription 11.18.

Apparatus: Spatula, beaker, glass rod, funnel, measuring cylinder.

Compounding: Use tared container. Dissolve ephedrine HCl in $\frac{3}{4}^{th}$ volume of syrup. Add syrup to make final volume.

Container and storage: Store in well-closed containers. Use within two weeks.

Category and dose: Bronchodilator, 3 mg per kg body weight every 24 hours.

Patient counselling: Avoid administering to heart patient and in diabetics. It may cause idiosyncrasy.

Proprietory preparations:

- Liq. ASMOTONE (East India): Each 5 ml contains, ephedrine HCl 10 mg, caffeine anhydrous 90mg, belladonna tincture 0.5 ml, alcohol 7 per cent.
- TENDRAL LIQUID (Parke Davis): Each 5ml contains, theophylline 32.5 mg, ephedrine HCl 6 mg, phenobarb 2mg, alcohol 9-10per cent, in syrup base.

Prescription No. 11.30

℞

Chlorpheniramine Maleate Syrup, USP

Chlorpheniramine Maleate — 40.0 mg

Glycerin — 2.5 ml

Syrup — 8.3 ml

Sorbitol Solution — 28.2 ml

Sodium Benzoate — 0.1 g

Alcohol — 6.0 ml

Water, colour, flavour to make — 100.0 ml

Principle :

Chlorpheniramine Maleate (CPM) is antihistaminic (H_1-receptor antagonist) and has potential value in the treatment of nasal allergies, vasomotor rhinitis and effective in nasal congestion. In addition, it is used to treat allergic rash, insect bites, and drug induced allergic reactions. CPM is widely used in proprietary antitussive formulations.

Drowsiness is the serious side effect of antihistaminics, but CPM has low incidences than promethazine, diphenhydramine. Newer antihistamines such as cetirizine and terfenadine cause very less sedation.

CPM is soluble in 4 ml of water and 10 ml alcohol. Glycerin, syrup and sorbitol have sweetening effect and they impart viscosity. Presence of syrup in smaller amounts makes the preparation less glycogenic. Sodium benzoate is the preservative.

Compounding:

i) Dissolve CPM in sufficient amount of water. Add sorbitol solution, syrup, glycerin and alcohol. Colour and flavour may be dissolved in water, or in alcohol.

ii) Add sodium benzoate. Filter the solution. Rinse the beaker with water and filter it in the same solution.

iii) Adjust final volume with remaining water.

Container and storage: Store in well-closed containers. Protect from light.

Category and dose: Antihistaminic, 10 ml 3 to 4 times a day. Child 1-2 yrs, 2.5 ml twice daily; 2-5 yrs, 2.5ml 3 to 4 times a day; 6-12 yrs, 5 ml 3 to 4 times a day.

Label: It may cause drowsiness.

Patient counselling: It may cause drowsiness. Interaction with alcohol could be dangerous. Since it causes either sedation, or excitation, avoid driving. Administrater with caution to patients with hepatic diseases and epilepsy.

Proprietary preparations:

- Syp ALERNYL–DC (Sigma): Each 10 ml contains, dextromethorphan HBr 20 mg, CPM 4 mg, phenylpropanolamine HCl 25 mg, menthol q.s. in syrup base.

- ALEX PAED DROPS (Lyka) : Each ml contains, phenylpropanolamine HCl 12.5mg, CPM 2mg.

- CAPEX EXPECTORANT (Seagull): Each 5 ml contains, CPM 4 mg, ammonium chloride 125 mg, sodium citrate 55 mg, menthol 1 mg in syrup base.

Prescription No. 11.31

R

Ferrous Sulphate Mixture, Paediatric BPC

Ferrous Sulphate	—	1.2 g
Ascorbic Acid	—	0.1 g
Orange Syrup	—	10.0 ml
Chloroform Water, DS	—	50.0 ml
Water, freshly boiled and cooled, to make	—	100.0 ml

Principle :

Ferrous sulphate, gluconate, fumarate, choline citrate, glycine sulphate and recently used Iron (III) hydroxide polymaltose complex are the choice of drugs in iron deficiency anemias. 1 per cent rise in haemoglobin content is expected to occur in an average adult by administration of 50 mg/ml of Iron. Actually, body requirement is 2 pmg daily but due to poor absorption a higher iron does is recomended. It may require six month's treatment for the restoration of body iron. The soluble ferrous salts are effective rather than the ferric salt. Ferrous sulphate contains 20 per cent of Fe (iron). The acidity of gastric content, proteins containing-SH groups, and ascorbic acid maintains iron in the ferrous state. Excess dose causes haemosiderosis. Iron may cause darkening of teeth and faeces. Swallowing of solution through straw prevents discolouration of teeth. The oral administration of iron sometimes produces GI irritation, abdominal pain, nausea and vomiting. To avoid GI irritation, the preparation should be given after meals and preferably well diluted with water. Ferrous sulphate tablets may cause more local GI irritation than the liquid dosage form. To avoid irritation and for chemical stability, iron tablets are coated. The coated tablets should release complete dose of the drug before duodenum, where iron has better absorption.

Ferrous sulphate is very soluble in water. Ferrous sulphate oxidises to brown coloured ferric sulphate. Use of hard water as vehicle accelerates oxidation, making preparation yellowish-brown. Ascorbic acid is antioxidant. Orange syrup is a flavoured sweetening agent. Chloroform water is a preservative and has flavouring properties. For infants, when dose of mixture is less than 5 ml, pharmacists should dispense diluted preparation, using chloroform water as diluent. For prolonged iron therapy, physicians may ask refill of prescription.

Apparatus: Spatula, beaker, glass rod, funnel, measuring cylinder.

Compounding:

i) Dissolve ferrous sulphate in 10 ml water. Add chloroform water and ascorbic acid. Add orange syrup. Filter.

ii) Rinse the beaker with water and filter it in the same solution.

iii) Adjust final volume with remaining water.

Container and storage: Use amber coloured glass bottles. Dropper or spoon should be provided when a dose is fraction of 5 ml. Store in tightly closed containers, in a cool place. Use within two weeks.

Category and dose: Haematinic. Child up to 1 year, 5 ml 3 times day; 1-5 years, 10 ml 3 times a day. Well diluted with water.

Label : Take with aid of water after meal.

Patient counselling : Preparation may stain the teeth and blacken faeces. Swallow the solution through straw. Do not co-administer antacid, tetracycline, ciprofloxacin. To avoid GI irritation, preparation should be given after meals with plenty of water. Ferrous preparations should not be taken with tea. Occasionally, it may cause constipation. Avoid administering to patients with peptic ulcer.

Proprietary preparations: Liquid preparations of Iron salt includes.

- Liq. IBEROL TONIC (Abbot): Ferrous sulphate ⟶ elemental Iron 26.25 mg/5ml with vit C and vit B.

- Liq. ASTYFER (Tablet India): Ferrous glycine sulphate (275 mg/10 ml) with amino acids.
- Syp. FEGEM (Torrent), Syp. CHERI (Indchemie): Iron (III) hydroxide polymaltose elemental Iron 50 mg/5 ml.
- Liq. DEXORANGE (Franco-India): Ferric ammonium citrate ≈ elemental Iron 32 mg/15 ml with folic acid, cyanocobalamine.
- Liq. FACICAP (Grandix), Syp. FEBEX (Sega Labs) : Ferrous gluconate (300 mg/15 ml).
- Syp. HAEMPLUS (Wings): Iron choline citrate 150 mg/15 ml with folic acid, vit–B.
- Susp. HEMSI (Serum Institute): Ferrous fumarate 300 mg with vit-B and amino acids.

Prescription No. 11.32

R

Strong Ammonium Acetate Solution, IP, BPC

Glacial acetic acid	— 45.3 g
Ammonium bicarbonate	— 47.0 g
Ammonia solution, Strong	— 10.0 ml
Purified water, to make	— 100.0 ml

Principle :

This is an example of a solution prepared by chemical reaction.

Dil. glacial acetic acid + Ammonium bicarbonate = Ammonium acetate + carbon dioxide + water. The reaction is allowed to complete in mortar. When gas evolution ceases, strong ammonia solution is added to neutralise unreacted acid.

It contains 57.5 per cent w/v of ammonium acetate. The weight per ml of the solution is 1.081 -1.091 g.

1 part of strong ammonia solution is diluted with 7 parts of water to produce dilute ammonium acetate solution. Ammonium acetate reacts with lead; therefore the container should be lead-free.

Apparatus : Spatula, beaker, glass rod, mortar, funnel, measuring cylinder.

Compounding :

i) Dilute the glacial acetic acid with about 35 ml of purified water.

ii) Dissolve ammonium bicarbonate portion by portion in dilute glacial acetic acid.

iii) Add sufficient quantity of the strong ammonia solution to achieve the following end point. Make final volume with purified water.

Dilute one drop of this reaction mixture ten times with water and test the colour change with indicator.

With 1 drop of solution of bromothymol blue = full blue colour,

With 1 drop of solution of thymol blue   = full yellow colour.

Container and storage: Store in well-closed lead-free, glass bottles. , in a cool place.

Category and direction to use: Diaphoretic, 1-4 ml.

Handling precaution: Handle glacial acetic acid and strong ammonia solution with care.

Monophasic Liquids

Prescription No. 11.33

℞

Piperazine Citrate Elixir IP, BPC

Piperazine Citrate	— 18.0 g
Chloroform Spirit	— 0.5 ml
Glycerin	— 10.0 ml
Orange Oil	— 0.02 ml
Syrup	— 50.0 ml
Water, freshly boiled and cooled make	— 100.0 ml

Principle :

Piperazine citrate is freely soluble in water. Orange oil, chloroform spirit and glycerol acts as flavour. Chloroform spirit and glycerol also have preservative properties. Syrup is sweetening agent. Piperazine citrate narcotises the worms thus enabling . To avoid reinfection, one it has to be administered over period of a week. When a preparation is prescribed for infant, in which case the dose is fraction of 5 ml; pharmacists should dispense solution after dilution with syrup. The dose of diluted solution should be changed to 5 ml and it should be used within two weeks. Alternatively, dropper or small capacity spoon should be provided to measure a small dose.

Apparatus: Spatula, beaker, glass rod, funnel, measuring cylinder.

Compounding :

i) Dissolve piperazine citrate in sufficient amount of water.

ii) Add orange oil, glycerin, syrup, chloroform spirit and alcohol. Filter the solution. Rinse the beaker with water and filter it in the same solution.

iii) Adjust final volume with the remaining water.

Container and storage: Store in well-closed amber-coloured, glass bottles. away from light.

Category and dose: Anthelmintic. For threadworms 5-15 ml daily in divided doses; for round worms as a single dose up to 30ml. Children: 9 to 12 months, 2.5 ml; 2 to 3 years, 5 ml; 4-6 years 7.5 ml; 7-12 years 10 ml.

Patient counselling: It may occasionally cause dizziness and GI disturbances. Avoid administering to epileptic patient and patient with impaired renal or hepatic functions. Avoid recommending it to patients who are pregnant pregnancy.

Proprietary preparations:

- Syp. PIPERAZINE CITRATE (Burroughs Wellcome) : 750 mg/5 ml.

Prescription No. 11.34

℞

Sodium Chloride Mouthwash, Compound BPC

Sodium chloride	— 1.5 g
Sodium bicarbonate	— 1.0 g
Peppermint emulsion, concentrated	— 2.5 ml
Chloroform water, double strength	— 50.0 ml
Water, freshly boiled & cooled, to make	— 100.0 ml

Principle :

The aqueous solubility of sodium chloride and sodium bicarbonate is 1 part of each in 3 and 11 parts of water respectively. Both of this should be stored in airtight containers. Since the salts create osmosis, a warm solution of sodium chloride is traditional household mouthwash and gargle to maintain general oral hygiene. Peppermint emulsion and chloroform water are flavours. The chloroform water also acts as preservative.

Apparatus: Spatula, beaker, glass rod, sintered glass filter, measuring cylinder.

Compounding:

i)   Dissolve sodium chloride and sodium bicarbonate in ¾th volume of water. Add peppermint emulsion and chloroform water.

ii) Filter. Rinse the beaker with water and filter it in the same solution.

iii) Adjust the final volume with the remaining water.

Container and storage: Store are tight fluted bottles. Store in airtight containers in a cool place.

Category and Direction to use: Mouthwash and gargle. Dilute with an equal volume of warm water before use.

Label: For external use only. Not to be swallowed in large amounts.

Patient counselling: Dilute with an equal amount of warm water before use. Not to be swallowed in excess.

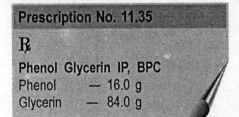

Prescription No. 11.35

℞

Phenol Glycerin IP, BPC
Phenol   — 16.0 g
Glycerin   — 84.0 g

Principle:

Phenol is soluble in water and glycerin. It is deliquescent and caustic to handle. Phenol is fungicide. The use of preparations containing phenol, sodium phenolate and menthol in glycerin is effective as throat paint, and, in diluted state, as gargle and mouthwash.

A 5 per cent solution in glycerin is useful in curing ear-ache. Today, such preparations are not much in use.

Apparatus: Porcelain dish, glass pestle, spatula, beaker, funnel, glass rod, water bath.

Compounding:

iii) Triturate the powdered phenol with glycerin to produce a smooth dispersion.

iv) Warm the mixture using water bath with constant stirring to get a solution. Filter if necessary.

Container and storage: Store in fluted well-closed bottles. in a dry place. Provide applicaiton brush.

Category and direction to use: Local analgesic and antiseptic.

Label : For external use only.

Handling precaution: Phenol is caustic, handle with care.

Patient counselling: It may be diluted with glycerin. Dilution with water may render phenol caustic. If accidentally spilt on healthy skin, it should be removed by swabbing with alcohol.

Prescription No. 11.36

℞

Sulphacetamide Ear Drops NFI, 1979
Sulpacetamide Sodium   — 4.5 g
Sodium metabisulphite   — 0.1 per cent
Phenyl mercuric nitrate   — 0.002 per cent
Water, freshly boiled and
cooled, to make   — 15.0 ml

Principle :

The BPC preparation contains 30 per cent w/v of drug. Sulphacetamide sodium is bacteriostatic. It competes with PABA for intake by bacterial enzyme. It is soluble in 1.5 parts of water. Sulphacetamide sodium is sensitive to oxidation. Freshly boiled and cooled water or purified water, which is free from dissolved oxygen should be used. Sodium metabisulphite is an antioxidant and phenyl mercuric nitrate is is preservative. Its topical application may cause skin sensitisation.

Apparatus: Glass pestle, spatula, beaker, funnel, glass rod.

Compounding: Dissolve sodium bicarbonate in ¾th volume of water. Add glycerin and make final volume with water.

Container and storage : Store in coloured fluted bottles fitted with a metal caps with rubber liner. A dropper fitted in a screw cap is provided separately. Store in an airtight container in a cool place. Protect from light. It should be used within 4 weeks after opening the container.

Category and direction to use : Bacteriostatic. 2-3 drops in each ear, repeat every 2-3 hours in a day.

Label : For external use only.

Patient counselling : Do not freeze the container. As described under Ear drops.

Prescription No. 11.37

℞

Turpentine Enema BNF 1957
Turpentine oil   — 5.0 ml
Soap enema, to make — 100.0 ml

Principle :

Turpentine oil is volatile oil. It is immiscible in water. Soap enema acts as vehicle and the soft soap present in it acts as o/w emulsifying agent. The evacuant action of the enema is due to local irritation and lubricating properties of the oil.

Apparatus : Spatula, beaker, funnel, glass rod, measuring cylinder.

Compounding : Mix turpentine oil with soap enema in a bottle. Close the bottle and shake vigorously to produce white creamy emulsion.

Category and direction to use: Bowel Cleaning. 600 ml by rectal injection. To be warmed at body temperature before use.

      Other information is the same as that described in the Prescription No. 11.20.

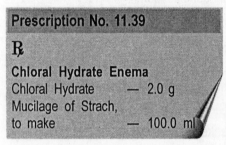

Prescription No. 11.38

℞

Magnesium Sulphate Enema INF 1979
Magnesium Sulphate   — 50.0 g.
Purified water, to make — 100.0 ml.

Principle :
Magnesium sulphate is soluble in 1.5 parts of water. An evacuant action of the enema is due to osmotic retention of water in rectal canal inducing evacuation.
Apparatus : Spatula, beaker, funnel, glass rod, measuring cylinder.

Compounding : Dissolve magnesium sulphate in water.

Category and direction to use : Bowel cleaning. 60-180 ml by rectal injection. To be warmed at body temperature before use.

Other information is same as that described in Prescription No. 11.20

Prescription No. 11.39

℞

Chloral Hydrate Enema
Chloral Hydrate   — 2.0 g
Mucilage of Strach,
to make   — 100.0 ml

Principle :
Chloral hydrate is a sedative, hypnotic. It is soluble in 0.25 parts of water. When taken orally, it is unpleasant to taste and causes local gastric irritation.
Apparatus : Spatula, beaker, funnel, glass rod, measuring cylinder.
Compounding : Dispense chloral hydrate in starch mucilage.

Category and direction to use : Sedative, hypnotic. 120 ml by rectal injection.

Other information is same as that described in Prescription No. 11.20

Prescription No. 11.40

℞

Weak Iodine Solution, I.P.
Iodine   — 2.0 g
Potassium Iodide   — 2.5 g
Alcohol(50 per cent),
to make   — 100.0 ml

Principle :
Tincture Iodine is synonym. Iodine is soluble in 13 parts of alcohol. Alcohol increases antiseptic action of the preparation. It is mainly used as skin disinfectant. It is used undiluted in treatment of superficial wounds. The alcohol containing solutions are more painful due to increased penetration. Each ml contains 20 mg of free iodine and about 35mg of total iodine.

Apparatus: Spatula, beaker, glass rod, funnel, measuring cylinder.

Compounding:
    i)   Dissolve potassium iodide and iodine in sufficient amount of water.
    ii)   Add alcohol and filter the solution. Rinse the beaker with alcohol and filter it in the same solution.
    iii) Adjust final volume with remaining alcohol.

Label : Alcohol content (45-48 per cent v/v), Inflammable. For external use only. Other conditions are same as Prescription No. 11.4

Prescription No. 11.41

℞

Strong Iodine Solution I.P.

Iodine	—	10.0 g
Potassium Iodide	—	6.0 g
Water	—	10.0 ml
Alcohol (90 per cent), to make	—	100.0 ml

Principle :

Tincture Iodine, Strong, is its synonym. Strong iodine shows slight absorption when preparations are applied on skin.

Container and storage: Store in fluted iodine-resistant containers. Cork Closure must not be used. It should be stored in tightly closed containers away from naked flame. Use within a week.

Category: Antiseptic.

Label : For external use only. Alcohol content, 74-79 per cent v/v; Inflammable.

Patient counselling : Inflammable, keep away from naked flame. Do not apply near eyes.

Other conditions are same as Prescription No. 11.4.

● ● ● ● ●

12 Suspensions

Suspensions are the mixtures containing insoluble solids. More precisely, suspensions are heterogeneous, biphasic, thermodynamically unstable liquid systems in which insoluble solid particles (as internal/discontinuous/dispersed phase) are uniformly distributed in liquid phase (external/continuous phase/dispersion medium). These may require inclusion of physical stabiliser or suspending agent. The pharmaceutical oral suspensions are mostly made in aqueous liquid phase. According to particle size, density of solid and solid phase arrangement, suspensions are classified in the following way:

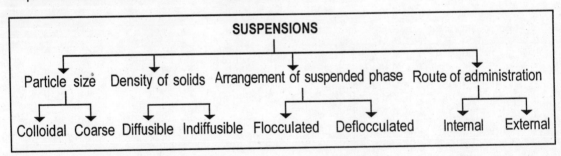

1) **Colloidal suspensions:** When the solid particles are less than 1μm in size, suspensions are called colloidal suspensions.

2) **Coarse suspensions:** When the size of solid particles is from 1μm to 50–75 μm, these suspensions are termed as coarse suspensions.

3) **Suspensions containing diffusible solids:** Many of the drug substances are light in weight and possess good wetting properties. After shaking, such drugs remain sufficiently suspended, at least till the time the required dose is removed. These drugs are called diffusible solids.

Examples of diffusible solids include bismuth carbonate, bismuth subnitrate, light kaolin, light magnesium carbonate, magnesium trisilicate, magnesium hydroxide, etc.

4) Suspensions containing indiffusible solids: Pharmaceutical substances, such as, aspirin, chalk, sulphadimidine, phenacetin, calamine, zinc oxide, etc., sediment rapidly after shaking and they do not remain uniformly distributed in the continuous phase. Such substances are called indiffusible solids. Such suspensions are compounded using suspending agents. Increased viscosity of continuous phase reduces the rate of sedimentation and keeps the indiffusible drug suspended for sufficient period of time. Generally, compound powder of tragacanth, (2 g/100 ml) or tragacanth mucilage (1/4 of volume of mixture) is used as suspending agents.

5) Route of administration: Suspensions may be for internal use, eg. Mixtures; suspensions not for internal use, eg. inhalations and enemas; or for topical application, eg. lotions and

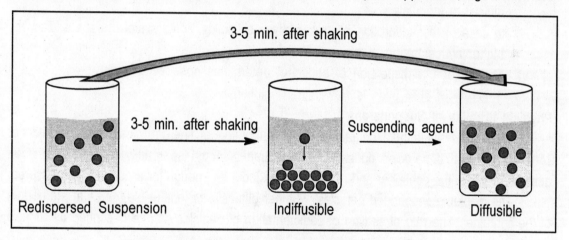

Figure 12.1: Diffusible and Indiffusible Suspensions

liniments.

Advantages of Suspensions

  i) Bio-availability of finely dispersed and wet drugs is faster than that of the solid dosage forms. Solid dosage forms require more time for disintegration and de-aggregation.

 ii) Large doses of insoluble drugs are easier to swallow in the form of suspensions, than solid dosage forms, eg. antacid and antidiarrhoeal preparations.

iii) The higher surface area of suspended phase is more effective to exert their effect, e.g. insoluble antacids, adsorbents such as kaolin, pectin, etc.

 iv) Drugs are chemically more stable in the insoluble state than in the soluble state.

  v) Liquid preparations are easy to swallow and are thus more useful for pediatric and geriatric use.

vi) Solid drugs are less unpleasant to taste than their solutions, eg. Paracetamol, chloramphenicol palmitate.

vii) Suspension is one of the techniques to attain slow and sustained drug release.

viii) It is the choice of dosage form to present an insoluble drug in the liquid form.

Disadvantages of Suspensions

i) A number of drugs have some solubility in commonly used solvents and this can lead to physical instability of the suspension.

ii) A drug in reduced state of particle size is thermodynamically less stable and tends to aggregate. Some drugs undergo physicochemical changes during milling and this makes it difficult to attain desired particle size.

iii) Though a drug in insoluble state is more palatable, due to higher surface free energy, fine drug particles could adsorb added flavours and colours and make a system difficult to formulate.

iv) In case of the adsorption of preservatives by solids, liquid system needs addition of higher concentration of preservative.

v) The uniform re-dispersion of sediment determines dose accuracy.

vi) The rate of absorption is slower than solutions.

Physical Stability of Suspensions

Suspensions should contain uniform distribution of fine particles, which should not settle rapidly and if particles do settle, the sediment should be readily re-dispersible upon gentle shaking of the container and remain suspended long enough for a dose to be measured.

The insoluble suspended particles, whether diffusible or indiffusible, settle at the bottom of the container. The rate of settling or sedimentation of particles can be described by Stoke's law:

$$V = \frac{d^2(\rho_s - \rho_p)g}{18\eta}$$

Where, V is the terminal velocity of a spherical particle,

d is the diameter of particle

ρ_s and ρ_p are the densities of dispersed phase and dispersed medium respectively,

g is the acceleration due to gravity, and

η is the viscosity of dispersed medium.

The rate of settling is directly proportional to the diameter of suspended particles. However, reduction in size is not always possible. Particles with size 2-5 μm show Brownian motion.

The suspended phase and medium should be of equal density. Vehicles such as syrup, IP, and sorbitol solution, are used to adjust the density. Increasing the viscosity of external phase is the usual approach to reduce the rate of sedimentation in pharmaceutical suspensions. Various types of suspending agents including gum acacia, tragacanth, methylcellulose, bentonite, carbomer, etc. are usually used for this purpose.

Suspensions containing diffusible drugs are formulated without the use of suspending agents. The indiffusible suspension requires suspending agent.

Concept Clear : Physical Stability of Suspensions

Suspensions should :
- Have uniform distribution of mono-sized fine particles with no change in it.
- Not sediment rapidly and if they do settle, it should be readily re-dispersible.
- Be viscous, but not be unpourable.
- Densites of drug and vehicle should be same.

FORMULATION

The ingredients employed in suspensions vary as per the nature of the drug, i.e., diffusible or indiffusible. Suspensions containing indiffusible solids require thickening agents. Suspensions for internal use are mostly aqueous, whereas, for other routes it may be aqueous, non-aqueous, hydroalcoholic or oily.

Drug

The drug should have minimum solubility, maximum chemical stability and good wettability in the vehicle. Drugs with some solubility in the vehicle, could result in the growth of crystals due to fluctuations in storage temperatures.

Formulation of suspensions containing diffusible solids is less complex than that of the Those with indiffusible solids. Incorporation of suspending agent in latter type may lead to problems such as, adsorption of flavours and preservatives, unpourability, etc.

The drug particles are also generated by chemical reaction or by precipitation, eg. milk of magnesia. The precipitation is done either by change in solvent or the pH of solvent systems. The precipitate formed should not be too fluid or too gelatinous. Rarely, active ingredients used in suspensions not in solid state, but it requires to be produced in suspension form, eg. volatile oils in inhalations in such cases, a suitable excipient is required for uniform distribution of such volatile oils.

Drug, should have pleasant organoleptic properties. Drugs in insoluble state have less objectionable taste than their solution.

Additives

1) Vehicle : Water is the choice of vehicle for oral liquids. Syrup, sorbitol, glycerin are usually used with water either to impart body to the preparation, as anti-gelling agents, or to improve palatability of the preparation. The added co-solvents or pH of system should not change the solubility of the drug in the vehicle. Suspensions administered by routes other than oral route may contain other non-aqueous or oily vehicles. Calamine lotion is official in two forms, aqueous form and oily form.

2) Wetting Agents : Some insoluble drugs do not wet readily with water and their lumps float on the surface of the liquid. This poor wetting is attributed to the presence of entrapped air on the surface of solid. To ensure satisfactory wetting and escape of entrapped air from liquid preparations, the solid-liquid interfacial energy must be reduced; and for this purpose, surfactants having HLB 7-9 are useful in concentrations up to 0.1 per cent. For oral administration, of non-ionic surfactants, tweens and spans are preferred and for products used externally, quillaia tincture and sodium lauryl sulphate are used. The second approach is levigation. Glycerin, propylene glycol, sorbitol are valuable levigating agents. These viscous solvents

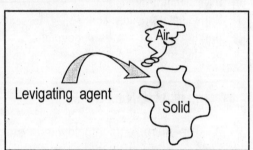

Figure 12.2: Mechanism of Levigation

flow into the voids/pores of the particles to displace air. e.g. sulphur lotion contains quillaia tincture, alcohol and glycerin to increase wettability of precipitated sulphur. Hydrocolloids, such as acacia, tragacanth and sodium alginate forms hydrophilic coat on the surface of hydrophobic particles.

Concept Clear : Drug and Wetting Agent

Drug for suspensions should :
- Have minimum solubility, maximum chemical stability and good wettability in the vehicle.
- Be light in weight, stable during milling and mixing.

Vehicle of choice for oral use is water.

Wetting agents acts by :
- Reducing interfacial tension: Surface active agents.
- Displacing adsorbed air from surface of the particle: polyhydric alcohols.
- Forming hydrophilic coat on surface of particle: hydrocolloids.

3) Suspending Agents: Suspending agents act mainly by increasing the viscosity of external phase, thus reducing the rate of sedimentation of dispersed particles. In addition, some suspending agents also form a protective coat around the individual particles, making them less sensitive to electrolyte concentration. Hydrocolloids like acacia, tragacanth, and cellulose increase the viscosity of water by binding water molecules and thereby limiting their mobility and fluidity. Many of them are protective colloids in low concentration (<0.1 per cent) and viscosity enhancers in relatively high concentration. Suspending agents are selected on the basis of viscosity thus produce. Table 12.1 summarises comparative viscosities of some suspending agents.

Table 12.1 Some commonly used Suspending Agents

Suspending agent	% w/v to give 800 cps	Usual concentration %
• Acacia	35 - 38	10
• Tragacanth	2.8 - 3	1 - 3
• Methylcellulose - 400	2.4	3 - 5
• Methylcellulose - 1500	1.7	2 - 3
• Carboxymethyl cellulose, low viscosity	4.0	2 - 3
• Carboxymethyl cellulose, high viscosity	0.7	1
• Bentonite	6 - 6.3	6

Types of Suspending Agents
I) Natural suspending agents (Natural hydrocolloids)
1) Acacia : Acacia is usually used as mucilage, which is 35 per cent dispersion of acacia in water. It increases viscosity of the water phase. Secondly, it is less sensitive to electrolyte concentration and forms protective coat around the dispersed particles. It is sticky to be used alone, and is thus, usually is combined with tragacanth. The viscosity of acacia solution is maximum between pH 3-9. Acacia is suitable for use in mixtures containing alcohol up to 35 per cent. Acacia often has high microbial count, therefore, use of preservative is necessary. It also contains a peroxidase enzyme which causes oxidation of oxygen-sensitive drugs. Heating the acacia mucilage for a few minutes at 100°C destroys the peroxidase enzymes.
2) Tragacanth: Tragacanth in 6 per cent concentrated mucilage is employed in quantities up to 10 ml/100 ml of mixture. It produces a viscous, but less sticky preparation. Viscosity of solution increases to maximum after several days. Tragacanth mucilage is effective over smaller ofrange pH 4 to 6. Like acacia, it is suitable for use in mixtures containing alcohol up to 35 per cent of the total volume. Advantage of tragacanth over acacia is its effectiveness in lesser amounts and it is free from the oxidase enzyme. Since material is from a natural source, preparations containing tragacanth require inclusion of preservative.
3) Starch : Starch mucilage is 2.5 per cent starch in water and it is used as ingredient of

compound powder of tragacanth.

4) Compound powder of tragacanth (CPT) : It is a mixture of 20 per cent of powdered acacia, 15 per cent of tragacanth, 20 per cent of starch and 45 per cent of sucrose. It has combined properties of all ingredients and used in quantities of 2 g/100 ml of mixture.

5) Sodium alginate : Sodium alginate forms a viscous colloidal solution with water. To avoid lump formation, sodium alginate should be wetted with alcohol, glycerin or propylene glycol and then mixed with water, using high speed mixer. It is stable in pH range of 4-10 and possesses maximum viscosity at pH 7.

6) Clays : Clays are naturally occurring minerals. Bentonite, hectorite and veegum are the different clays used as suspending agents. Bentonite is natural colloidal hydrated aluminum silicate. It hydrates readily, absorbing many times of their volume of water and swell up to about twelve times its original volume. 5per cent dispersion is generally used as suspending agent. Hectorite absorbs more water than bentonite does and exhibits thixotropy.

Properties of Veegum are intermediatery between bentonite and hectorite.

The pH of aqueous clay dispersion is somewhat alkaline in nature and they are most stable between pH 9 and 11. Clays require adequate preservation and non-ionic preservatives are most suitable.

II) Semi-synthetic suspending agents

1) Methyl cellulose (MC) : Methyl cellulose is soluble in cold water, but insoluble in hot water. It can be used in mixtures containing 70 per cent alcohol. Methyl cellulose is resistant to bacterial attack.

2) Sodium Carboxymethyl cellulose (Sodium CMC): It is soluble in both cold and hot water. Sodium CMC is generally used in 0.25 to 1 per cent concentration as suspending agent. Being anionic, it is incompatible with cationic compounds. It can tolerate alcohol concentration upto 50 per cent.

3) Hydroxyethyl cellulose (HEC) : It is soluble in both cold and hot water. It can be used successfully in mixtures containing alcohol upto 80 per cent.

4) Microcrystalline cellulose (MCC) : MCC disperse readily in water to produce thixotropic gels.

III) Synthetic suspending agents

1) Carbopols : Carbopols are synthetic, high molecular weight carboxyvinyl polymers. Thus dissolve in water and the dispersion is acidic in nature. Its advantage as a suspending agent is its effectiveness in low concentration, resistant to microbial attack and uniformity in composition.

2) Colloidal silicon dioxide : It is used in concentration of 1.5 – 4 per cent to stabilise suspensions.

4) Density Modifiers : Ideally, the density of suspended phase and medium should be equal. Although it is difficult, the density of vehicle can be increased by replacing water totally or partly with syrup, sorbitol, etc.

5) Preservative : Preservatives employed in suspensions are the same as that of monophasic liquids. However, suspended particles with high surface-free energy may adsorb preservatives, e.g. benzalkonium chloride adsorbed by kaolin.

6) Organoleptic Additives : Flavouring agents, colours and sweeteners are selected in association with each other on the basis of the age of the patient and the route of administration. Both dyes and lakes, are used in combination to overcome limitations of individual. The other selection criteria are the same as that for monophasic liquids.

Concept Clear : **Formulation of suspensions**

Suspending agents increase viscosity of external phase, in turn reduce the rate of sedimentation of dispersed particles. It is required when a drug is indiffusible.
- Natural hydrocolloids : Acacia mucilage, tragacanth mucilage, sodium alginate, clays.
- Semi-synthetic suspending agents : MC, Sodium CMC, HEC, MCC.
- Synthetic suspending agents : Carbopols, Colloidal silicon dioxide.

Density Modifiers : Density of dispersion medium = Density of suspended phase.
Preservative : Should not get adsorbed on drug surface.
Flavouring agent, colouring agents (dyes and lakes) and sweetening agents.

COMPOUNDING OF SUSPENSIONS

Diffusible Solids : Fine powder of drug is mixed with other solid additives by the doubling up method. Powder blend is levigated with small amount of vehicles or suitable levigating agent, to produce a smooth paste. Soluble additives are first dissolved in the vehicle and solution is added as smooth paste in small amounts, triturating after each addition. The resultant uniform dispersion made free from foreign particle is poured in a tared bottle. The final volume is adjusted with the remaining vehicle.

If formula contains colouring agent, it is usually triturated with a smooth paste of drug before its dilution with the vehicle. This technique allows uniform distribution and penetration of colouring agent into the powder.

Indiffusible Solids : The procedure to prepare suspension containing indiffusible solids differs from the one given above in that, that it requires a suspending agent. Suspending agent in dry powder form is mixed with drug. Otherwise the drug is triturated with gum mucilage to produces smooth paste which is further diluted with the vehicle.

Addition of Tinctures : Tinctures are hydroalcoholic solutions of drug having low water solubility. Precipitation of such substances may occur when tinctures are added to water. The resultant precipitate may be diffusible (myrrh tincture) or non-dispersible clot. The formation of non-dispersible precipitate can be prevented by the addition of well-diluted tincture in small amounts in dispersion of protective colloid, triturating well after each addition. Coating of the resultant fine precipitate with protective colloid avoids formation of clot.

Final Volume Adjustment : Uniform dispersion is made free from any foreign particle by straining. The apparatus used for straining is very simple. It generally consists of a strainer medium (muslin, wool or cheese cloth) and a frame to hold it. A plug of absorbent cotton wool or cotton gauze placed in a funnel is also used for straining. The strainer medium must be washed before use to remove loose fibres. It is poured in a tared bottle to adjust to the final volume. The mortar and pestle should be rinsed, using remaining amount of vehicle before making the final volume.

The final volume is adjusted using a tared container. Since biphasic liquid contains insoluble internal phase, there are chances of loss of settled or adhered drug in measuring cylinder; secondly suspensions are comparatively more viscous preparations.

Dilution: Reasons and processes are same as in solutions.

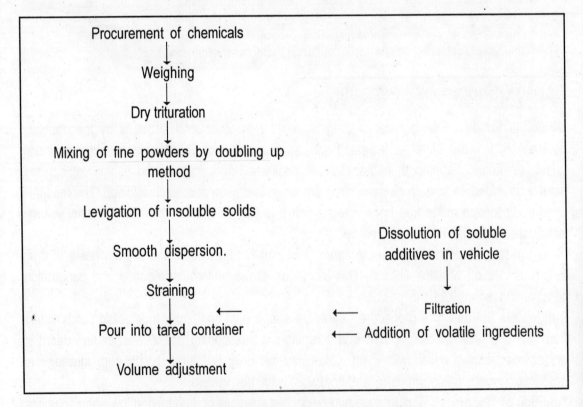

Figure 12.3: Compounding of Suspensions

Container and Storage: Oral suspensions are dispersed in screw–capped plain or amber glass bottles. The suspensions not meant for oral use are dispensed in fluted bottles. The products should be stored in a cool place, but not in a refrigerator.

Label : The suspensions should be labelled "Shake well before use". In addition, label should include directions for use incase of inhalations, lotions, etc.

Dispensing : Suspensions that show non-dispersible cake, increase or decrease in viscosity, large particles, or change in colour, flavour and taste should not be dispensed.

Patient counselling and Documentation: Patient should be instructed to shake the bottles before use, and about storage, and health related parameters. The PMR and CDR should be maintained as part of good compounding and dispensing practices.

ORAL SUSPENSIONS

Oral suspensions mostly contain water as vehicle. These should be supplied with 5 ml measure for measurement of dose. If dose is less than 5 ml, these should be diluted with vehicle or any other suitable liquid, maintaining the quality of suspensions. Supply of small capacity spoon or dropper is an alternative to dilution. Suspensions are labelled as 'Shake well before use'.

Proprietary preparations :

- ACTIFIED PLUS PAEDITRIC SUSPENSION (Burroughs Wellcome) : Paracetamol 125 mg, Triprolidine HCl 0.625 mg, Phenylpropanolamine HCl 6.25 mg, per 5 ml. For upper respiratory tract congestion with pyrexia.

- ARINAC SUSPENSION (Knoll Pharma) : Ibuprofen 100 mg, Pseudoephedrine HCl 15 mg, per 5 ml. For nasal congestion, common cold and bodyache.

- CISADE (Unichem), CIZA (Intas) : Cisapride 1 mg/ml: In chronic constipation.

- TINI-F SUSP (Kopran) : Tinidazole 100 mg, furazolidone 35 mg, per 5 ml. In amoebiasis.

- ZUPAR (Glaxo Allenburys) : Ibuprofen 100 mg, paracetamol 125 mg per 5ml. PONSTAN (Park-Davis) : Mefenamic acid 50 mg/5 ml. ANAFEBRIN (Themis), N-LID (Orchid) : Nimesulide 50mg/ml. Analgesic, antipyretic, anti-inflammatory.

- AZIWOK (Wockhardt) : Azithromycin 200 mg/2.5 ml, KEFLOR (Ranbaxy) : Cefaclor 187 mg/ 5 ml. CEFADUR (Protec) : Cefadroxil 250 mg/5 ml. CHLORAMPHENICOL (Boehringer Mannheim) : Chloramphenicol 125 mg/5 ml : Antibiotics as antibacterial.

- SEPTRAN (Burroughs Wellcome), ALCORIM (Albert David) : Trimethoprim 40 mg, sulphamethoxazole 200 mg/5 ml. Sulpha antibacterial.

R

Magnesium Trisilicate Mixture, BPC

Magnesium Trisilicate	— 5.0 g
Light magnesium carbonate	— 5.0 g
Sodium bicarbonate	— 5.0 g
Peppermint emulsion, concentrated	— 2.5 ml
Chloroform Water, DS	— 50.0 ml
Water, freshly boiled & cooled, to make	— 100.0 ml

Principle :

Magnesium trisilicate is a weak antacid with acid consuming capacity of 15 mEq of HCl per gram and usually it is used in combination with other antacids. The unreacted magnesium trisilicate provides a protective coat over ulcerated area. Magnesium carbonate is more effective with acid neutralising capacity of 20.6 mEq of HCl per gram. Due to release of carbon dioxide, it may cause flatulence.

Magnesium trisilicate is insoluble in water; whereas, light magnesium carbonate is slightly soluble in water. Sodium bicarbonate is soluble in 11 parts of water. Magnesium trisilicate and light magnesium carbonate are diffusible, because of which the suspension does not require suspending agent. Peppermint oil is a flavouring agent and for miscibility it is added in the form of its emulsion. This example explains the selection of flavour in association with category. Peppermint oil and chloroform have carminative action. Chloroform water additionally acts as vehicle and preservative. Since that preservative is volatile in nature, preparation should be recently prepared. A preparation containing chloroform should be protected from light.

Apparatus : Mortar and pestle, beaker, glass rod, spatula., funnel, measuring cylinder.

Compounding :

i)   Sift the powders. Mix these by the doubling up method to ensure uniform distribution. Gradually add enough quantity of water and triturate after each addition to get smooth pourable dispersion.

ii) Transfer the mixture to tared bottle. Add peppermint emulsion, chloroform water.

iii) Rinse the mortar and pestle with remaining amount of water and adjust the volume with it.

Container and storage : Store in airtight, amber coloured glass bottles. in a cool place. Protect from light. Use within two weeks.

Category and dose : Antacid. Dose : 10 ml 3 times a day with water.

Label : Shake well before use.

Patient counselling : Avoid giving to patients with hypophosphataemia and impairment of renal function. If diarrhoea occurs discontinue the use and contact the physician. Do not co-administer with antidepressants, antiepileptic drugs, and enteric coated dosage forms. Take food regularly. Drink enough water, avoid spices. Avoid smoking, alcohol, tea and coffee. Take enough sleep.

Proprietary preparations :

- Susp. GELUSIL LIQUID (Parke Davis) : Magnesium trisilicate 625 mg, dried aluminium hydroxide gel 312 mg, per 5 ml.

- Susp. ACIGON (Boehringer Mannheim) : Magnesium trisilicate 80 mg, sodium bicarbonate 140mg, sodium alginate 440 mg, dried aluminium hydroxide gel 160 mg/10 ml.

- Susp. AIGIFLUX (Panacea) : Magnesium trisilicate 125 mg, sodium alginate 200 mg, aluminium hydroxide gel 300 mg, activated simethicone 50 mg/10 ml.

- Susp. GASTRACID (Meyer Organics) : Magnesium trisilicate 50 mg, magnesium hydroxide 120 mg, calcium carbonate 400 mg, simethicone 5 mg/5 ml.

Note 2 : Antacids : Hyperacidity is the excessive secretion of gastric fluid. The common reasons are irregular eating habits consuming spicy food, carbonated drinks and alcohol. Smoking, stress, and bacterial infections also cause hyperacidity. Antacids are the agents, which maintain gastric pH near to 4. Sodium bicarbonate, magnesium salts such as oxide, carbonate, hydroxide, and calcium carbonate act chemically to cause acid neutralisation. Though heavy magnesium carbonate has similar actions as that of the ight variety, light variety is used to formulate suspensions and the heavy variety is used in antacid powders. Sodium bicarbonate, a water soluble antacid shows rapid action and relieves feeling of distension. The continuous use of these powders may cause alkalosis. Magnesium salts increase bowel movement and they are laxative in higher doses whereas aluminium salts cause constipating. Calcium carbonate also has constipation effect. The carbonate and bicarbonate type of antacids have disadvantage of liberation of carbon dioxide in GI tract.

Magnesium trisilicate and aluminium hydroxide are adsorbant type of antacids. Alunimium hydroxide also has some neutralisation capacities. Magnesium trisilicate is converted into magnesium chloride and colloidal silica. Colloidal silica in the gel form adsorbs acid. Unlike oxide, carbonate or bicarbonate salts, magnesium trisilicate is slow acting, does not cause alkalosis and is more useful in dyspepsia. Liquid antacid preparations are usually more effective than solid preparations.

Prescription No. 12.2

℞

Chalk Mixture, Paediatric, BPC

Chalk	— 2.0 g
Tragacanth Powder	— 0.2 g
Concentrated Cinnamon Water	— 0.4 ml
Syrup	— 10.0 ml
Chloroform Water, DS	— 50.0 ml
Water, freshly boiled &	— 100.0 ml

Principle :

Chalk is adsorbent type of antidiarrhoeal. It quickly raises pH above pH 3. It also has constipating effect at higher doses. Diarrhoea is mainly due to poor hygiene, or due to bacterial infection, or drug induced. The risk in diarrhoea is rapid dehydration.

Chalk mixture is a suspension containing indiffusible solid. Tragacanth acts as suspending agent. Cinnamon water and syrup are used as flavouring agents and sweetening agents respectively. Syrup also gives body to the preparation. Chloroform water is a preservative vehicle and it also has flavouring properties.

Apparatus : Mortar and pestle, beaker, glass rod, spatula, funnel, measuring cylinder.

Compounding :

i)   Sift the chalk. Triturate chalk and tragacanth with syrup.

ii) Add water to get a smooth pourable dispersion. Transfer the mixture to a tared bottle. Add chloroform water and cinnamon water.

iii) Rinse the mortar and pestle with the remaining amount of water, and adjust the volume with it.

Container and storage : Store in amber-coloured glass bottles in a cool place. Protect from light. Use within two weeks.

Category and Dose : Antidiarrhoeal : Children : Up to 1 yr, 5 ml; 1 to 5 yrs, 10 ml; 3 times a day with water.

Label : Shake well before use.

Patient counselling : Take oral rehydration salt and maintain water intake. Avoid fatty and dairy food. Wash hands after each bowel movement to avoid spread of infection.

Prescription No. 12.3

R

Sulphadimidine Mixture, Paediatric, BPC

Sulphadimidine	— 10.0 g
Compound powder of tragacanth	— 4.0 g
Amaranth solution	— 1.0 g
Benzoic acid solution	— 2.0 ml
Raspberry syrup	— 20.0 ml
Chloroform water, DS	— 50.0 ml
Water, freshly boiled & cooled, to make	— 100.0 ml

Principle :

Sulphadimidine is bactericidal. It competes with PABA and is preferentially taken up by bacterial enzymes.

Sulphadimidine is very slightly soluble in water and it is an indiffusible solid. The compound powder of tragacanth (CPT) acts as suspending agent. Benzoic acid is a preservative. Amaranth is a colouring agent. Raspberry syrup is used as flavouring agent and sweetening agents. It also gives body to the preparation. Chloroform water, DS, is preservative, vehicle and also has flavouring properties. CPT is 'natural product' and increases chances of microbial contamination. Though this mixture contains mixture of volatile and non-volatile preservative, it should be recently prepared. When a preparation is prescribed for infants below 6 months, it should be dispensed after dilution with chloroform water, making the minimum dose of 5 ml.

Apparatus : Mortar and pestle, beaker, glass rod, spatula, funnel, measuring cylinder.

Compounding :

i)   Sift the sulphadimidine. Triturate sulphadimidine and CPT with syrup to produce a smooth dispersion.

ii) Add amaranth solution and mix well. Add chloroform water and benzoic acid solution.

iii) Transfer the mixture to tared bottle and add cinnamon water.

iv) Rinse the mortar and pestle with remaining amount of water and adjust the volume with it.

Container and storage : Store in amber coloured glass bottle. Store in airtight containers in a cool place. Protect from light. Use within two weeks.

Category and dose : Bactericidal. Children Dose : Infant 6 months to 1 yr, 5 ml; 1 to 5 yrs, 10 ml; 3 times a day with water.

Label : Shake well before use.

Patient counselling : It may cause allergy, avoid administering to hypersensitive patients. In case of allergic reaction, stop the treatment and drink abundant water. During treatment patients should avoid exposure to direct sunlight. In case of mild nausea or vomiting, contact the physician.

Milks and Gels

These are viscous aqueous suspensions containing precipitate of inorganic drugs having particle size closer to colloidal range prepared without the addition of any suspending agent. These are also termed as shake preparations. Milks and magmas differ from gels in that, the solid phase is larger in size. These are prepared by hydration of inorganic substance or by chemical reaction. The microcrystalline particles of the precipitate holds appreciable amount of water. These suspensions remain fairly uniformly dispersed with slow settling of the suspended phase. The sediment formed is easily redispersible by moderate shaking. Rheologically, these are thixotropic in nature.

Milk of bismuth is aqueous suspension of bismuth hydroxide and bismuth subcarbonate. It involves two reactions, viz., bismuth subnitrate with nitric acid and ammonium carbonate with ammonia and then mixing the resulting two products. It is an antacid, astringent and forms a protective coat on the inflamed lining of the GI mucosa. Bentonite magma is mainly used as suspending agent. It is a 5 per cent aqueous dispersion of bentonite. The bentonite is allowed to hydrate under slow stirring to produce viscous magma.

Aluminium hydroxide gel is aqueous suspension of aluminium hydroxide and the hydrated aluminum oxide produced from aluminium chloride or aluminium alum. It is capable of neutralising 29.4 mEq of hydrochloric acid per gram and it has the ability to buffer gastric pH between 3 and 4.

Milk of magnesia is aqueous suspension of magnesium hydroxide, which can be prepared by hydration of magnesium oxide, or by reaction between magnesium sulphate or magnesium chloride with sodium hydroxide. Magnesium hydroxide acts by acid neutralisation, eg. 34.3 mEq of acid neutralises per gram. It also forms a protective and soothing coat on ulcerated gastric mucosa. Magnesium salts increase bowel movement and are laxative in higher doses and these are therefore combined with aluminium hydroxide gel, which is constipating. Milk of magnesia raises the pH from 8 to 9, which may cause acid rebound. In combination with aluminum hydroxide, it buffers gastric content between pH 3 and 5. Excess gelling due to the electrostatic interaction between magnesium hydroxide gel and aluminium hydroxide gel, is prevented by addition of antigelling agents.

Proprietary preparations :

- Susp. GELUSIL PLUS (Parke Davis) : Magnesium hydroxide paste (equiv. to magnesium hydroxide 150 mg) 0.75 g, Aluminium hydroxide gel (equiv. to dried aluminium hydroxide gel 300 mg) 1.88 g, dimethicon 0.125 g per 5 ml.

- Susp. LOGASCID (Astra Zeneca) : Magnesium hydroxide 200 mg, dried aluminium hydroxide gel 200mg, activated dimethicon 20 mg, 5 ml.

- Susp. DIGENE GEL (Knoll Pharma) : Magnesium hydroxide 18 5mg, dried aluminium hydroxide gel 830mg, methylpolysiloxane 25 mg, 10 ml.

Prescription No. 12.4

℞

Magnesium Hydroxide Mixture, BP 1973
Magnesium Sulphate — 4.75 g
Magnesium Oxide, light — 5.25 g
Sodium Hydroxide — 1.50 g
Chloroform — 2.5 ml
Water, freshly boiled &
cooled, to make — 100.0 ml

Principle :

The synonyms are milk of magnesia and cream of magnesia. This is an example of suspensions that involves generation of solute in required particle size by chemical reaction. Magnesium hydroxide is formed by hydration of magnesium oxide or chemical reaction.

Fluid, easily settling precipitate : $2NaOH + MgSO_4 = Mg(OH)_2 + Na_2SO_4$

Gelatinous precipitate : $2MgO + 2H_2O = 2Mg(OH)_2$

The product is more economically produced by the direct hydration of magnesium oxide. The product of only hydration reaction becomes unpourable gel on standing. In the second reaction, magnesium sulphate or magnesium chloride is allowed to react with alkali hydroxide to give magnesium hydroxide and alkali sulphate. The resultant precipitate should be made sulphate free by washing it with warm water. The product of combined reactions, namely, hydration and precipitation is of intermediate and required quality; diffusible and not too fluid or not too viscous.

Milk of magnesia is white, opaque, more or less viscous, suspension from which varying proportion of water separates on standing. Milk of magnesia suspension contains 7.0 to 8.5 per cent $Mg(OH)_2$. It is alkaline with pH 10 and citric acid (0.1per cent) is added to minimise interaction with glass container. Volatile oils up to 0.5 ml per 1000 ml are added as flavour. Volatile oils are also carminative in action. Chloroform water acts as vehicle, preservative and flavouring agent.

Apparatus : Mortar and pestle, beaker, glass rod, spatula, funnel, measuring cylinder.

Compounding :

i) Dissolve sodium hydroxide in 15 ml and magnesium sulphate in 25 ml of water.

ii) Add light magnesium oxide in solution of sodium hydroxide and mix it well to produce a smooth dispersion.

iii) Dilute the dispersion with 10 ml water and pour it in a thin stream in solution of magnesium sulphate. Stir continuously during mixing.

iv) Keep the dispersion aside. Decant the clear liquid. Strain the residue using calico strainer.

v) Wash the precipitate with warm water to make it sulphate-free. The sulphate-containing washing produces a white precipitate with barium chloride solution; which disappears on addition of hydrochloric acid.

vi) Disperse the sulphate-free precipitate in 50 ml water. Add chloroform.

vii) Make the final volume in tared container with water.

Container and storage : Store in tightly closed coloured glass bottles in a cool place. Use within two weeks.

Category and dose : Antacid. Dose, 10 ml 3 times a day with water. Laxative, 25 ml 3 times a day with water.

Label : Shake well before use.

Patient counselling : Avoid giving it to patients with hypophosphataemia and impairment of renal function. Do not co-administer with antidepressants, antiepileptic drugs, and with enteric coated dosage forms. Otherwise, take enteric dosage forms at least two hours before antacid. Do not store in a cool place.

Proprietary preparations :

• DEY'S MILK OF MAGNESIA: Hydrated magnesium oxide, 8 per cent w/w, calculated as magnesium hydroxide, I.P.

Dry Powders for Suspensions

Dry powders for oral suspensions are powder mixtures that require the addition of water (reconstitution) at the time of dispensing and are mostly for paediatric use. These are called dry syrups or reconstitutable oral suspensions.

Advantages of dry suspensions :

1) Poor chemical stability of drug in aqueous vehicle, eg. antibiotics can be formulated as dry suspensions. (2) The dry powders may have a shelf life of 2 years, but the reconstituted suspension should be used within two weeks.

3) The other advantages includes-minimising physical stability problems of liquid suspension and easy handling of the light-weight products.

Formulation : The basic requirement of dry suspensions is that, they must disperse quickly and completely during reconstitution. Majority of the drugs are antibiotics for paediatric use. Mostly drugs are in insoluble state and the reconstituted products are suspensions, and rarely are they solutions of soluble drugs. The Penicillin V potassium is soluble and the reconstituted liquid is solutions. The suspension types of formulations require suspending agents. The other additives include wetting agents, sweeteners, flavours, preservative and colours. The dry mixture is either powder blend, granules or mixture of them.

Dispensing : Pharmacists should counsel the patients in the following manner.

i)   Tap the container lightly to loosen the powder.

ii)   Add freshly boiled and cooled water up to the volume adjustment mark in the bottle and shake it for uniform distribution of powder.

iii)   Shake well before use.

iv)   Use within the prescribed period, i.e; 2 weeks, after reconstitution.

Proprietary preparations :

* AMOXIPEN (PCI), GLAMOXIN (Glaxo),
  MOX (Rexcel) : Amoxycillin 125 mg/5 ml.
* RESPIMOX (Wockhardt) : Amoxycillin 250 mg,
  bromhexine HCl 8mg/ml.
* ZITHROCIN (Biochem),
  AZIWIN (Bal Pharma) : Azithromycin 200 mg/5 ml.
* CEFADROL (J.K.Ind),
  SAFEDROX (Lincoin) : Cefadroxil 125 mg/5 ml.
* SEPEXIN (Lyka), SANCEPH (Uni Sankyo),
  BLUCEF (Blue Cross) : Cephalexin 125 mg/5 ml.

INHALATIONS

Inhalations are liquid preparations of volatile ingredients, whose vapours are intended to be inhaled after adding it to hot water. The liquid may be aqueous or alcoholic solution, or aqueous dispersion of a drug.

The benzoin inhalation and, menthol inhalation are solutions of respective volatile substance in industrial methylated spirit. Menthol and benzoin inhalation is 2 per cent w/v menthol dissolved in benzoin inhalation. Menthol and eucalyptus inhalation, and terebene inhalation are aqueous dispersions containing light magnesium carbonate as dispersing agent.

The insoluble or immiscible volatile drugs such as camphor, menthol, eucalyptol, eucalyptus oil and clove oil are difficult to produce in a uniform dispersion. Adsorption of such drugs on inert solids having high surface areas is an alternative to improve uniform distribution. Adsorption of drug on fine powders also increases its surface area and rate of vaporisation of drug. The dispersing agent should fulfill the following criteria :

i) It should have higher surface area for adsorption but adsorption, should not be too strong to hamper vaporisation during inhalation.

ii) It should be light and diffusible. The dispersion formed using the indiffusible powder will be difficult to re-disperse and require suspending agent, which will increase viscosity of the preparation, resulting in reduced vaporisation of drug.

iii) Formulations of oil-in-water emulsions is second alternative to improve dispersibility of volatile oils. But emulsions are physically less stable, secondly the interfacial film produced by the surfactant around the oil droplets will also interferes with vaporisation of the drug.

Therefore, diffusible solids, such as light magnesium carbonate, is the best choice as dispersing agent in inhalations.

The common household vaporiser, producing a fine mist of steam, is often used for administration of inhalation.

Inhalants are different from inhalations. The container of an inhalant consists of drug(s) that are adsorbed / impregnated on cotton/wool substrate. The substrate is dipped in an emulsion of volatile substances in viscous, non-volatile vehicle, such as liquid paraffin. The forceful inhalation carries the vapours of the volatile substances into the nasal passage, where they exert their effect.

Container and storage : Store in airtight, colourless glass bottles in a cool place.

Label : For external use only. Shake well before use.

Patient counselling : Add 5 ml to a litre of hot water and inhale the vapours whenever necessary. The use of 'Rub' as decongestants may be hazardous to infants.

Proprietary preparations :

● BROVON INHALANT (Briddle Sawyer) : Atropine methonitrate 0.14 per centw/v, Papaverine HCl 0.88 per cent w/v, total adrenalin 0.9 per centw/v, chlorbutol 0.5 per cent w/v. Drops for inhalation for relief from bronchospasm.

Prescription No. 12.5
℞
Menthol and Eucalyptus Inhalation, BPC
Menthol — 2.0 g
Eucalyptus oil — 10.0 ml
Light Magnesium carbonate — 7.0 ml
Water, freshly boiled & cooled, to make — 100.0 ml

Principle :

Inhalation of warm vapours containing volatile principles, causes liquefaction of the viscous mucus. It is useful in relieving cough. Menthol, eucalyptus, camphor and benzoin are commonly used aromatic substances in treatment of tracheitis, bronchitis and sinusitis. Oily solution, if instilled in the nasal mucosa, may cause lipoid pneumonia.

Menthol is slightly soluble in water and eucalyptus oil is immiscible with water. The solution of menthol in eucalyptus oil can be distributed in water by formulating a suspension. Fine powder of diffusible substance such as light magnesium carbonate is the best-suited excipient for inhalations. Adsorption of oil on to the fine powder in the form of minute droplets, will ensure both its uniform distribution in the vehicle and the ease of vaporisation when placed in hot water.

Apparatus: Mortar and pestle, beaker, glass rod, spatula, funnel, measuring cylinder.

Compounding:

i) Dissolve the fine powder of menthol in eucalyptus oil. Pass magnesium carbonate through sieve no.80. Triturate oil with magnesium carbonate.

ii) Add water to get a smooth pourable dispersion. Transfer the mixture to a tared bottle. Adjust the volume with remaining amount of water.

Container and storage: Store in airtight clear glass bottles in a cool place. Protect from light.

Category and directions for use: Nasal decongestant. Add 5 ml to a litre of hot water and inhale the vapours whenever necessary.

Label : For external use only. Shake well before use.

Patient counselling : Use hot, but not boiling water for generation of vapours. Avoid touching The nose frequently. Use soft hankie for blowing the nose. Apply protective creams around the nose to avoid irritation. Take rest. Take diet rich in vitamin C.

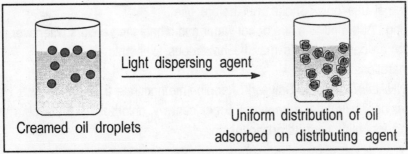

Figure 12.4: Role of Distributing Agent in Inhalation

TOPICAL SUSPENSIONS

Lotions

Lotions are solutions or suspensions for external use. Suspensions type of lotions are also termed as 'Shake Lotions'. The evaporation of the vehicle after, its application deposits a thin coat of powder on the skin. Topical application of a suspension with massage may cause inflammation or redness of skin depending on hardness and roughness of particles, therefore should not be applied with friction. The suspensions must be labelled as 'Shake well before use'.

Prescription No. 12.6

℞

Calamine Lotion I.P, B.P.

Calamine	—	15.0 g
Zinc Oxide	—	5.0 g
Bentonite	—	3.0 g
Sodium Citrate	—	0.5 g
Liquid Phenol	—	0.5 ml
Glycerin	—	5.0 ml
Rose water, to make	—	100.0 ml

Principle :

Calamines and zinc oxide act as skin-protective and astringent. Phenol 0.2-2.5 per cent, acts as antipruritic. Calamine lotion is used for relief from itching, which may be due to allergy, diabet, worm infection, or anxiety. It is indicated in case of prickly heat, sunburn, insect bite and all other allergies. About 250 ml of calamine lotion will cover the entire skin of an adult.

Calamine is chemically zinc oxide coloured pink or reddish-brown with ferric oxide and the shade depends on the amount of ferric oxide. It is insoluble in water and indiffusible. The aqueous dispersion shows pH 9. Bentonite is native colloidal hydrated aluminium silicate having capacity to absorb water to form either sol or gel, depending on its concentration. Because of thixotropic nature of bentonite in water, vigorous shaking breaks the gel structure to produce thin pourable suspension and, on standing, reformation of structure occurs. Drug particles remain entrapped in the gel structure. It is negatively charged and in the presence of cationic drugs it forms flocculation, or aggregation, and such aggregated suspensions are more viscous. Sodium citrate acts on the principle of controlled flocculation and produces a pourable suspension. It also acts as antioxidant and buffer.

Sodium citrate is very soluble in water. Liquefied phenol is antipruritic and mixture of it with glycerin is water-miscible. Phenol and glycerin are preservatives. Glycerin is humectant. After evaporation of water, glycerin holds the fine powders on the skin. It also increases viscosity of the suspension.

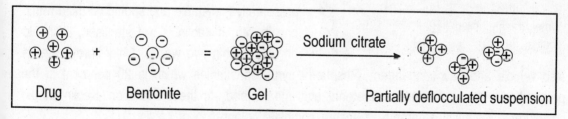

Drug   Bentonite   Gel   Sodium citrate   Partially deflocculated suspension

Figure 12.5: Role of Sodium Citrate

Apparatus : Mortar and pestle, beaker, glass rod, spatula, funnel, measuring cylinder.

Compounding :

i) Sift powdered drugs. Mix these by the doubling up method.

ii) Dissolve sodium citrate in ¾th volume of rose water. Triturate calamine, zinc oxide and bentonite with it.

iii) Add liquefied phenol in glycerin. Mix it well with calamine mixture.

iv) Transfer the mixture to a bottle with the aid of rose water. Rinse the mortar and pestle with rose water. Adjust the volume in a tared container.

Container and storage : It should be packed in well-closed, amber colored, fluted bottles.

Category and direction for use : Protective, Astringent. Apply on affected area without friction.

Label : Shake well before use. For external use only.

Handling precaution : Liquid phenol is caustic, deliquescent and efflorescent.

Patient counselling : Apply on affected area without friction and allow evaporation of vehicle. Do not apply near the eyes.

Proprietary preparations :

• CALADRYL LOTION (Parke Davis) : Calamine 8per cent w/v, diphenhydramine HCl 1 per cent w/v, camphor 0.1 per cent wv, specially denatured spirit 2.37 per cent w/v.

• CALAK LOTION (Shalaks) : Calamine 15 per cent, Zinc oxide 5per cent, glycerin 5 per cent.

ADDITIONAL EXERCISE

Prescription No. 12.7

℞

Kaolin Mixture, Paediatric, BPC

Light Kaolin	— 20.0 g
Amaranth Solution	— 1.0 ml
Benzoic acid Solution	— 2.0 ml
Raspberry Syrup	— 20.0 ml
Chloroform Water, DS	— 50.0 ml
Water, freshly boiled & cooled, to make	— 100.0 ml

Principle :

Kaolin is adsorbant type of antidiarrhoeal. Kaolin is of two types, heavy and light. Due to diffusible nature, light kaolin is used in suspensions. Kaolin should be dry heat sterilised. The preparation containing sterilised kaolin in the presence of benzoic acid and chloroform water as preservative, is stable and should be used within one month. If kaolin is not sterilised, it should be used within two weeks. Chloroform water is also vehicle and flavouring agent. Raspberry syrup constittules which is 20 per cent of the preparation, acts as flavoured sweetener and imparts body to the preparation. Kaolin should be triturated well with amaranth to ensure complete colouration of kaolin.

Apparatus : Mortar and pestle, beaker, glass rod, spatula, funnel, measuring cylinder.

Compounding :

i) Sift the kaolin. Triturate kaolin with raspberry syrup and some water to produce a smooth dispersion. Add amaranth solution and mix well till no white particle is visible.

ii) Add water to get a smooth pourable dispersion. Transfer the mixture to tared bottle. Add benzoic acid and chloroform water.

iii) Adjust the volume with remaining amount of water.

Container and storage : Store in aritight, amber coloured, glass bottles in cool place. Protect from light. Use within two weeks.

Category and dose : Antidiarrhoeal : Children Dose : Up to 1 yr, 5 ml; 1 to 5 yrs , 10 ml; 3 times a day with water.

Label : Shake well before use.

Patient counselling : Take oral rehydration salt and maintain water intake.

Proprietary preparations :

- Susp. CHLORAMBIN (AFD) : Light kaolin 1 g, pectin 50 mg, neomycin sulphate 50 mg and others, per 5 ml.

- Gel STREPTOMAGMA (Wyeth) : Light kaolin 1.5 g, pectin 135 mg, aluminium hydroxide 200 mg, streptomycin sulphate 150 mg, per 5 ml.

Prescription No. 12.8

℞

Paracetamol Suspension (MEP 1973)

Paracetamol	—	2.40 g
Compound Powder of Tragacanth	—	2.0 g
Saccharin sodium	—	150.0 mg
Compound Tatrazine solution	—	0.1 ml
Orange syrup	—	50.0 ml
Chloroform water, to make	—	100.0 ml

Principle :

As discussed in Prescription No. 4.4, paracetamol suspension is devoid of alcohol The commercial production of Paracetamol elixir is less due to the cost of the solvent. To avoid use of alcohol in syrups, number of commercial paracetamol brands have been recently prepared as suspensions. Being in the insoluble state, the bitter taste of paracetamol is a less intense. The CPT is suspending agent. Orange syrup has a sweet-viscous flavour. Sodium saccharin is an artificial water-soluble sweetener. Compound tatrazine solution is the colour. Chloroform water is volatile and, due to dilute in nature, its preservative property is not too effective; therefore, the suspension for large scale manufacturing should contain, primary suspending agent and, suitable preservative. It can be formulated as drops and should be supplied with a dropper.

Apparatus : Spatula, beaker, glass rod, measuring cylinder.

Compounding :

i) Sift paracetamol. Triturate it with CPT, using orange syrup to produce asmooth dispersion.

ii) Add compound tartrazine solution and sodium saccharin and mix well.

iii) Transfer the mixture to a tared bottle and add chloroform water.

iv) Rinse the mortar and pestle with remaining amount of water and adjust the volume with it.

Label : Shake well before use.

Refer prescription No. 11.7 for other information.

Proprietary preparations :

- CROCIN (GlaxoSmithKline); CALPOL (Burroughs Wellcome); 120 mg/5 ml, FEBREX (Indoco) : 250 mg/5 ml
- CROCIN DROPS (Glaxo SmithKline) : 100 mg/ml.
- CALPOL (Burroughs Wellcome), LOTEMP SUSP (Raptakos): Paracetamol 120 mg and 250 mg per 5 ml, respectively.

Prescription No. 12.9

℞

Sulphur Lotion BPC

Precipitated sulphur	—	4.0 g
Quillaia tincture	—	0.5 ml
Glycerin	—	2.0 ml
Alcohol (90 per cent)	—	6.0 ml
Calcium hydroxide solution, to make	—	100.0 ml

Principle :

Sulphur is antiseptic and keratolytic. It is useful in treatment of acne vulgaris. Precipitated sulphur is very slightly soluble in water and alcohol. It dissolves in hot calcium hydroxide solution. The alkaline pH increases keratolytic activity and thus penetration of the drug. Precipitated sulphur is hydrophobic substance having poor wetting properties. Its fine powder floats on the surface. Glycerin, alcohol and quillaia tincture increase the wettability. When sulphur is levigated with glycerin-alcohol mixture, these vehicles displace air present in the porous surface of the powder. Saponins in quillaia act by lowering surface tension. The improvement in wettability not only keeps the diffusible sulphur well distributed in the vehicle, but also enhances contact on the affected area. Alcohol also increases penetration of drug after application and produces cooling effect. Glycerin gives body to the preparation and helps to adhere drug powder onto the skin after evaporation of vehiclel. It is humectant.

Apparatus : Mortar and pestle, beaker, glass rod, spatula, funnel, measuring cylinder.

Compounding :

i) Sift sulphur powder. Triturate it with mixture of glycerin–alcohol.

ii) Add quillaia tincture. Triturate it well. Add little calcium hydroxide solution and make the mass pourable.

iii) Transfer the mixture to a bottle. Rinse the mortar and pestle with calcium hydroxide solution.

iv) Adjust the volume with the remaining amount of calcium hydroxide solution in a tared container.

Container and storage : It should be packed in amber coloured fluted bottles. Store in a well closed container.

Category and direction to use : Anti-acne. Apply on acne without friction.

Label : For external use only. Shake well before use.

Handling precaution : Sulphur is an irritant, avoid contact with skin.

Patient counselling : Apply on affected area without friction. Gradually increase the length of residence of lotion on the affected part depending on tolerance. If skin irritation persists, discontinue the use. Do not apply near the eyes.

Proprietary preparations :

- PERSOL FORTE Cream (Wallace): Precipitated sulphur 5 per cent, benzoyl peroxide 10 percent.

•••••

13 Emulsions

INTRODUCTION

Emulsions are thermodynamically unstable heterogeneous biphasic systems consisting of at least one immiscible liquid, which is dispersed as globules (the internal, discontinuous or dispersed phase) in the other liquid phase (the external, continuous phase or dispersion medium), which is stabilised by the presence of an emulsifying agent. Internal phase droplets are generally in the range of diameter 0.1 mm - 100 mm. Emulsions are of the following types:

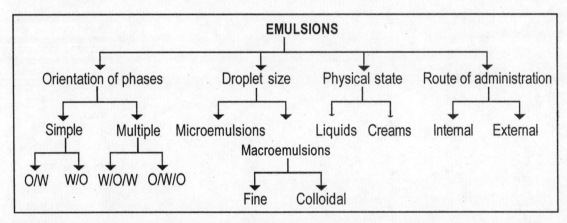

1) **Oil-in-water (o/w) emulsions:** Emulsions are biphasic liquid systems, one phase of which is usually polar (i.e. aqueous), while the other is relatively non-polar (i.e. oil). When oil droplets are dispersed in the continuous aqueous phase, the emulsion is termed as oil-in-water (o/w) emulsion.

2) **Water-in-oil (w/o) emulsions:** When oil phase serves as the continuous phase and water droplets as internal phase, the emulsion is water-in-oil (w/o) emulsion.

3) Multiple emulsions: These are of two types, o/w/o and w/o/w type. The oil-in-water-in-oil (o/w/o) emulsions are these emulsions in which the water droplets of the w/o emulsion enclose small oil droplets as internal phase. In water-in-oil-in-water (w/o/w) emulsions, water droplets are enclosed in internal oil phase of o/w emulsion.

4) Micro-emulsions: As per the globule size, emulsions can be classified into micro-emulsions and macro-emulsions. When the globule diameter is as small as 10-200 nm, the emulsions are termed micro-emulsions or micellar emulsions and they appear as clear transparent solutions.

5) Macro-emulsions: Emulsions with globules of mean diameters between 0.1 mm-5 mm are considered to be fine emulsions and those with predominantly large globules (up to 100 mm) are referred to as coarse emulsions. Unlike micro-emulsions, macro-emulsions are generally milky in appearance. This topic deals with macro-emulsions.

6) Physical state: Emulsions may be in the liquid form for internal or external use or semisolid form for external application, The latter is termed creams. Most of the pharmaceutical emulsions designed for oral administrations, are of o/w type; whereas, liniments, lotions and creams are either o/w or w/o type.

Pharmaceutical Applications of Emulsions

i)   Emodsions for oral use, help mask the taste of unpalatable oils/oil-soluble medicinal agents. For example, the external water phase in cod liver oil emulsion masks the unpleasant taste of the oil. The external phase can also be suitably flavoured to enhance the masking effect.

ii)   Emulsions permit the administration of a liquid drug in a subdivided form, which enhances the rate and extent of drug absorption.

iii) Water sensitive drugs can be formulated as liquid dosage form in the form of o/w emulsions.

iv)   Oily emulsions provide unfavourable conditions for microbial growth.

v)   For topical application, creams are preferable to ointments due to their spreading ability and easy washability, their less greasy nature and improved appearance.

vi)   Parenterally, o/w emulsions containing fats, vitamins and carbohydrates are administered intravenously to patients who cannot take food by mouth. W/o emulsions containing oil-soluble drug provide an effective sustained release mechanism. These are injected by intramuscular route.

vii) It is economical to administer costly oil phase in emulsion form, where it is diluted with water, provided the therapeutic value and stability remain unaffected.

      However, liquid emulsions are physically less stable and have less acceptability compared to solutions and suspensions.

Modern Dispensing Pharmacy

Formation of an emulsion

The emulsion, immiscible liquids are triturated to produce small droplets of both the phases. This step involves two processes, first, the dispersion of one liquid throughout another in the form of droplets and second, the coalescence (rejoining) of droplets of similar phases to form initial bulk liquids. The higher surface-free energy of droplets makes the system thermodynamically unstable. When two or more drops of the same liquid come in contact with one another, they tend to coalescence, making one larger drop having a lesser surface free energy than the total surface free energy of an individual drop.

The physically stable emulsion contains uniform distribution of droplets of either phase throughout the continuous medium. It means any one phase remains as droplets and the other phase undergoes coalescence to form a continuous medium. The third agent, an emulsifying agent, is required to maintain the integrity of the individual droplets of either of the phases, formed during compounding, by preventing coalescence.

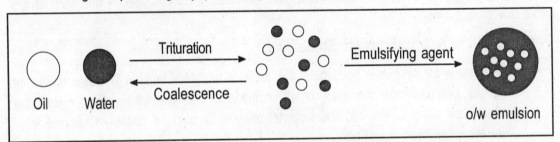

Figure 13.1: Formation of Emulsion

Concept Clear : Emulsions

Emulsions are thermodynamically unstable heterogeneous biphasic systems consisting of immiscible liquids, where one phase is dispersed in other liquid phase, which is stabilised by the presence of an emulsifying agent.

- Types : o/w, w/o, multiple, micro and macro emulsions, creams.
- Emulsifying agent : Prevent coalescence, determine the type of emulsion.

INSTABILITY OF EMULSIONS

Cracking (Coalescence)

When two or more globules of internal phase approach each other, they may undergo coalescence and separate out as a distinct layer.

1) Interfacial tension: Dispersion of immiscible liquids makes the system more energetic due to the increase in surface free energy (ΔG).

$$\Delta G = \gamma \Delta A$$

Where, Y interfacial tension and ΔA increase in total surface area. Such thermodynamically unstable emulsions tend to aggregate, to decrease the total energy, but it makes the emulsions physically unstable. Lowering interfacial tension can lower the increased energy, ΔG, and in turn the rate of coalescence. Surface-active agents reduce interfacial tension.

2) Interfacial film: Droplets come closer shaking or vibration, or which allows the content of the droplets to combine to form larger droplets. The flexible interfacial film of sufficient mechanical strength, formed by an emulsifier can minimise the coalescence.

3) Electrostatic forces: A system with higher inter-droplet electrostatic repulsion does not allow dispersed globules to coalesce and, this repulsion between droplets, results in a stable emulsion. Electrostatic forces can be adjusted by addition of electrolytes in optimum concentration.

4) Physicochemical interaction: The emulsion containing incompatible ingredients could lead to cracking of an emulsion. For example,

  i)   Addition of polyvalent soaps, or use of hard water, to prepare emulsion-containing monovalent soap as emulsifying agent.

  ii) Combination of cationic and anionic emulsifying agents will produce a cracked emulsion due to neutralisation.

  iii) Hydrophilic emulsifiers, such as acacia, tragacanth and gelatin precipitate by the addition of organic solvent, like alcohol.

  iv) Alkali soap emulsifying agents tend to decompose in acidic pH.

  v)   Electrolytes, if used in other than optimum concentrations, change electrostatic forces.

  vi) Dispersed phase and dispersed medium dissolve in a common solvent to form a monophasic system, i.e., Soap liniment.

5) Microbial degradation: Moulds, yeasts and bacteria can bring about the decomposition of an emulsifying agent, producing a weak interfacial film. This can be avoided by addition of preservatives.

6) Excess of dispersed phase: Chances of collision are of droplets more in concentrated emulsions, which in turn increase probability of coalescence.

Creaming of Emulsion

Creaming of emulsion is the separation of dispersed globules in the form of a concentrated layer on the top of emulsion. Mostly, oils are light and hence move upwards to form a cream layer. Creaming is not a serious instability problem, if uniform re-dispersion can be achieved by shaking the emulsion. Creaming can be explained by Stoke's law (Refer Chapter 12).

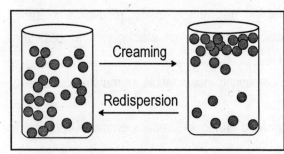

Figure 13.2 : Creaming of emulsions

1) **Small particle size:** Larger dispersed globules (>10 m) cream much more rapidly than smaller globules. Aggregates of globules formed by coalescence or flocculation have a greater tendency to cream than individual globules.

2) **Viscous external phase:** Rate of creaming is inversely proportional to the viscosity of external phase. The viscosity of water as external phase can be improved by use of hydrophilic colloids such as gum acacia, sodium carboxymethyl cellulose, agar, tragacanth, etc. In case of w/o emulsions, viscosity of oil phase can be increased by use of polyvalent metal soaps, high melting waxes, etc.

3) **Equalisation of density:** To reduce the rate of creaming, the density difference between the dispersed phase and dispersed medium should be minimum.

4) **Storage temperature:** The viscosity and solubility of an emulsifying agent is influenced by the cycling in storage temperature. At high temperature, due to reduction in viscosity, rate of creaming is greater. At refrigeration temperature, due to ice formation, deformation of oil globules under pressure of ice particles increases chances of coalescence. Hence, an optimum temperature should be maintained.

Phase Inversion

Phase inversion is the change in type of emulsion from o/w to w/o and vice versa. Some reasons of phase inversions are as follows:

1) Change in phase volume ratio: Theoretically, the maximum volume that can be occupied by mono-sized spherical droplets of the dispersed phase of an emulsion is 74 per cent of the total volume. If the proportion of internal phase is increased above 74 per cent, it would become the external phase. In general, emulsions containing 30-60 per cent of internal phase are less prone to phase inversion.

2) Changing the emulsifier: Monovalent soaps like sodium and potassium oleate favour, o/w emulsion, but addition of divalent soaps like magnesium or calcium soap to such emulsions will cause the emulsion to invert. Similarly, addition of electrolytes into the emulsion prepared using soap emulsifiers, may cause phase inversion due to the change in degree of ionisation, thereby changing HLB (Hydrophilic–lipophilic balance) of the emulsifying agent.

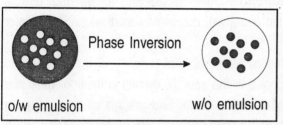

o/w emulsion   w/o emulsion

Figure 13.3: Phase Inversion

3) Change in temperature: Phase inversion can also occur when solubility of emulsifier is temperature dependant. The temperature at which phase inversion occurs is termed as phase inversion temperature (PIT). If phase inversion is unintentional, i.e., it takes place during storage, then it is a sign of instability.

Concept Clear : **Creaming and Phase Inversion**

Creaming of emulsion is the separation of dispersed globules in the form of a concentrated layer at the surface of an emulsion. Reasons for creaming are:
- Large and light droplets.
- Thin external phase.
- Difference in density
- Storage temperature

Phase inversion is the change in type of emulsion from o/w to w/o and vice versa.
Reasons for phase inversion are:
- Excess internal phase.
- Change in HLB or solubility of emulsifying agent.
- Change in temperature

FORMULATION

Suspensions and emulsions are biphasic liquid systems, where an insoluble solid and an immiscible liquid, respectively, are internal phases. When the dispersed phase is diffusible solid, suspension may not require suspending agent; but in case of an emulsion, oil and aqueous phases have to be blended with an emulsifying agent.

Drug

In emulsions, the drug component is either oil or drug soluble in either of the liquid phases, and it is rarely an insoluble solid. Mang of oils themselves act as active ingredients.

Oil Phase

Oil phase plays various roles in an emulsion. The oil phase is either used for its therapeutic value, or for auxiliary uses, such as soap formation, carrier for oil-soluble drug or as an emollient, lubricant, etc. The most commonly used oils for their therapeutic value are as given below:

i)   Turpentine oil (counter irritant) and benzyl benzoate (scabicide) for external use.

ii) Fish oils (vitamin source), liquid paraffin (laxative), castor oil (laxative) and arachis oil (nutrient) for internal use.

iii) Soya bean oil and sunflower oil (nutrition) for parenteral use.

The examples of auxiliary uses of oil phase in the specific emulsion include- oleic acid for soap formation in white liniment and in oily calamine lotion; and arachis oil as lubricant in oily calamine lotion. Sesame oil, peanut oil and cottonseed oil are used as vehicles for injections.

The oil phase, which varies in consistency, is used to adjust consistency of the final product. The oil phase should be liquid at the time of emulsification. Examples of oils of different consistency are:

1) Liquids   : Mineral oil, vegetable oils.

2) Semisolids : Soft paraffin, wool fat.

3) Solids   : Paraffin wax, bees wax.

Additives

Aqueous phase: Freshly boiled and cooled water is an aqueous phase for emulsion. When the drug, or additive, is soluble in water, it is dissolved in it before mixing with the oil phase.

Emulsifying agent: Emulsifying agents act mainly in two ways:

a) Reducing interfacial tension and/or

b) Forming interfacial film.

The emulsifying agents can be classified in the following ways:

I)   According to physicochemical nature

a) Polysaccharides   :   i)   Natural: Acacia, tragacanth, starch.

ii)   Semi-synthetic: Methylcellulose, sodium CMC.

b) Surfactants	:	i)	Anionic: Alkali soaps, Alkyl sulphates.
		ii)	Cationic: Quaternary ammonium compounds.
		iii)	Non-ionic: Spans and Tweens.
c) Finely divided solids	:		Clays, milk of magnesia, aluminum hydroxide gel.
d) Sterol containing substances	:		Beeswax, wool fat, wool alcohols.

II) According to the nature of interfacial films formed

a) Monomolecular interfacial films produced by surface-active agents.

b) Multi-molecular interfacial film produced by hydrocolloids.

c) Solid particulate films produced by fine powders, such as bentonite, magnesium hydroxide.

a) Polysaccharides: These hydrocolloids are o/w type of emulsifying agents. They act by forming multi-molecular interfacial film and by increasing viscosity of water phase. Acacia is most frequently used extemporaneously compounded oral emulsions. Initially, emulsions are stable due to viscosity and stickiness produced by acacia, but acacia emulsions cream rather quickly. Emulsion stabilisers such as tragacanth, sodium alginate, or agar are used in combination with acacia to increase the viscosity of aqueous phase. Due to their sticky natures acacia emulsions are not suitable for external use. Irish moss is considered as primary emulsifier, but preparation of its mucilage is time consuming and requires high shear equipments.

The low viscosity grades of methylcellulose and sodium carboxy methylcellulose are usually used as o/w emulsifying agents, or emulsion stabilisers.

b) Surfactants: In majority of the emulsions, surfactants are used as primary emulsifying agents. Surfactants are ionic, non-ionic and ampholytics. Due to toxicity, ionic surfactants are restricted to topical use. Ampholytics are not commonly used as emulsifying agents. Surfactants act by two mechanisms, by forming monomolecular interfacial film and by reducing interfacial tension. Hydrophilic surfactants produce o/w type of emulsions, whereas, lipophilic surfactants are used to produce w/o type of products.

Soap emulsifying agents are of two types, soft soap and hard soap. The free fatty acid or oil containing them is chemically reacted with sodium or potassium hydroxide or triethanolamine to produce soft soap. Hard soaps are salts of fatty acids with divalent or trivalent cations. The oils used for soap formation include olive oil, almond oil, and linseed oil. The other vegetable oils, such as cottonseed oil, corn oil, peanut oil and mineral oil do not form soap. Monovalent soaps are soluble or dispersible in water and produce o/w emulsion and divalent soaps are w/o type. Soap emulsifying agents are alkaline. These are only suitable for the preparations that are externally used, especially on unbroken skin.

---

c) **Finely divided solids:** Fine solid particles act as emulsifying agents by forming thick impenetrable particulate interfacial film. As compared to emulsifying agents mentioned above, these types of emulsions require more mechanical energy to form. Magnesium hydroxide acts as both antacid and emulsifying agent in its emulsion with liquid paraffin. Clays like betonite and hectorite are used to produce emulsions for topical use.

d) **Sterol-containing substances:** Beeswax, wool fat, wool alcohols are w/o type of emulsifying agents; but, in most cases, these are used as emulsion stabilisers. Beeswax is used with borax to form sodium cerotate, which is an emulsifying agent in cold cream. Wool fat absorbs 50 per cent of its weight of water and produces w/o type of emulsion. Wool alcohol is nothing but emulsifying fraction of wool fat, used as w/o emulsion stabiliser and as emollient.

Antioxidants: Rancidity is the usual problem associated with emulsions containing unsaturated fats and oils. Oil-soluble antioxidants, such as, tocopherol, butylated hydroxy anisole (BHA), butylated hydroxy toluene (BHT) is more suitable. Other antioxidants include, citric acid, tartaric acid, ascorbic acid, sodium bisulphate, etc.

Preservative: The aqueous phase is more sensitive to microbial growth and hence the preservative should be concentrated more in that phase. It should remain in its unionised form and should have oil-water partition coefficient less than one.

Organoleptic additives: In the o/w emulsions, water phase itself masks the, unpleasant taste of the oil phase. Secondly, both the oil and water phases can be flavoured. As Pharmaceutical emulsions have acceptable milky appearance, for this reason colouring agents are not required to be addied in an them.

Concept Clear : Formulation of Emulsion

Oil, water and emulsifying agents are three basic components of the emulsion.

Oil phase plays various roles in the emulsion. It acts as active ingredient, helps in soap formation, acts as vehicle for drug or is an emollient, lubricant, etc. Oil phase must be liquid at the time of emulsification.

Emulsifying Agents act by reducing interfacial tension and/or by forming interfacial film.

- Surfactants are primary emulsifying agents acting by forming monomolecular interfacial film and by reducing interfacial tension.
- Polysaccharides are o/w type of emulsifying agents forming multi-molecular interfacial film and by increasing viscosity of water phase.
- Finely divided solids form thick impenetrable particulate interfacial film.

Antioxidants soluble in oil are more suitable. These include tocopherol, BHT, BHA.

Preservatives should remain in unionised form and should have oil-water partition coefficient less than one.

Emulsions have an acceptable milky appearance. The water phase of o/w emulsions itself masks the unpleasant taste of an oil phase; secondly, both oil and water phases can be pleasantly flavoured.

Selection of Emulsifying Agent

Emulsifying agents are selected on the basis of route of administration of product, type of emulsion and stability of emulsion.

1) Type of emulsion: Emulsifying agents, as per their affinity towards immiscible liquid phases are generally classified into hydrophilic and lipophilic emulsifiers. Hydrophilic emulsifiers are preferentially soluble in aqueous phase, but have some solubility in oil phase and reverse is also true for lipophilic emulsifiers. The Bancroft rule states that hydrophilic emulsifying agent produces o/w emulsions, whereas lipophilic emulsifying agent produces w/o type of emulsions.

Table 13.1: HLB values of some emulsifying agents

No.	Emulsifying Agent	HLB
1)	Acacia	8.0
2)	Tragacanth	13.2
3)	Gelatin	9.8
4)	Sorbitan tristearate (Span 65)	2.1
5)	Sorbitan monooleate (Span 80)	4.3
6)	Sorbitan monostearate (Span 60)	4.7
7)	Polyoxyethylene sorbitan monostearate (Tween 60)	14.9
8)	Polyoxyethylene sorbitan monooleate (Tween 80)	15.0
9)	Triethanolamine oleate	12.0
10)	Sodium oleate	18.0
11)	Potassium oleate	20.0
12)	Sodium lauryl sulphate (SLS)	40.0

2) Route of administration: Majority of the oral emulsions are o/w type. For external use, aqueous emulsions are selected for wet skin and oily emulsions for dry skin. Polysaccharides and non-ionic surfactants, due to their non-toxicity, are the choice of emulsifying agents for oral use. Soap emulsifying agents, due to their toxicity and objectionable taste, are unsuitable for oral use, and due to their alkaline nature, are not suitable for application on broken skin. The cationic surfactants, because of their antimicrobial action, are most suitable for topical use. Emulsifying agents used in external emulsions should provide additional properties such as emollient, lubrication and protection after application.

3) Emulsion stabilisers: Auxilliary emulsifying agents can be used with preliminary emulsifying agents as emulsion stabilisers, e.g. the creaming of acacia emulsions is reduced by combining acacia with tragacanth or sodium alginate. Combination of two or more emulsifying agents is preferred over single emulsifying agent. For example, emulsifying ointment bases, such as emulsifying wax and cetrimide wax, contain mixture of ionic surfactant with non-ionic surfactant (Refer Prescription No. 14.4). The w/o emulsions are comparatively physically less stable than o/w emulsions. The stability of w/o emulsions can be improved by use of emulsion stabiliser (wool fat in oily calamine lotion) or by preparing emulsion through phase inversion (White liniment).

Concept Clear : Selection of Emulsifier

- Hydrophilic surfactants produce o/w type of emulsions whereas lipophilic surfactants are used to produce w/o type of products.
- Non-ionic surfactants and hydrocolloids are non-toxic as compared to ionic surfactants.
- Monovalent soap are o/w emulsion and divalent soaps are w/o type.
- The o/w emulsions are comparatively physically more stable than w/o emulsions.

COMPOUNDING OF EMULSIONS

Emulsions are compounded by several methods, depending on the nature of ingredients, equipment available and quantity of emulsion to be prepared. Emulsions are compounded using mortar and pestle, electric mixers, hand homogeniser or by bottle method. The immiscible liquids and emulsifying agents are triturated in a porcelain mortar, using flat - headed pestle. Glass mortars, due to their smooth surface, will not produce emulsions with finely divided internal phase.

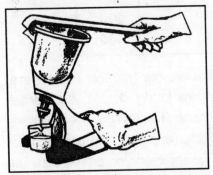

Figure 13.4 : Hand Homogeniser

Electric mixers can be used, but high chances of them entrapping air are their limitations. Hand homogenisers are used to produce finer globules, and emulsions of improved quantity.

Bottle Method

Bottle method is employed for extemporaneous preparation of emulsions containing volatile oils or oleaginous substances of low viscosity. The oil phase and emulsifying agent are added in a dry bottle of double capacity than the final volume of emulsion. After addition of the aqueous phase, the bottle is shaken vigorously to produce an emulsion. The soap emulsions for external use may contain soap, or in situ soap is allowed to form between higher free fatty acid and alkali. Volatile oils, due their low viscosity, require high proportion of gum; but the gum selected should be an easily dispersible fine powder.

Gum Emulsions

Among the polysaccharides, gum acacia is frequently used for extemporaneous preparation of oral emulsions. As compared to surfactants, gums are weak emulsifying agents. Gums mainly act by forming multi-molecular interfacial film and by increasing viscosity of the water phase. These require more mechanical energy to produce emulsions. Pre-emulsion or primary emulsion is an intermediate step to produce physically stable emulsion. The primary emulsion is then diluted with external phase to produce required amount of final emulsion. Instead of triturating the whole amount of oil phase, aqueous phase and emulsifying agent, in primary emulsion, part of the external phase is triturated with the internal phase and emulsifying agent. Since the volume of liquid is small, the shearing force required to produce fine emulsion is easily attended to the milky white appearance and clicking sound indicates the formation of primary emulsion. This technique is also termed as low energy emulsification.

The gum emulsions are o/w type and the quantity of aqueous phase and emulsifying agent required to prepare primary emulsion, is determined by the nature of the oil phase, (Table 13.2). The volatile oils and oleoresins require more gum due to their low viscosity and tendency to form w/o emulsions. When an emulsion contains two or more oil components, the quantity of gum for each is calculated separately and total of the amounts thus obtained, is used. Tragacath is 10 times more effective than acacia.

Table 13.2: Proportions of emulsion components to prepare Primary Emulsion

Type of Oil		Proportion of components			
		Oil	Water	Acacia	Tragacanth
Fixed oils	: Castor oil, Cod liver oil, Almond oil, Liquid paraffin.	4	2	1	0.1
Volatile oils	: Turpentine oil, Cinnamon oil, Peppermint oil.	2	2	1	0.1
Oleo resins	: Balsum of peru, Male fern extract	2	4	2	0.2

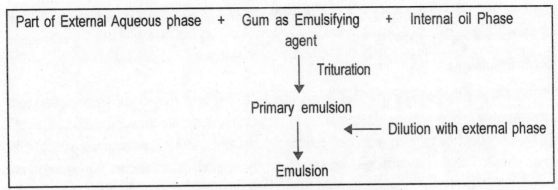

Figure 13.5: Principle of Primary Emulsion

Dry Gum and Wet Gum Method

Primary emulsion is compounded either by dry gum method or by wet gum method. In dry gum method, the oil phase is triturated with gum powder to form a lump-free dispersion. A portion of the aqueous phase is added in it and triturated to produce the primary emulsion. In wet gum method, the emulsifying agent is triturated with twice its weight of water. The oil phase is triturated with resultant mucilage to form the primary emulsion. The primary emulsion is then diluted with remaining amount of aqueous phase. The oleoresins are viscous and sticky, therefore to avoid losses during compounding, thus it should be weighed by difference method or 5 per cent excess quantity should be calculated.

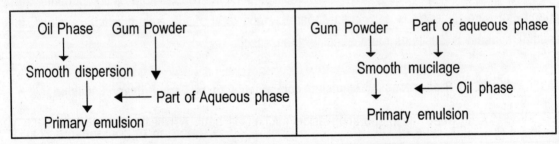

Figure 13.6: Dry Gum and Wet Gum Method

Emulsions Containing Surfactants

Surface-active agents and soaps are primary emulsifying agents. These require comparatively low mechanical energy to produce a stable emulsion. Unlike hydrocolloids and fine solid particles, surfactants greatly reduce interfacial tension, reducing rate of coalescence during dispersion. Though it is not essential to make a primary emulsion, emulsions are better compounded, using part of external phase, followed by dilution with the remaining of external phase. Drug and other additives are dissolved in respective phases as per their solubility. The internal phase is usually added in the external phase. When phase inversion is expected during compounding, the external phase is gradually added in the internal phase. The semisolid emulsifying agents, like wool fat and emulsifying wax, are melted and mixed with aqueous phase in warm condition.

Emulsions Containing Fine Solid Particles

High energy equipment, such as homogenisers are required for emulsions containing irish moss, clays, magnesium hydroxide and other fine solids.

Incorporation of Medicament

i) Drugs are dissolved in respective phases as per their solubility. The miscible liquids or soluble drugs are dissolved in the external phase before emulsifications, or such solutions are added to the primary emulsion during dilution.

ii) Drugs soluble in the internal phase may be dissolved in it before emulsification, or solution of to the drug in internal phase is added in portions, with trituration, to the in primary emulsion using excess of emulsifying agents.

iii) Alcoholic drug solutions are added below alcohol tolerance limit of emulsifying agent and dilute alcoholic solutions are added in smaller amounts, with trituration after each addition, in an emulsion.

Container and storage: Oral emulsions should be packed in screw-capped plain or amber coloured glass, or plastic bottles. The viscous emulsions should be packed in wide mouth jars. Emulsions for external use are dispensed in fluted bottles, or plastic bottles, of various shapes. These should be stored in a cool place but not in the refrigerator.

Dispensing: Emulsions showing cracks, development of odour, or bigger droplets, should not be dispensed. The PMR and CDR should be maintained.

Concept Clear : Method of Emulsification

- Bottle method is employed for compounding of emulsions of low viscosity oils, such as volatile oils.
- Gums are weak emulsifying agents and such emulsions are prepared through primary emulsions either by dry gum or wet gum method.
- Primary emulsion is low energy emulsification technique, which involves formation of stable emulsions with minimum energy by mixing of part of external phase with oil and gum. Volatile oils and oleoresins require more gum than fixed oils.
- Formation of emulsions using surfactant requires comparatively low mechanical energy because they act by two mechanisms, forming monomolecular interfacial film and by reducing interfacial tension. The reduction in interfacial tension slows the rate of coalescence of internal phase.

Several tests are available to identify type of emulsion. Some of the more common methods are given below.

1) Miscibility Test

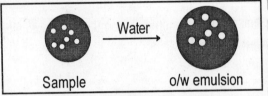

Figure 13.7: Miscibility Test

Principle:
Dilution of emulsion with external phase maintains physical stability of the emulsion.
Method: Dilute the test emulsion with water, if emulsion does not show separation of phases, it indicates oil-in-water type of emulsion.

2) Fluorescence Test

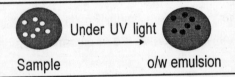

Figure 13.8: Fluorescence Test

Principle:
Many oils show fluorescence when exposed to UV light.
Method: Emulsion is observed against UV light under microscope. Fluorescence of entire field indicates oil as external phase and spotted fluorescence is observed when water is external phase.

3) Colour Test

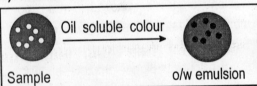

Figure 13.9: Colour Test

Principle:
Water phase or oil phase shows colouration when an emulsion is triturated with water or oil soluble colouring agent respectively.
Method: Triturate emulsion with oil-soluble dye and observe under microscope. If internal phase (globules) appears coloured against colourless background, it indicates oil-in-water type of emulsion. If droplets remain colourless, it indicates w/o emulsion.

4) Conductivity Test

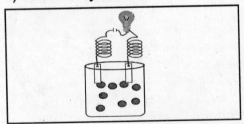

Figure 13.10 : Conductivity Test

Principle:
Water as continuous phase is good conductor of electrical current.
Method: Immerse a pair of electrodes in an emulsion and complete the circuit by connecting them to a lamp to create an electric potential. Under

Emulsions

the applied current, if the lamp glows, it indicates water as continuous phase.

5) Cobalt Paper Test

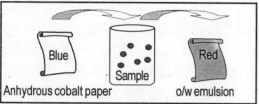

Figure 13.11: Cobalt Paper Test

Principle:

Anhydrous cobalt is blue and hydrated cobalt is red.

Method: Treat filter paper with cobalt chloride solution and dry it. Dip the dry treated paper in an emulsion. The change in colour of paper from blue to pink-red indicates oil-in-water type of emulsion.

PHARMACEUTICAL EMULSIONS

Oral Emulsions

Stable emulsions represent an effective liquid formulation for oral administration of disagreeable tasting drugs. The drugs's improved palatability, in the form of emulsion can be obtained by enveloping the internal phase containing the drug, by an inert external phase. Gastrointestinal absorption of poorly water-soluble compounds can often be improved by formulating an emulsion. Majority of oral emulsions are o/w type.

Prescription No. 13.1

R

Castor oil emulsion, NFI
Castor oil   — 37.5 ml
Acacia powder   — 10.0 g
Cinnamon water, to make — 100.0 ml

Principle:

Ricinoleic acid present in castor oil is an irritant and causes rapid evacuation of bowels. The increase in intestinal motility often causes abdominal cramps. It is contraindicated in case of intestinal obstruction. It should be used with caution during menstruation and in pregnancy. Castor oil is best administered with milk or fruit juice. Castor oil has highest density among the fatty oils; therefore, little excess gum should be used. The primary emulsion formula is 4 : 2 : 1, i.e., use 20 ml of cinnamon water with oil and gum quantities of the formula. Cinnamon water is a carminative and flavouring agent.

Apparatus: Spatula, beaker, mortar and pestle, glass rod, funnel, measuring cylinder.

Compounding: Dry gum method

i) Triturate castor oil with acacia powder. Add 20 ml of water and triturate to produce creamy primary emulsion.

ii) Dilute the primary emulsion with cinnamon water, triturating after each addition.

iii) Pour the mixture in a tared bottle. Adjust the volume with remaining amount of cinnamon water.

Container and storage: Store in well-closed containers, in cool a place.

Category and dose: Laxative, 30 to 60 ml.

Instruction on label: Shake well before use.

Patient counselling: Take with milk or fruit juice. Take fibrous food. Drink 2 liters of water per day. Alcoholic drinks cause dehydration making defecation dry and difficult. Avoid repeated and excess dosing. Avoid administering to children less than 3 years of age and give them a diet of fruit pulp and excess water.

Note 3: Laxatives: Laxatives are drugs used to treat constipation. Constipation is abnormally infrequent bowel motion. Poor diet habits, hormonal disturbances, pregnancy, medicines like narcotics, aluminium, iron, etc., may cause constipation. Laxatives should be prescribed only in extreme canditions, such as:

a) Condition of excessive straining required during defecation (such as that occuring in angina).
b) Increased risk of rectal bleeding as in hemorrhoids (piles).
c) Drug-induced constipation.
d) For expulsion of worms after anthelmintic treatment.
e) To clear the GI tract before radiological diagnosis and surgery.
f) To relieve acute constipation during pregnancy.

Laxatives act by following mechanisms:

i) Bulk forming agents relieve constipation by increasing faecal mass, which stimulates peristalsis, eg. ispaghula and methylcellulose.
ii) Stimulant laxatives increase intestinal motility, eg. senna, cascara, docusate sodium, bisacodyl. Rectal administration of glycerin and soft soap causes mild irritation and act as laxatives.
iii) Softners such as methylcellulose, liquid paraffin and rectally administered glycerin and arachis oil cause softening of faecal matter.
iv) Osmotic laxatives act by retaining fluid in the bowel by osmosis, eg. magnesium sulphate, magnesium hydroxide, lactulose.

Prescription No. 13.2

℞

Liquid Paraffin Emulsion I.P.

Liquid Paraffin	— 50.0 ml
Indian Gum Powder	— 12.5 g
Tragacanth Powder	— 0.5 g
Sodium Benzoate	— 0.5 g
Vanillin	— 0.05 g
Glycerin	— 12.5 g
Chloroform	— 0.25 ml
Water, freshly boiled & cooled, to make	— 100.0 ml

Principle:

Liquid paraffin is a mixture of liquid hydrocarbons obtained from mineral source. It is a laxative, which after oral administration, softens the faecal contents and retards absorption of water. The usual dose of un-emulsified mineral oil is 15 ml and dose of this emulsion is 30 ml. The water phase in o/w emulsion masks unpleasant taste of liquid paraffin. The smaller droplets of liquid paraffin in emulsion have more surface area; hence, their enhanced distribution in faecal content contributes to produce effective

Emulsions

lubrication and stool softening. It is given in small doses, two to three times a day. Large doses of liquid paraffin leads to leakage from the anus, impaired appetite and reduced absorption of fat-soluble vitamins. Heavy liquid paraffin is less likely to cause leakage. The absorption of smaller droplets of highly emulsified liquid paraffin from the alimentary tract, results in deposition of liquid paraffin in the mesenteric lymph nodes, liver and spleen. Administration of mineral oil should be discouraged in elderly, debilitated patients, because of the danger of lipoid pneumonia.

Liquid paraffin is practically insoluble in water and in alcohol and soluble in chloroform and volatile oils. Indian gum is an emulsifying agent, it acts by forming multimolecular interfacial film and by increasing viscosity of water phase. Acacia emulsions cream rather quickly, hence, tragacanth an emulsion stabiliser, is used in combination with acacia, to increase the viscosity of aqueous phase. Chloroform enhances dispersion of gums. Glycerin increases viscosity. Sodium benzoate is the preservative and Vanillin is the flavouring agent. The primary emulsion proportion of oil : water : gum is 4 : 2 : 1.

Apparatus: Spatula, beaker, mortar and pestle, glass rod, funnel, measuring cylinder.

Compounding: Dry gum method.

i) Triturate liquid paraffin, chloroform, with powder mixture of Indian gum, tragacanth and vanillin. Add 25 ml water and triturate to produce a creamy primary emulsion.

ii) Dissolve sodium benzoate in water. Add glycerin and sodium benzoate solution in the primary emulsion by triturating well-and making it liquid enough to pour.

iii) Pour the mixture in a tared bottle. Adjust volume with the remaining amount of water.

Container and storage: Store in well-closed, amber coloured, glass bottles. Protect from light.

Category and dose: Laxative, 30 ml once daily at bed time; Children does- 5-12 yrs, 8 ml daily.

Instruction on label: Shake well before use.

Patient counselling: Avoid repeated and excess dosing. Include fibrous foods and excess water in the diet. Should not be given to children under 3 years of age.

Proprietary preparations:

• AGAROL (Warner): Liquid paraffin 9.54 ml, phenolphthalein 400 mg, agar 60 mg, per 30 ml.

Topical Emulsions

Formulations for topical application are more acceptable as emulsions than as oils, because the oil phase has poor skin feel, cannot be spread easily, or washed easily either and can stain clothes. In general, aqueous emulsions are preferred for moist skin and oily emulsions for dry skin. Emulsions for topical use can be formulated in the form of liniments, lotions or applications.

Proprietary Preparations:

• LINIMENT MYOSTAL (Solumiks Piramal): Mahanarayan tel 4 ml, nirgudi tel 4 ml, gandapuro tel 1 ml, deodar tel 0.5 ml, gandhabiroja 0.2 g, per 10 ml. Counter irritant, topical analgesic.

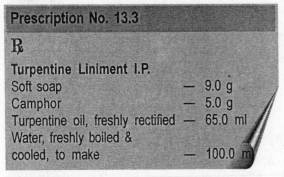

Prescription No. 13.3

℞

Turpentine Liniment I.P.

Soft soap	—	9.0 g
Camphor	—	5.0 g
Turpentine oil, freshly rectified	—	65.0 ml
Water, freshly boiled & cooled, to make	—	100.0 ml

Principle:

Turpentine oil and camphor are counter irritants and rubefacient. Counter irritants are the agents that themselves produce slight irritation on the skin thereby causing skin stimulation. These are useful in treatment of painful lesions of muscle, tendons and joints. Iodine ointment is another example of counterirritant formulation.

Turpentine liniment is o/w type of soap emulsion. Soft soap is monovalent soap produced by saponification between sodium or potassium hydroxide and higher fatty acids. In addition to emulsifying property, soft soap acts as detergent, lubricant and contributes to penetration of drugs into the skin. Since turpentine oil is less viscous and soft soap is easy to disperse, bottle container is best suited for compounding. Turpentine oil should not be exposed to air for a prolonged period of time, otherwise it becomes viscous, yellow and acidic. Freshly rectified oil should be used.

Apparatus: Spatula, beaker, measuring cylinder.

Method:

i) Mix soft soap with small portion of water. Dissolve camphor in turpentine oil.

ii) Gradually add the turpentine oil to soap mixture, mixing well after each addition.

iii) Transfer the mixture to a tared bottle with the aid of purified water and shake the mixture thoroughly until a creamy emulsion is obtained.

iv) Keep the preparation aside for half an hour. Adjust the volume with water. Mix well.

Container and storage: It should be packed in amber coloured, fluted glass bottles. Store in well-closed containers, in a cool place. Protect from light.

Category: Counterirritant, rubefacient.

Instruction on label: Shake well before use. For external use only. Apply by rubbing well on intact skin.

Patient counselling: Shake the container before use. Do not apply around the eyes.

R

Calamine Lotion, Oily BPC

Calamine	—	5.0 g
Wool Fat	—	1.0 g
Oleic Acid	—	0.5 ml
Arachis Oil	—	50.0 ml
Lime water, to make	—	100.0 ml

Principle:

Calamine liniment is synonym of this preparation. Calamine acts as protective and astringent. The official preparations are of two types, viz., aqueous suspensions (calamine lotion) and oily emulsions, containing suspended calamine (oily calamine lotion). The external oil phase improves adhesion of calamine on the skin. The oil acts as emollient and smoothening agent and it is best suited for dry skin. The calcium oleate formed by *in situ* reaction between oleic acid and calcium hydroxide is divalent soap type of emulsifying agent. Since the w/o emulsions are physically less stable, wool fat is used as emulsion stabiliser to improve the stability of this particular w/o emulsion.

Apparatus: Porcelain dish, glass rod, mortar, pestle, spatula, beaker, measuring cylinder.

Compounding:

i) Melt wool fat, arachis oil and oleic acid together.

ii) Triturate the calamine and mix it with base mixture above. Pour mixture in a tared container.

iii) Add calcium hydroxide solution and shake vigorously. Adjust the final volume.

Container and storage: It should be packed in fluted bottles. Store in well-closed containers, in a cool place.

Category: Protective.

Instruction on label: Shake well before use. For external use only. Apply without rubbing on intact skin.

Patient counselling: Shake the container before use. Apply without rubbing, on intact skin. Do not apply around the eyes.

Applications

Applications are liquid, or semi-liquid, preparations for application on the skin. Applications are mainly meant to keep the drug in contact with skin for prolonged periods of time and to help apply on larger portions of the skin. The easily spreadable liquid preparation, of slightly higher viscosity can fulfill these requirements and 'applications' is the better option for such treatments. Like lotions, these should be applied without rubbing, but are more viscous. These are solutions, suspensions or emulsions. Betamethasone valerate scalp application is the solution of betamethasone valerate in isopropyl alcohol, thickened to render the preparation slightly viscous. Compound calamine application is viscous dispersion of calamine, zinc oxide and zinc stearate in paraffin base. DDT application and gamma benzene hexachloride application are solutions of drug in xylene, emulsified and thickened, using emulsifying wax. Benzyl benzoate application is o/w emulsion prepared using emulsifying wax.

Prescription No. 13.5

℞

Benzyl Benzoate Application, IP

Benzyl benzoate	—	25.0 g
Emulsifying wax	—	2.0 g
Purified water, to make	—	100.0 ml

Principle:

Its synonym is Benzyl benzoate lotion. Benzyl benzoate is used in treatment of scabies and pediculosis. Benzyl benzoate is efficient and easier to apply than insoluble drugs like sulphur.

When the topical administration of medicament on the affected area needs to be light, not lead to irritation and the applied drug to remain on the affected area for prolonged periods, then applications is choice of dosage form. The medicament is applied after drying the skin properly after a hot bath. It is re-applied on the next day and washed off the third day. More than one such course may be required depending on the state of infection. Adults require about 120-180 ml and children require 60-90 ml of Benzyl benzoate application.

Benzyl benzoate is immiscible in water. Emulsifying wax acts as o/w emulsifying agent and stiffening agent.

Apparatus: Porcelain dish, glass rod, mortar and pestle, spatula, beaker and measuring cylinder.

Compounding:

i) Melt the emulsifying wax. Add Benzyl benzoate and mix.

ii) Pour the mass in a warm mortar. To it add ½ the warm water with trituration, to produce a smooth milky dispersion. The consistency should be such that it can be poured.

iii) Transfer it to a tared wide-mouth jar and adjust the final volume with water.

Container and storage: It should be packed in amber-coloured, wide mouth, bottles. Store in well closed containers, in a cool place. Protect from light.

Category: Antiparasitic (Scabicide).

Instruction on label: Shake well before use. For external use only.

Patient counselling: Shake the container before use. Scrub the area with soft soap in a hot bath to open up the pores. After drying, immediately apply the medication with a brush on the body from the neck down; make a second application on the following day and wash off on the third day. Protect the eyes during application. At the end of the course, the patient should thoroughly bathe and dress in clean clothes. Family members should be treated simultaneously.

Proprietary preparations: Ointment

• SCABINDON (Indon): Benzyl benzoate 25 per cent, benzocaine 2 per cent, DDT 1 per cent.

Prescription No. 13.6

℞

Liquid Paraffin and Magnesium Hydroxide
Emulsion BPC, NFI
Liquid Paraffin — 25 ml
Magnesium Hydroxide Mixture — 70 ml
Chloroform Spirit — 5 ml

Principle:

Mixture of Magnesium Hydroxide and Liquid Paraffin is synonym for this. Liquid paraffin acts as laxative due to its lubricating and stool softening effect. Magnesium hydroxide is a saline purgative. As compared to individual drugs, combination of these drugs possesses effective laxative action. Magnesium hydroxide also acts as emulsifying agent by formation of solid particulate interfacial film. Such emulsions require high mechanical energy and it is better produced using a homogeniser. Chloroform spirit is a flavouring agent and preservative.

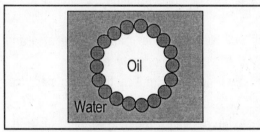

Figure 13.12: Solid Particulate Interfacial

Apparatus: Spatula, beaker, mortar and pestle, glass rod, funnel, measuring cylinder.

Compounding:

i) Triturate magnesium hydroxide mixture with chloroform spirit.

ii) Add liquid paraffin and homogenise the mixture.

iii) Pour the mixture in a tared bottle.

Container and storage: Store in wide mouthed, amber coloured bottles. Store in well-closed containers. Protect from light.

Category and dose: Strain free Laxative, 5-20 ml when required.

Instruction on label: Shake well before use.

Patient counselling: Avoid repeated and excess dosing. Intake of fibrous food is essential. Avoid administering to children below 3 years of age. Avoid administering to patients with renal impairment and intestinal obstructions.

Proprietary preparations:

- CREMAFIN (Knoll Pharma): Milk of magnesia 11.25 ml, liquid paraffin 3.75 ml, per 15 ml.
- LAXIT (Duckbill): Magnesium hydroxide 300 mg, liquid paraffin 1.25 ml, sodium carboxymethyl cellulose 50 mg, Simethicone 15 mg, per 15 ml.

Prescription No. 13.7

℞

Cod-liver Oil Emulsion, BPC 1959

Cod-liver oil	—	50.0 ml
Acacia	—	12.5 ml
Tragacanth	—	0.70 g
Bitter almond oil, volatile	—	0.10 ml
Saccharin Sodium	—	10.0 mg
Chloroform	—	0.20 ml
Water, freshly boiled & cooled, to make	—	100.00 ml

Principle:

Cod-liver oil is a source of vitamin A and vitamin D. It is used as a dietary supplement for pediatric patients, to prevent rickets and for helping calcification of bones.

Cod-liver oil is practically insoluble in water, but miscible chloroform. Acacia gum is an emulsifying agent. Tragacanth is an emulsion stabiliser. Chloroform enhances dispersion of gums. Sodium saccharin is a water-soluble sweetening agent. Almond oil is used as flavouring agent. The primary emulsion formula is: oil : water : gum in 4 : 2 : 1 ratio.

Apparatus: Spatula, beaker, mortar and pestle, glass rod, funnel, measuring cylinder.

Compounding: Dry gum method

i) Triturate cod-liver oil, chloroform and bitter almond oil with a powder mixture of acacia and tragacanth. Add 25 ml of water and triturate to produce a creamy primary emulsion.

ii) Dissolve sodium saccharin in water. Dilute the primary emulsion with it by triturating well. The consistency should be such that it can be poured.

vi) Pour the mixture in a tared bottle. Adjust the final volume with remaining amount of water.

Container and storage: Store in amber-coloured bottles. For pediatric use, it should be dispensed as drops. Store in airtight containers, in a cool place. Protect from light.

Category and dose: Vitamin A and D supplement, 8 ml to 24 ml daily in divided doses. For children up to 1 year, 2.5 ml daily is essential and for 1 to 5 years, 5 ml daily.

Instruction on label: Shake well before use.

Precaution: When exposed to sunlight, vitamin A is rapidly destroyed and on absorption of air, the oil becomes thick.

Prescription No. 13.8

℞

White Liniment, BPC

Turpentine Oil	—	25.0 ml
Oleic acid	—	8.5 ml
Dilute Ammonia solution	—	4.5 ml
Ammonium Chloride	—	1.25 ml
Water, freshly boiled and cooled	—	62.5 ml

Principle:

Turpentine oil is counterirritant and rubefacient. Turpentine liniment is o/w type of emulsion. It contains 65 per cent v/v of turpentine oil, with 5 per cent w/v camphor. The o/w emulsions are non-staining and easily washable. White liniment is w/o type of soap emulsion containing 25 per cent v/v of turpentine oil. The external oil phase facilitates application with massage. However, the w/o emulsions have comparatively poor physical stability; and hence phase inversion is attempted to improve the same.

Oleic acid and dilute ammonia solution react *in-situ* to produce monovalent soap. The hydrophilic nature of monovalent soap contributes the formation of the initial o/w type of emulsion. The phase inversion is attributed to the addition of ammonium chloride. Ammonium chloride increases the rate of forward reaction, producing an excess of soap and ultimately reducing ionisation. The non-ionisable precipitate of soap makes surfactant-water interface comparatively less hydrophilic and increased number of free hydrocarbon chains make surfactant-oil interface more lipophilic.

$$R\text{-}COOH + NH_4 \longrightarrow R\text{-}COONH_4 \text{ (Ionisable)} \qquad : \text{o/w emulsion.}$$

$$R\text{-}COOH + NH_4 \xrightarrow{NH_4Cl} R\text{-}COONH_4 \text{ (Excess and un-ionisable)} \qquad : \text{w/o emulsion}$$

Figure 13.13: Phase Inversion in White liniment

Apparatus: Mortar, pestle, spatula, beaker, measuring cylinder.

Method:

i) Mix dilute ammonia solution with equal volume of previously warmed water.

ii) Mix this in a mixture of oleic acid and turpentine oil in a tared bottle and shake it to produce a milky white emulsion.

iii) Dissolve ammonium chloride in remaining amount of water. Add this drop by drop in the emulsion, shaking after each addition. Adjust the final volume.

Step: It should be packed in well-closed, amber coloured, fluted glass bottles,. in a cool place. Protect from light.

Category: Counter irritant, rubefacient.

Instruction on label: Shake well before use. For external use only. Rub on intact skin.

Patient counselling: Shake the container before use. Rub on intact skin. Do not apply around the eyes.

●●●●●

14 Semisolids

INTRODUCTION

Semisolid dosage forms are dermatological preparations intended for application externally on the skin, to produce local or systemic effect. These are ointments, creams, pastes, gels, poultices and plasters.

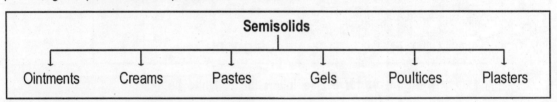

OINTMENTS

Definition and Uses

Ointments are semisolid preparations with or without medicaments, intended for external applications. Due to their plastic flow property, during application, there is a definite yield value and the resistance to flow drops as its application on the skin is continued.

Classification of Ointments: Depending on their use, ingredients present and methods of compounding, ointments are classified into the following types:

i) According to the state of Medicaments:

   a) Medicated ointments: Ointments, which contain medicament or mixture of medicaments in dissolved or dispersed form, when applied, produce local or systemic effect.

   b) Non-Medicated ointments: Non-medicated ointments are mixtures of ointment bases used for emollient, protective and lubricating effect on the skin.

ii) According to the type of ointment bases:

a) Oleaginous bases: Ointments prepared by using petrolatum, waxes, vegetable/mineral oils, eg. calamine ointment, coal tar and zinc oxide ointment.

b) Absorption bases: Ointments prepared by using wool fat, lanolin or wool alcohols, eg. simple ointment, wool alcohols ointment and salicylic acid ointment.

c) Emulsifying bases: Ointments prepared by using bases containing surface-active agent, eg. emulsifying ointment, cetrimide emulsifying ointment and whitfield ointment.

d) Water-soluble bases: Ointments prepared by using polyethylene glycol bases, eg. macrogol ointment.

iii) According to the method of preparation:

a) Incorporation method: Sulphur Ointment.

b) Fusion Method: Simple Ointment.

Advantages:

i) They provide means of site-specific application of drug on affected area, which avoids unnecessary exposure of drug and thus side effects.

ii) They avoid first pass metabolism of drug.

iii) They are convenient for administering to unconscious patients or patients experiencing difficulty on oral administration.

iv) As compared to solid and liquid dermatological preparations, semisolid dosage forms have better adhesion and prolonged residence after application.

v) Comparatively, they are chemically more stable and easy to handle than liquid dosage forms.

vi) They are a suitable dosage form for bitter-tasting drugs.

Disadvantages :

i) The oily semisolid preparations can cause staining and are cosmetically less aesthetic.

ii) Application with the finger tip may contaminate the ointment, or cause irritation when applied.

iii) As compared to solid dosage forms, semisolid preparations are bulky to handle.

iv) Though semisolids allow more flexibility in dose, dose accuracy is determined by accuracy in the quantity to be applied.

v) Physicochemically less stable than solid dosage forms.

FORMULATION OF OINTMENTS

1) Drug

Drugs can be formulated in semisolid dosage forms for their local or systemic effect. They should have sufficient solubility in their respective vehicles but must not possess higher affinity towards it. Percutaneous absorption occurs by passive diffusion and depends on the concentration of formulation.

2) Ointment Bases

i) Properties of ideal ointment bases

i)   They should be inert, non-irritating and non-sensitising.

ii) They should be compatible with skin pH (pH 5.5) and skin secretions and should not dehydrate the skin, retard wound healing or interfere with normal skin functions.

iii) They should be pharmaceutically elegant and should possess good stability throughout their shelf life.

iv) They should be compatible with common medicaments and should be easy to compound.

v)   They should have good solvent and/or emulsifying property, but should not increase affinity of the drug towards the vehicle.

vi) They should produce an ointment of the right consistency, which is neither too hard nor too soft and should melt or become soft at body temperature.

vii) They should enhance contact of medicament with skin and should have longer residence when applied.

viii) They should be emollient, protective, non-greasy and easily removable.

ix) They should release medicament readily at the site of application and should not interfere with drug penetration through skin.

ii) Types of semisolid bases:

a) Oleaginous bases: These are water-insoluble bases. They form an occlusive film on the skin.

i) Hydrocarbon bases are available as liquid paraffin, soft paraffin and hard paraffin blend of which can produce ointment of required consistency. These form an occlusive film on the skin, absorb no or less water, are stable to heat, resistant to rancidity and microbial growth and due to saturation, possess wide range of compatibilities. White petrolatum is the bleached product of yellow petrolatum. Unbleached petrolatum is used as ointment base mainly for coloured drugs and white petrolatum for white or colourless ingredients. The bleached form is not used for application on broken skin and is also not suitable for use in eye ointments. Liquid paraffin is used to soften the ointment; whereas, hard paraffin is used as stiffening agent.

ii) Fixed oils such as almond oil, castor oil and cottonseed oil, because of their emollient effect and solvent properties, are often used in ointments.

iii) Synthetic esters of fatty acids, such as glycerol monostearate, isopropyl myristate, isopropyl palmitate and butyl strearate are more uniform in composition and resistant to rancidity.

iv) Longer-chain alcohols and acids including stearic acid, stearyl alcohol, cetyl alcohol and cetostearyl alcohol are commonly used in combination with other bases, either to improve both emollient property and water absorption capacity, or as w/o emulsion stabilisers.

v) Hydrocarbon waxes are auxiliary bases, used to hold oils within their matrix structure without bleeding, such as ozokerite and ceresin.

b) Absorption bases: These are oleaginous bases capable of absorbing several times their own weight of water to form water-in-oil (w/o) emulsion. These are anhydrous, water insoluble and not washable by water, but permit easy inclusion of water or an aqueous solution of drug. These have good emollient, but poor occlusive properties.

i) Anhydrous base: Wool fat is anhydrous base; it absorbs twice its weight of water to produce w/o emulsion. Wool fat is sticky to use.

ii) W/o emulsifying bases : Lanolin (hydrous wool fat) is product of wool fat formed by addition of 30 per cent water, which can absorb further water, forming w/o emulsion. Wool alcohol is emulsifying fraction of wool fat and ointment containing wool alcohol, absorbs an equal weight of water to form w/o emulsion.

c) Emulsifying bases: They are water-insoluble, but miscible and washable type of o/w emulsions. They contain hydrophilic surfactants, which are of anionic, cationic or non-ionic type. The presence of surfactant enhances percutaneous absorption of drug. However, high concentration of surfactant may form complex with the drug, reducing its release. Emulsifying wax is anionic type of ointment base. It is composed of 10 per cent sodium lauryl sulphate and 90 per cent cetosteryl alcohol. Emulsifying ointment consists of 30 per cent w/w emulsifying wax in paraffin base. Cetrimide is cationic surfactant having self medicinal value, bactericidal action. Cetrimide wax is composed of 10 per cent cetrimide and 90 per cent cetosteryl alcohol. Cetrimide emulsifying ointment contains 3 per cent cetrimide in paraffin base. Cetomacrogol is non-ionic and cetamacrogol emulsifying wax consists of 20 per cent cetamacrogol 1000 with 80 per cent cetostearyl alcohol and cetamacrogol ointment contains 30 per cent cetamacrogol emulsifying wax in paraffin base.

d) Water-soluble bases These are polyethylene glycols, macrogols or carbowaxes. The low molecular weight PEG is liquid, whereas, high molecular weight PEG is waxy solid at room temperature. Product of required consistency can be produced using combination of PEG of various molecular weights. These have limited capacity to absorb water without physical change but incorporation of about 5 per cent of acetyl alcohol or stearyl alcohol increases water absorption up to 25 per cent. These are water-soluble, washable, non-occlusive bases and they do not produce protective and emollient effect. Being easy to wash, makes them readily removable by perspiration. Increased percutaneous absorption of drug is mainly attributed to its solubilising effect. Dehydration of stratum corneum by PEG bases may irritate the skin or retard drug penetration.

Table 14.1: Various grades of PEG bases

Base	Consistency	Melting point (^{0}C)
PEG 200, 300, 400	Liquid	—
PEG 1000	Soft semisolid	37 - 40
PEG 1500	Semisolid	38 - 41
PEG 4000	Waxy solid	50 - 56
PEG 6000	Waxy solid	60 - 63

e) **Other bases :** Bases such as polyols are hygroscopic substances like glycerin, sorbitol (70 per cent) and propylene glycol. They are used for their humectant, emollient, antidrying and antirolling properties.

3) Other Additives

i) **Buffers:** The buffers are added in semisolid dosage forms for various purposes such as compatibility with skin, drug solubility and stability. Skin, due to its weak acidic nature, tolerates weak acidic medicines to greater extent than alkaline formulations. Sodium acetate, sodium citrate, potassium metaphosphate are some of the examples of buffers.

ii) **Antioxidants:** Unsaturated oily phase is more prone to oxidation and oil-soluble antioxidants such as BHT, BHA, tocopherol and propyl or methyl gallates are more suitable. The water soluble antioxidants are useful to prevent oxidation of drugs when it is formulated in water soluble/water-washable bases.

iii) **Preservatives:** Oil based preparations do not provide good media for microbial growth. Ointments containing water require protection against microbial contamination. In addition to the safe for consumption, preservatives such as methyl and propyl paraben, benzoic acid, sodium benzoate; phenol, cresol, benzalkonium chloride, Dowicil®, phenyl mercuric salts, thiomersal like orally toxic preservatives, are also suitable in topical preparations.

iv) **Organoleptic additives:** The cosmetic value of topical preparations is a major criterion for acceptance of the product. The semisolid preparations should be creamy white or of a faint, appealing colour, soft and smooth to touch and pleasantly perfumed; at the same time, it should be easy to spread and easy to wash. In most of the cases, the colour of the preparation is the result of the colour of the drug used in it. Both, natural colours and certified dyes and lakes, are useful colours for topical preparations. e.g. D & C Red No. 22 (Eosin), D & C yellow No.7 (Fluorescine), Ext. D & C yellow No. 7 (Naphtol Yellow S). Flower-based perfumes such as lavender, rose and jasmine are preferred.

Concept Clear : **Formulation of Ointment**

Drug: Soluble or insoluble. Produce local or systemic effect.

Oleaginous base: Liquid, soft and hard paraffin. Occlusive, water immiscible; It acts as an emollient and protective. It is greasy, sticky and difficult to wash.

Absorption bases: Oleaginous bases are capable of absorbing water. They are water-insoluble and hence unwashable in water. They permit inclusion of aqueous phase; have emollient, but poor occlusive properties.

Wool fat absorbs water to form w/o emulsion. Lanolin is hydrous wool fat

Emulsifying bases: Water miscible and washable type of o/w emulsions. They have emollient properties and allow addition of water-phase. Emulsifying wax is anionic; cetrimide wax is cationic, whereas cetamacrogol emulsifying wax is non-ionic.

Water-soluble bases: PEG, water-soluble, washable, non-greasy, non-occlusive bases, increase solubility of insoluble drug. Do not produce protective and emollient effect.

Buffers: Skin compatibility, solubility, stability and transdermal penetration of drug.

Antioxidants: Oil-souble and water-soluble.

Preservative: Orally safe preservatives and additional preservatives like phenol, cresol, Dowicil, benzalkonium chloride, phenyl mercuric salts, thiomersal, etc.

Colours: Natural, certified dyes and lakes. Flowery perfumes, etc.

COMPOUNDING OF OINTMENTS

1) Incorporation method: It is also termed as levigation, trituration or mechanical mixing method.

i) Insoluble substances should first be reduced to fine powder and passed through sieve no. 85. It is levigated with some drops of levigating agent to produce a smooth dispersion. The levigating agent may be a melted base, or any other liquid, miscible with base. Mineral oil is suitable for oleaginous, absorption or w/o emulsifying bases while, water and glycerin serve well with water-miscible and water-soluble bases. The rest of the base is then added in geometrical dilution.

---

ii) If any drug is soluble in water or oil, it is dissolved in the smallest possible amount of the respective phase liquid the resulting solution is incorporated into oily, or water miscible base. It is not advisable to use co-solvents like alcohol or chloroform, to dissolve the drug, because drug may crystallise out as the solvent evaporates. The use of glycerin, propylene glycol can minimise the crystallisations of the drug during storage.

iii) Ointments containing small quantities of powders can be produced by spatulation. Lumpy particles are more easily pressed out by a spatula and it is easy to transfer the product completely from the ointment slab than mortar and pestle. White, or light, coloured ointments are preferably compounded using a dark background slab and dark coloured ointments are rompounded using white background slab. Stainless steel spatula is commonly used, but it interacts with drugs like iodine, salicylic acid, tannic acid and mercuric salts. Hard rubber spatula is used in such cases.

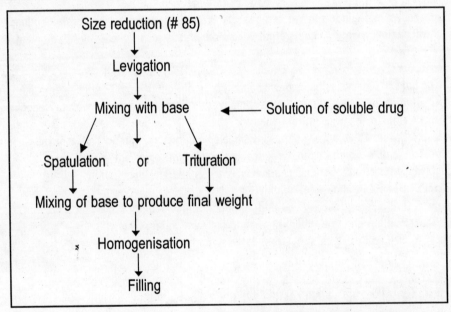

Figure 14.1: Compounding of Ointments by Incorporation Method

Mortar and pestle is preferred when quantity of ointment is large or when relatively large amount of liquid is to be incorporated. Compounded ointment may be forced through triple roller mill for further uniformity and fineness.

2) Fusion Method: Melting and mixing is the most suitable technique in the following cases:
- Ingredients that are solid at room temperature and that do not lend themselves well to mixing by incorporation, e.g. hard paraffin, beeswax, wool alcohols, stearyl alcohol, cetyl alcohol and high molecular weight PEG.

- Solid drugs that are readily soluble in the melted base.
- Incorporation of a significant amount of water into the absorption base or emulsifying base.

The steps involved in fusion method are given below.

i) Grate the waxy solids : The ingredients having highest melting point are melted first using a porcelain dish. Other oil phase ingredients are then added in the decreasing order of their melting points. Alternatively, all the bases are melted together? The hot molten liquid of low melting component hastens the melting of higher melting point component. Excess heating of the low melting point substance is limitation of the latter method.

ii) Aqueous phase containing heat stable and soluble ingredients is warmed to a temperature at least 2°C above that of the oil phase.

iii) A phase having smaller volume is added in hot condition into another phase of same temperature with agitation. Agitation is continued during cooling to obtain a semisolid mass. Vigorous stirring should be avoided to minimise air entrapment.

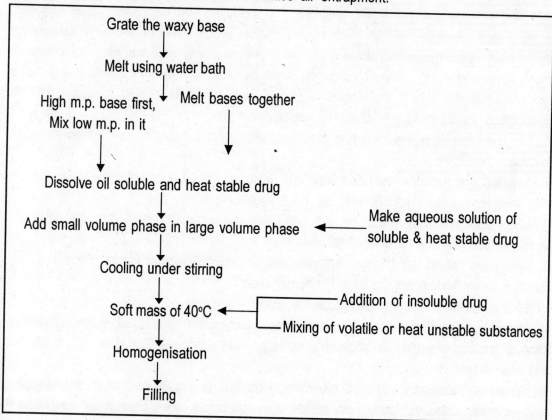

Figure 14.2 : Compounding of Ointments by Fusion Method

iv) Soluble and heat-stable medicaments are dissolved either in oil or water phase before heating, or in hot vehicle before mixing. Fine powder of insoluble drug is levigated with soft base and it is processed like incorporation method. Volatile and heat sensitive drugs such as menthol, camphor, methyl salicylate, iodine and perfumes are added at low temperature, below 40° C, during cooling, by stirring. The rapid vaporisation of volatile substances may cause local chilling effect, which is a worse form of localised cooling.

v) Proper stirring during the cooling stage avoids localised cooling, otherwise. The product adjacent to the cool surface (mixing rod, spatula, wall of the container) congeals first and the product in the bulk remains as soft mass. Such non-uniform cooling may result in separation of high melting point substances in the form of granular particles.

3) Dilution: The dilution of semisolid dosage form involves either dilution of existing marketed semisolid preparation with suitable ointment base, or non-medicated/cosmetic semisolid product. For example, cetrimide cream of 1 to 5 per cent concentration is used in seborrhoea of the scalp; whereas, creams of strengths 0.5-1 per cent are suitable for the treatment of superficial wounds and minor skin infections. For paediatric skin care products, low strength formulation is essential, and in such cases, doctors recommend to dilute the proprietary antibacterial, antifungal ointment/cream with white petroleum jelly/vanishing cream. The mixing, mainly of the potent drug above by patients, above by patients, may not be uniform and hance hence pharmacists should themselves dispense such mixed, or diluted, products, Diluted preparations should be used within two weeks.

The following points should be considered while compounding diluted semisolid dosage forms:

i) In general, for wet skin, cuts and infections, water-miscible base should be used. For dry skin, allergic conditions and itching, oily base should be used.

ii) Base used for dilution should be compatible with the original product, e.g. change in pH, presence of oppositely charged surfactant/ions.

iii) Base used should not change the, physicochemical properties of drug/dosage form, eg. aqueous cream should not be diluted with oily base.

iv) Dilution with base should not reduce the drug release rate.

v) For medications to be applied on small specific area, the base used should produce a viscous; product, whereas, for application on larger skin surface, the product should be thin, and non-sticky.

Containers and storage: Ointments, creams and pastes are usually packed in screw-capped, plain or amber coloured, wide-mouth bottles or in collapsible tubes. Semisolids are stored in a cool place Most of these are stable for one month.

Label: For external use only.

Dispensing: Ointments showing lumps or grittiness, crystal growth, bleeding or change in consistency should not be dispensed. The PMR and CDR should be maintained.

Proprietary preparations:

- DERMAL OINT (Amrutanjan): Salicylic acid 10 per cent, boric acid 5per cent, camphor 1 per, perfumed base 84 per cent. Used against eczema, ringworm.
- MICODOL (Dolphin): Miconazole 2 per cent. Antifungal.
- GAB Ointment (Gufic), GAMASCAB Cream (Nulife): Gamma benzene hexachloride 1 per cent. Scabicidal.
- ETHNORUB (Ethnor): Methyl salicylate 4per cent, mephenesin 5 per cent, iodine 0.5 per cent. For cramps, sprains and medical massage.
- PARAMINOL (Franco-Indian): Para aminobenzoic acid 10 per cent. Sunscreen.

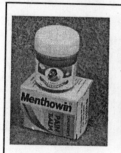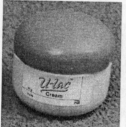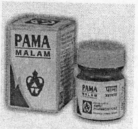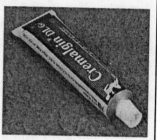

Wide-mouth bottles and collapsible tubes

(Courtesy of Sanjivani Remedies, NuLife Pharmaceuticals and Amrut Pharmaceuticals).

Figure 14.3: Containers for Semisolid Dosage Forms

Prescription No. 14.1

℞

Sulphur Ointment IP
Sublimed Sulphur — 10.0 g
Simple ointment,
white — 90.0 g

Principle:

Sulphur is antiseptic and keratolytic. It is useful in the treatment of acne vulgaris. Sublimed sulphur is very slightly soluble in water. It is obtained by sublimation of native sulphur. It is a gritty powder and should be finely sifted. Precipitated sulphur is free from grittiness; it is prepared by precipitation from sublimed Sulphur. The sulphur Ointment BP contains precipitated sulphur. Prolonged use of sulphur may cause dermatitis.

Apparatus: Ointment slab, spatula, sieves.

Method: Trituration

i) Sift the sublimed sulphur through sieve no. 85.

ii) Triturate the fine powder geometrically with simple ointment, using an ointment slab, to produce a smooth mass.

iii) Gradually, incorporate remainder of the simple ointment to obtain the final weight.

Container and storage: Store in well-closed wide-mouth bottles in a cool place.

Category and Direction to use: Scabicide. Apply every night for 3 nights.

Patient counselling: Do not apply on broken skin and near the eyes as it causes irritation.

Proprietary preparations:

PERSOL FORTE (Wallace): Precipitated Sulphur 5 per cent w/w, benzoyl peroxide 10 per cent. Antiacne.

Prescription No. 14.2

℞

Compound Benzoic Acid Ointment BPC
Benzoic Acid	—	6.0 g
Salicylic Acid	—	3.0 g
Emulsifying Ointment	—	91.0 g

Principle: -

Whitfield's ointment. It is antifungal. Fungi grows and prospers in the stratum corneum. Gradual desquamation of the stratum corneum, in which the fungus embeds, is essential for the antifungal treatment in tinea pedis (athlete's foot) and tinea capitis (ringworm of the scalp). Whitfield's ointment combines the fungistatic activity of benzoic acid and keratolytic activity of salicylic acid. Salicylic acid causes desquamation of the stratum corneum; thereby removing the infected stratum corneum and enhancing the penetration of benzoic acid.

Benzoic acid is soluble in 275 parts of water and salicylic acid in 460 parts of water. The emulsifying ointment is water-miscible base prepared by fusion.

Apparatus: Ointment slab, spatula, sieves, water bath.

Compounding: Trituration

i) Sift the benzoic acid and salicylic acid through sieve no. 85 and mix these fine powders.

ii) Levigate these fine powders geometrically with emulsifying ointment using ointment slab to produce a smooth mass.

iii) Gradually incorporate remainder of emulsifying ointment to obtain final weight.

Container and storage: Store in well-closed wide-mouth bottles in a cool place.

Category and direction to use: Fungicidal. In treatment of athlete's foot and ringworms. Apply on affected area twice daily.

Handling precaution: i) Salicylic acid is very irritant if inhaled. ii) Use stainless steel sieve for sifting salicylic acid.

Patient counselling: Do not apply on broken skin and near the eyes; it causes irritation. Take

---

a bath or clean and dry the skin twice daily. Do not share towels. Use cotton under-garments. In case of Athelete's foot, use antifungal powder in shoes and socks as preventive measure and to minimise proliferation of the infection. Continue the application of Whitfield's ointment for next two weeks after recovery.

Proprietary preparations:

- PRAGMATAR (SmithKline Beecham): Benzoic acid 6 per cent, Salicylic acid 3 per cent, menthol 0.5 per cent, camphor 2 per cent. Antifungal.

- EXSORA (Nulife): Benzoic acid 6 per cent, Salicylic acid 3 per cent, Icthammol 2 per cent, Triamcinolone acetonide 0.01 per cent. Antifungal, anti psoriasis and for chronic dermatitis.

Prescription No. 14.3

℞

Methyl Salicylate Ointment BPC
Methyl Salicylate   — 50.0 g
White Beeswax   — 25.0 g
Hydrous Wool Fat   — 25.0 g

Principle:

Topically, methyl salicylate is used for relief of pain in sciatica, lumbago and rheumatic conditions. It is volatile and should be added at low temperature. Lanolin or hydrous wool fat is a water absorption base. The water content of lanolin accomodates water-soluble methyl salicylate. Beeswax acts as stiffening agent to counteract softening due to higher content of liquid phase, methyl salicylate. Methyl salicylate causes softening of plastic container.

Apparatus: Porcelain dish, glass rod, water bath, spatula, ointment slab.

Compounding: Fusion method.

i) Melt grated beeswax in porcelain dish on a water bath. Add hydrous wool fat in melt of bees wax and continue heating till complete melting of bases occurs.

ii) Allow it to solidify by stirring. At 40-45 °C add methyl salicylate, by stirring.

iii) Homogenise the mass on ointment slab.

Container and storage: Store in tightly closed amber-coloured, glass jars. in a cool place. Protect from light.

Category and direction to use: Gives relief from pain. Apply with massage.

Handling precaution: It is volatile and should be added at low temperature. Methyl salicylate causes softening of plastic container.

Patient Counselling: Apply it by rubbing in. Keep container tightly closed. Do not apply on broken skin. Methyl salicylate has odour of wintergreen candy, so keep it away from children. Maintain proper posture while working, standing, sitting or driving. Avoid heavy physical work. To avoid back pain and pain of lower limbs, maintain a proportionate weight. Avoid wearing high heeled shoes.

Proprietary preparations:

- KILPANE CREAM (Biddle): Methyl salicylate 15 per cent, menthol 6 per cent, Eucalyptus oil 1.5 per cent;
- WORFAST CREAM (Emil): Methyl salicylate 14.8 per cent, Menthol 5.5 per cent, Eucalyptus oil 1.8 per cent, Turpentine oil 7.9per cent;

CREAMS

Definition and Uses

Creams are semisolid emulsions intended for application on the skin or mucous membrane. Creams possess pseudoplastic flow properties with very little yield value. Pharmaceutically, creams are of two types, viz., oily creams and aqueous creams:

i) The oily creams are w/o emulsions containing lipophilic emulsifying agents, such as wool fat, wool alcohols, divalent soap of fatty acids, or fatty acid esters of sorbitan (Span). These creams are employed as emollients and cleansing agents.

ii) The aqueous creams are o/w emulsions containing an oil-in-water emulsifying agent like, monovalent soaps of fatty acids, hydrophilic surfactants or a polyethylene glycol derivative of sorbitan fatty acid ester (Tween). Aqueous creams are most useful as water washable bases. On application to the skin, water phase evaporates depositing the water-soluble drug on the skin. The increased concentration gradient across stratum corneum promotes percutaneous absorption of the drug.

Creams are often preferred over an ointment, because, creams are less greasy and easier to apply. The cool feeling due to evaporation of water sooth of the inflamed area. Additionally, creams interfere less with skin functions and have more skin contact than ointments. Creams are physically more stable than liquid emulsions, because of the reduced chances of creaming and coalescence at semisolid state.

Formulation of creams

Creams are the extension of oleaginous ointments. Like liquid emulsions, these contain oil phase, water phase and emulsifying agent, but are made semisolid by addition of stiffening base. The creamy white appearance and soft texture is more appealing and it is not necessary to add colouring agents. According to the bases used, the composition of creams is as follows:

1) **Absorption base type:** As discussed above, these are anhydrous bases having capacity to absorb water resulting in w/o emulsions. Lanolin or hydrous wool fat is w/o cream, which contains 70 per cent wool fat and 30 per cent water. It has further capacity to absorb water. Oily

cream, IP, contains equal parts of wool alcohol and water.

2) Surfactant base type: The ionic and non-ionic surfactants are used to form creams. The aqueous Cream, BP, is o/w semisolid emulsion contains 30 per cent emulsifying ointment in aqueous phase, i.e., Emulsifying ointment — 30.0 g, Chlorocresol — 0.1 g and Purified water — 69.9 g.

The cetrimide cream is o/w cream, which is an example of cationic surface active agent. It is self antiseptic. The non-ionic creams are non-toxic and suitable to apply on broken skin. Cetamicrogol cream is non-ionic type, it is o/w cream containing 30 per cent cetamicrogol emulsifying ointment and 0.1 per cent chlorocresol in water.

3) Soap type: These are semisolid soap emulsions. As discussed under liquid emulsions, most soaps are alkaline and suitable only for unbroken skin. Soap made using triethanolamine is almost neutral. Cold cream is beeswax borax cream. The cerotic acid from beeswax reacts with sodium borate (borax), producing monovalent soap. The w/o type of cold cream is the choice of cosmetic for dry skin; and such oily cream is produced by phase inversion. The oily layer produced by cream prevents transepidermal water loss and it is emollient. The vanishing cream is general purpose aqueous cream based on the formation of stearate soap between stearic acid and sodium and potassium hydroxide. The other alkalis used for these include triethanolamine, borax, dilute ammonia solution and sodium bicarbonate. Like oily calamine Liniment BPC, Zinc Cream, BP, is w/o emulsion based on *in situ* formation of calcium oleate. These include wool fat as w/o emulsion stabiliser.

Compounding of Creams

Cream consists of oil phase, aqueous phase and emulsifying agent. The oil phase (oils, fats and waxes) should be mixed in its liquid form with water in the presence of the emulsifying agent. Emulsification is possible only when two immiscible phases are liquid. Creams are prepared by fusion method. Usually, internal phase is added in external phase, but when phase inversion is desired, external phase can be incorporated in internal phase. Container and storage: In addition to wide-mouth glass, or plastic containers, creams can be packed in collapsible tubes. Creams should be stored in a cool place.

Filling a collapsible tube: The soft semisolids such as ointments prepared by fusion, creams and extrudable pastes are more aesthetic to fill in collapsible tubes. The extemporaneous filling of semisolids in collapsible tube involves the following steps:

i) Cut the butter paper slightly longer than the tube with width such that, when rolled into a cylinder, made up it slightly lesser in diameter than the diameter of tube.

ii) Place the semisolid on the paper, the length of which should be the same as length of tube.

Roll it into a cylinder.

iii) Puncture the nozzle seal of tube and keep it open to permit the of air to escape.

iv) Insert the roll from the open end of tube up to the nozzle end. Hold the rolled extra paper in one hand and press the open end of tube with spatula. Gently pull the paper out, leaving the semisolid cream behind in the tube.

v) Flat ten about ½ inch of the bottom of the tube with the spatula. Make two fold of this flattened end and press it firmly (crimp).

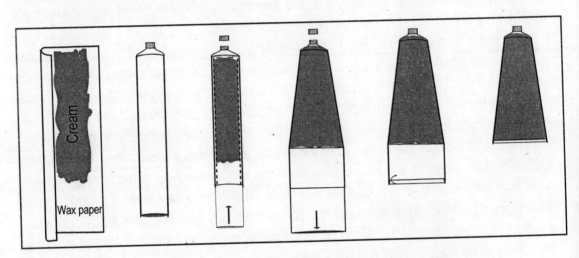

Figure 14.4: Filling of Semisolid In Collapsible Tube

Dispensing: If cream shows breaking, lumps or grittiness, crystal growth, contraction due to loss of water, it should not be dispensed.

Proprietary preparations:

- EVION CREAM (E Merck): Tocopherol acetate 1 per cent w/w, Propylene glycol 5 per cent w/w, liquid paraffin q.s. used in case of eczema, dermatitis and pruritis.

- MYCOCID (Chemo Pharma), CANESTEN (Bayer): Clotrimazole 1 per cent. Antifungal.

- ZOVATE CREAM (Glaxo), BAYCORT (Bayer): Beclomethasone 0.025 per cent. Steriodal anti-inflammatory, dermatitis.

- SILVER SULFA (Indol), SILVIRIN (Raptakos): Silver Suphadiazine 1 per cent. Applied on burns.

- BECLOCORTIN –N (Sun), BEC-N (Remedies India): Betamethasone dipropionate 0.025 per cent, neomycin sulphate 0.5 per cent. Used in case of allergic dermatitis and Psoriasis.

Principle:

Cetrimide is a cationic surfactant; chemically it is quaternary ammonium compound. It is used as cleansing agent in seborrhoea and acne vulgaris and as antiseptic in treatment of superficial wounds, burns and minor skin infections. Activity of cetrimide is greatly reduced in the presence of soaps, anionic compounds and organic matter.

Cetrimide is cationic hydrophilic emulsifying agent. Cetostearyl alcohol is a non-ionic hydrophobic agent. The mixed emulsifying agent improves physical stability of emulsion in two ways: a) The mixed emulsifier consisting of optimum proportion of hydrophilic and lipophilic agents is more effective to reduce interfacial tension. Secondly, the ionic emulsifying agent alone may result in the formation of a weak interfacial film due to electrostatic repulsion. The presence of non-ionic surfactant contributes to the formation of closely packed complex interfacial film. The cetosteryl alcohol also increases viscosity and it improves emollient properties.

Apparatus: Porcelain dish, spatula, waterbath, beaker, glass rod, mortar and pestle.

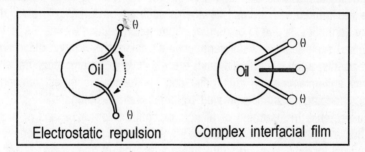

Electrostatic repulsion   Complex interfacial film

Figure 14.5: Electrical Concept of Mixed Emulsifier System

Compounding:

i) Dissolve cetrimide in freshly boiled and cooled water (aqueous phase).

ii) Melt cetostearyl alcohol, add liquid paraffin. Keep the solution warm (oily phase).

iii) Add warm aqueous phase in warm oily phase at the same temperature. Stir gently until cooled. Homogenise the cream in mortar.

Container and storage: Store in wide-mouth glass bottles. Do not use rubber or plastic containers. Store in a cool place.

Category and label: Antiseptic. For external use only.

Patient counselling: Avoid repetitive use of cetrimide and avoid contact of wet dressing with the skin, it may cause hypersensitivity. Avoid contact with eyes and body cavities.

- SILODERM (Vardhaman): Dimethicone (20) 20 per cent, zinc oxide 5 per cent, Calamine 1.5 per cent w/w. Cetrimide 1.125 per cent w/w, Chlorocresol 0.09 per cent. Gives relief in contact dermatitis, bed sores, minor burns and itching.

Note 3: Topical Remedies:

Emollients: These agents soothe, smooth and hydrate the skin. Emollients are indicated in dry skin disorders such as ichthyosis. The effect of emollients is short lived and need frequent application. Ointments based on water absorption and emulsifying base are often effective for these purposes.

Barrier and Protective: These contain water repellant substances and they are useful to give protection against irritation, or repeated hydration, such as napkin rash, bedsores. These include zinc oxide, silicone cream and paraffin cream.

Sunscreens: These agents protect the skin from harmful radiations. The reflectant barrier preparations produce an opaque, thick layer and minimise contact between the sun's rays and skin. These include titanium dioxide, zinc oxide and calamine based preparations. The substances such as aminobenzoic acid and padimate O absorb the radiations that cause sunburn.

Skin cleansers: Saline solution is general cleansing agent for skin and wounds. Cetrimide, povidone-iodine, chlorhexidine, potassium permanganate, hydrogen peroxide, benzalkonium chloride are cleansers, skin disinfectants and antiseptics. Soft soap is useful in removal of adherent crusts. Emulsifying ointments and aqueous creams are used in case scaling occurs.

Keratolytics: Dry and hyperkeratotic skin and skin disorders, involving such conditions as eczema, psoriasis and warts are treated with keratolytic agents such as urea, salicylic acid, dithranol.

Eczema: Eczema, or dermatitis, is due to epidermal inflammation caused by various factors. Emollients are effective on dry and scaly lesions. Astringents such as calamine and zinc oxide are used in mild eczema. Keratolytic agents, such as salicylic acid, are effective in chronic eczema with pronounced scaling. Coal tar has anti-inflammatory, antipruritic and keratolytic properties. Ichthamol has milder action than coal tar. Weeping eczema is treated by potassium permanganate.

Steroid responsive eczema: In treatment of allergic or contact dermatitis and seborrhic dermatitis, steroids, such as beclomethasone, betamethasone, fluticasone and hydrocortisone are used.

Anti-dandruff: Dandruff is excessive non-inflammatory scaling of the scalp. Cleansing with mild detergent, shampoos containing antimicrobial agents and Selenium sulphide is usual treatment.

Antipruritic: Pruritus may be caused by systemic diseases such as hypersensitivity, malignant diseases, jaundice, as well as by skin diseases such as psoriasis, eczema and scabies. Phenol, camphor and menthol have a mild antipruritic effect when prepared in emollient base. Calamine preparations, coaltar extract and local anesthetics are widely used.

Anti-acne: Cleansing the skin with detergent solution, or cetrimide solution followed by application of antiseptic and keratolytic, is usual treatment of acne. Abrasive agents, benzoyl peroxide, sulphur and antibiotics such as erythromycin and tetracycline are commonly used in anti-acne therapy.

Topical antibacterial: The commonly used antibacterials for skin infections includes, povidone iodine, framycetin sulphate, neomycin sulphate, gentamycin, oxytetracyclin. Silver sulphadiazine and nitrofurazone are choice antibacterial agents useful for burns.

Topical antifungal: Fungal infections, including tinea pedis, are treated with benzoic acid, salicylic acid, benzoyl peroxide, clotrimazole and econazole nitrate. Nystatin, natamycin, amphotericin are more effective in skin infection due to *Candida* species.

Semisolids

Antiviral: Acyclovir is more effective than idoxuridine.

Paraciticidal: Benzyl benzoate, gamma benzene hexachloride are common scabicide drugs.

Topical anti-inflammatory agents: Diclofenac, ibuprofen, flurbiprofen, ketoprofen and nimesulide are topical non-steroidal anti-inflammatory drugs. Methyl salicylate, camphor and iodine are rubefacient, counter irritants. Mephenesin is muscle relaxant. Topical corticosteroids are used for the treatment of inflammatory conditions of skin except inflammation due to eczematous disorders.

PASTES

Definition and Uses

Pastes are basically ointments containing high percentage of insoluble solids (usually 20-50 per cent or higher). When packed, these should be soft enough to extrude from the tube and firm enough to retain their form when emerging from the tube. They have good adhesion on skin and they form a thick coat. As compared to ointment, they are stiffer, less greasy and more absorptive.

Pastes are preferred over ointments for the treatment of oozing lesions to absorb serious secretion. Due to the heavy consistency, they produce protective barrier on the skin and also they are used to localise the action without spreading drug onto healthy skin. Pastes are less macerating than ointments because of their porous nature, which allows perspiration to escape.

Formulation of Pastes

Drug is mostly insoluble solid; the size, shape and fracture of drug determines its distribution also the and texture of the, final product. The powder passing through mesh no. 85 is mostly used. Pastes for topical use are prepared using the following bases:

1) Oleaginous base: Lassar's paste, BP, Zinc Oxide Coal Tar paste, BPC and Zinc Oxide paste compound, IP.

2) Water miscible base: Resorcinol and sulphur paste, BPC, magnesium sulphate paste BPC, titanium dioxide paste, BPC.

3) Hydrocolloid base: Toothpaste, Unna's paste, IP.

The zinc oxide paste compound, IP, contains 25per cent each of zinc oxide and starch in white soft paraffin. As compared to ointment, stiffer paste is stiffer, and hance used for circumscribed lesions such as chronic eczema or psoriasis. Resorcinol and sulphur paste is used for treatment of acne and dandruff. The emulsifying base, which is less occlusive, easily washable and has cleansing properties, is suitable for it. Magnesium sulphate paste is prepared in anhydrous glycerin; the powerful osmotic effect of these two is used to treat boils. The titanium dioxide paste prepared in glycerin is useful to apply on weeping lesions.

Table 14.2: Differences between Ointment, Creams and Pastes

No.	Ointments	Creams	Pastes
1)	Ointments are semisolid solutions or dispersions prepared using oleaginous, water absorption, emulsifying or water-soluble base.	Creams are aqueous or oily semisolid emulsions. Drug is mostly in soluble state.	Pastes are semisolid suspensions containing high solid content, prepared using ointment bases or in hydrocolloids.
2)	Possesses plastic flow with definite yield value.	Creams are pseudo-plastic.	Concentrated pastes are dilatant, otherwise plastic or pseudoplastic.
3)	Ointments are sticky with poor spreadability. May spread on unaffected area.	Soft, less greasy creams have good spreadability. may spread on unaffected area.	Due to their stiffness, pastes are suitable to apply on circumscribed affected area.
4)	Long skin residence, but PEG ointments get washed off with sweat.	Intermediate residence with good skin penetration.	Longer residence on skin with no skin penetration.
5)	Occlusiveness order- Oleaginous >Absorption> Emulsifying (w/o>o/w) > Water-soluble.	The w/o emulsions are more occlusive than o/w emulsions.	No or very less occlusive.
6)	Cosmetically less appealing. Oily, sticky, staining and poor washability, except PEG bases.	High cosmetic value. Creamy white, soft and smooth. Non-staining with good washability.	Low cosmetic value. Deposits thick visible coat. Removable from skin but unsuitable for scalp treatment.
7)	Oily ointments are emollient and protective.	Emollient, but poor protective.	Good protective and may be emollient.
8)	Occlusive ointments interfere with normal skin function.	Miscible with skin secretions; o/w creams have less effect on skin function.	Unlike ointments and creams , pastes are porous, absorptive and less macerating.
9)	Examples : Sulphur ointment, Whitfield ointment, Iodine ointment.	Cetrimide cream, cold cream, zinc cream.	Unna's paste, Lassar's paste Morisan's paste

In toothpaste, thickening agents such as sodium carboxymethylcellulose, methylcellulose, gum tragacanth, gum karaya, sodium alginate, clays and carbomer are used to maintain the liquid and solid constituents in the form of a smooth paste. Other components include humectants, such as glycerin, sorbitol, propylene glycol; surfactants, detergents, preservatives, sweeteners and flavours.

Compounding of Pastes

Pastes containing oleaginous and emulsifying bases are prepared similar to ointments prepared by trituration method. The drug is mixed with a portion of congealed base, either directly or after levigation. The remainder of the base is then added by trituration, ensuring uniform dispersion of drug.

When the formula contains hydrocolloids as thickening agents, these are sprinkled on humectants under agitation. Water phase containing soluble additives is then added to this mixture. Drug is mixed with it and homogenised to produce a smooth paste. In Unna's paste the drug is dispersed in warm glycerol-gelatin mass, which is allowed to set.

Container and storage : Pastes are usually packed in collapsible tubes, or in jars. Pastes for topical use are applied liberally, either with a spatula, or spread on lint or other dressing.

Proprietary preparations :

- Desent (Indoco): Strontium chloride 10 per cent, EMOFORM (JL Morison): Potassium nitrate. Toothpaste for sensitive teeth.

Prescription No. 14.5

℞

Unna's Paste, IP

Zinc oxide	— 15.0 g
Gelatin	— 15.0 g
Glycerin	— 35.0 g
Purified water, to make	— 100.0 g

Principle:

It is official as zinc gelatin. Zinc oxide is water-insoluble powder having mild astringent, protective and antiseptic action. Gelatin is insoluble, but softens and swells in cold water. It dissolves in hot glycerin, forming plastic gel on cooling. The resulting paste has protective and absorptive properties.

The plastic preparations containing astringents, such as zinc oxide alone or in combination with starch or kaolin, are used as mechanical protectives. After melting, the warm preparation is applied as soft mass on the affected area with a brush and covered with a bandage. It is useful as a protective and pressure bandage for varicose lesions of lower limbs. It is called 'gelatin boot', or 'Unna's boot'. To avoid settling of zinc oxide in molten paste during application, the paste is dispensed in the form of small sheets, which are melted just before application.

Apparatus: Porcelain dish, spatula, water-bath, beaker, glass rod, mortar and pestle.

Compounding:

i) Cut the gelatin in small pieces and sift the zinc oxide through mesh no. 85.

ii) Soak the gelatin in water; add glycerin and heat on a water-bath at 100°C to dissolve gelatin. Keep it at this temperature for 1 hour to destroy microorganisms. Check and adjust the weight with water.

iii) Add zinc oxide in warm glycerol-gelatin mass by stirring, and continue stirring till it becomes just pourable.

---

iv) Pour the mass in a shallow tray and allow it to set. Cut into smaller pieces.

Container and storage: Store in wide-mouthed jars and supply a brush and bandage along with it. Store in well-closed containers in a cool place.

Category and label: Protective. Occlusive boot. For external use only.

Patient counselling: Melt the paste and apply the soft mass on the affected area with a brush; cover it with the bandage. Remove the dressing after 2-6 weeks by soaking with warm water.

Prescription No. 14.6

R

Lassar's Paste, NFI, 1979

Zinc oxide	—	24.0 g
Salicylic acid	—	2.0 g
Starch	—	24.0 g
White soft paraffin	—	50.0 g

Principle:

It is official as zinc oxide and salicylic acid paste. Zinc oxide is mild astringent, protective and antiseptic in action. Due to the presence of starch, this paste is capable of absorbing moisture to a greater extent than only zinc oxide paste. Salicylic acid is used in all hyperkeratonic and scaling disorders. White soft paraffin is used as emollient and it is preferred over the yellow form, because other ingredients are white in colour.

Apparatus: Porcelain dish, spatula, ointment slab, glass rod.

Compounding:

i) Sift the zinc oxide and starch through mesh no. 85. Mix all powders by doubling up method.

ii) Melt white soft paraffin on water bath. Cool by stirring.

iii) Triturate gradually the powder mixture with equal amount of soft base each time using an ointment slab.

Container and storage: Store in well-closed, wide mouth bottles in a cool place.

Category and label: For Athlete's foot and other dermatomycoses. Apply twice daily. For external use only.

Handling precaution:

a) Salicylic acid is highly irritant if inhaled.

b) Use stainless steel sieve for sifting salicylic acid.

Patient counselling: Causes irritation if applied on broken or inflamed skin. Use for prolonged periods of time may cause sensitivity or systemic side effects.

TOPICAL GELS AND JELLIES

Definition and Uses

Gels and jellies are transparent to opaque semisolids, being suspensions either of small inorganic particles, or large organic molecules dispersed in solvent, forming a three dimensional colloidal network structure. Gel network limits flow by entrapment and immobilisation of solvent molecules and exhibit characteristics intermediate to those of liquids and solids. Most of the times, the distinction between the terms gels and jellies is not clear. Generally, gels are considered to be more rigid than jellies. Jellies contain more fluid and less cross-linking.

Gels have viscoelastic properties. The solid-like matrix structure formed during storage breaks easily on shaking a bottle or squeezing a tube. Thinning under pressure allows its easy application on the skin; and its solid-like matrix makes it adhere onto the skin after application. Topically, gels have been employed in a wide variety of products, including drugs applied on skin, mucous membranes and eyes and cosmetically as dentifrices, skin and hair care preparations.

Types of gels

1) According to nature of colloidal phase: Inorganic gel contains gelling agents, such as bentonite, hectorite and aluminum hydroxide. Gels containing polymers like carbomer, poloxamer and polyvinyl alcohol are called organic gels.

2) According to solvent: Hydrogels are aqueous gels containing an insoluble polymer. These hydrophilic gels consist of water, glycerin and propylene glycol gelled with hydrocolloids. Organogels contain a non-aqueous solvent as the continuous phase, these hydrophobic gels consist of liquid paraffin with colloidal silica, metallic stearates, polyethylene glycol. Solid gels with low solvent concentration are termed as xerogels.

3) According to use: Gels are used as lubricating agent for catheters, rubber gloves and thermometers. These gels should adhere to the surface of the instrument and be able to minimise friction during surgical procedures.

Medicated gels, such as hydrophilic gels, contain high proportion of water and provide vehicle for water-soluble drugs. Depending on the site of application, these are classified as dental, dermatological, nasal, ophthalmic and vaginal gels. Greaseless, and more porous nature of gels, allows good release of medicament.

Gelling Agents: Most of the recent topical semisolids are formulated in the form of gels. The topical gels should not be tacky, should be easy to apply and should have high optical clarity. The following are the commonly used gelling agents:

i) Natural polymers, such as gelatin, sodium alginates, agar, tragacanth, guar gum, starch, carrageenan and clays. Most of these are anionic; chitosan is cationic; whereas, guar gum is neutral. Such gels require inclusion of preservatives.

ii) Semi-synthetic polymers: Sodium carboxymethyl cellulose, methylcellulose, hydroxypropyl cellulose, hydroxypropylmethyl cellulose. These resist growth of microorganisms, but undergo enzymatic degradation.

iii) Synthetic polymers like carbomer 934P, poloxamer 407 and acrylic polymers. A 25 percent solution of Poloxamer is liquid at refrigeration temperatures but a gel at room temperature.

Compounding of Gels

The gelling agents are dissolved in either aqueous, or alcohol, solvent, as per their solubility. These miscible vehicles are mixed and allowed to form gel. Gelling can also be achieved by warming aqueous solution, or keeping the solution overnight for complete solubility of polymer. Carbomer produces gel by neutralisation with suitable base.

Containers and storage: Gels are usually packed in collapsible tubes. Viscous gels for topical use can be packed in plastic, or wide-mouthed glass, bottles. A special type of applicator (nozzle) should be supplied with dental, nasal or vaginal gels. Gels filled in roll - on are less viscous gels, filled in tubes having a rolling ball at the moutn of the tube. opening. It improves the application of gel by producing a thin uniform gel layer without direct contact with tingers. Gels should be stored in a cool place.

Proprietary preparations:

- PERSOL GEL (Wallace), BENZAC AC (Galderma): Benzoyl peroxide 2.5 and 5 per cent; ACNECILLIN GEL (Themis): Clindamycin 1 per cent, ACNESOL (Systopic): Erythromycin 4 per cent. It is anti-acne.

- CLENORA GEL (DWD): Tannic acid 5 per cent, Choline salicylate 8 per cent; Cetrimide 0.01 per cent in glycerin; GELORA (Reckitt & Colman): Choline salicylate 8.7 percent, Cetalonium chloride 0.01 per cent, Ethyl alcohol 39 per cent. Cures mouth ulcers.

- VOVERAN EMULGEL (Novartis), DICLOFAM GEL(Max): Diclofenac 1 per cent w/v; RIBUFEN GEL (Knoll Pharma): Ibuprofen 10 per cent w/w; NAPROSYN GEL (RPG): Naproxen 10 per cent w/w, DOLONEX GEL (Pfizer): Piroxicam 0.5 per cent, NIMULID TRANSGEL (Panacea), EMSULIDE (Emcure): Nimesulide 1 per centw/w. NSAID.

- E2 GEL (Sun): 17-beta estradiol 0.06 per cent. For treatment in menopause, vaginal atropy.

- K-Y LUBRICATING JELLY (Johnson & Johnson): Jelly for endoscopy catheterisation.

Prescription No. 14.7

℞

Lubricating Gel, (APF)
Tragacanth	—	3.0 g
Glycerol	—	25.0 ml
Methyl paraben	—	70.0 mg
Propyl paraben	—	30.0 mg
Water, to make	—	100.0 g

Principle:

Tragacanth jellies are also referred to as bassorin paste. For lubricating purposes, gels containing 2-3 per cent tragacanth is used whereas for topical use it may be increased up to 5 per cent. Glycerin is used as dispersing agent and it is mixed with tragacanth to prevent lumps. Tragacanth produces effective viscosity in pH range 4.5-7.Tragacanth produces gels of different viscosities. It is susceptible to microbial growth, therefore, gel should be sterilised by autoclaving.

Apparatus: Mortar and pestle, beaker, measuring cylinder.

Compounding:

i) Make powder of tragacanth. Triturate with glycerin to produce a smooth dispersion.

ii) Add sufficient water and continue trituration. Dissolve the preservative in a little water and add in it.

iii) Pour in tared wide-mouth bottles. Adjust weight by water. Mix well.

Container and storage: Store in well-closed wide mouth, jars/bottles.

Category: Catheter lubricant.

Label: For external use only.

POULTICES

Poultices are viscous pasty preparations, applied hot onto the skin, to reduce inflammation, or to act as counter irritants. The material possesses the properties of heat-retention and absorption; due to the latter property, they draw infected fluid from the tissue when used on boils.

Prescription No. 14.8

℞

Kaolin Poultice ,I.P.

Heavy Kaolin, fine	— 5.27 g
Boric Acid, fine	— 4.5 g
Methyl Salicylate	— 0.2 ml
Mentha Oil	— 0.05 ml
Thymol	— 0.05 ml
Glycerin	— 4.25 g

Principle:

Kaolin poultice is a well known example of poultice, consisting of around 50 per cent heavy kaolin and 40 per cent glycerin. Heavy kaolin is an active ingredient of poultice, because of its low cost and negligible sedimentation in thick poultice preparation (Pharmaceutical liquid preparations contain light kaolin to minimise the problem of sedimentation). The kaolin-glycerin mixture has the qualities of good heat retention and absorption. Other ingredients include methyl salicylate as anti-rheumatic, thymol as bactericide and boric acid as weak anti-microbial agent. The mentha oil is used as perfume.

For preparing of kaolin poultice, heavy kaolin is first sifted and dried at 100°C to remove moisture. It is then mixed with boric acid and gradually triturated with glycerin to form a smooth paste. The mixture is then heated to 120°C for 1 hour with occasional stirring. The applied heat and the glycerin present in it, destroy the bacterial spores and *Clostridium tetani* that are present in kaolin. The temperature is limited to 120°C to prevent decomposition of glycerin in acroline or acetaldehyde. After cooling, volatile ingredients are added and mixed thoroughly.

Container and storage: Poultice should be packed in metal or glass jars and stored in airtight containers in a cool and dry place.

Direction to Use: The hot poultice is spread thickly on the dressing and applied to the affected area. Poultice should be stored in well-closed containers in a cool and dry place, to prevent absorption of moisture by the glycerin and loss of volatile constituents.

PLASTERS

Plasters are solid, or semisolid, masses made by incorporating medicaments in resinous or waxy bases, which are melted and spread on a suitable backing material. They are intended for external application to provide protection, mechanical support, or for local or systemic effects.

Formulation

Medicaments, which are usually incorporated in plasters, are salicylic acid, belladonna extract, capsicum oleoresin, zinc oxide, menthol, thymol, etc. The bases used include gum resins, oleoresins and waxes, which impart cohesiveness and firmness to the product. The backing material may be paper wool, cotton, rayon, muslin, silk, linen, rubber or plastic. The cotton alone, or cotton-wool backing material, provides support and the feeling of warmth. The porous plastic plasters are completely permissible to air and water vapours. When these are used, the wound does not become macerated; otherwise it consequently delays healing. The waterproof plastic adhesive plasters are used when complete exclusion of water vapour and air is desired. The plasters are available in different shapes and sizes as per the area of application. Commonly used plasters are back plasters, breast plasters, shoulder plaster, chest plasters, ear plasters and kidney plasters.

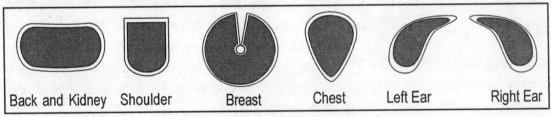

Back and Kidney   Shoulder   Breast   Chest   Left Ear   Right Ear

Figure 14.6: Shapes of Plasters

Adhesive plaster is composed of an adhesive base containing about 30 per cent of pure rubber mixed with fillers such as zinc oxide. It is frequently employed to secure dressings and for support. Salicylic acid plaster is a uniform mixture of 20-40 per cent salicylic acid in a suitable base, spread on a backing material like paper or cotton cloth. This is used as corn plaster for the keratolytic action of salicylic acid. Belladonna plaster is widely used as counter irritant in rheumatism. For preparation of belladonna plaster, mass containing approximately 22 per cent of belladonna extract is spread on a cotton cloth.

Compounding

The backing material onto which the mass is to be placed is cut into the required shape and size. Plastic mass is usually prepared by fusion method. Lump-free mass at moderate temperature is then spread upon a backing material with a spatula. Margin of half an inch is kept around the mass and it is allowed to solidify or dry.

Container and storage: Plaster should be covered with a waxed paper and dispensed in flat boxes, or individual plaster is wrapped and sealed. It should be stored in a cool place.

RECTAL AND VAGINAL SEMISOLIDS

Rectal ointments: Drugs are frequently administered rectally as enema, suppositories, and ointments. Drugs are administered rectally mainly for local effect and rarely for their systemic effect. The treatment of hemorrhoids and anal fissures mainly involves use of local anesthetics, vasoconstrictors, astringents, antiseptics and wound healing agents. These include, hydrocortisone acetate, lignocaine, zinc oxide, allantoin, heparin, framycetin sulphate, etc.

Rectal route for systemic effect may also be indicated as an alternative to oral route. Rectd routes are inducated in such conductors as, nausea, vomiting, gastrointestinal irritation, degradation of drug in GI tract, etc.

The rectal ointments are packed in collapsible tubes along with a rectal applicator.

Patient counselling:

i) Remove the cap and pierce the protective seal.

ii) Attach the applicator to the nozzle of the tube.

iii) Patient should lie on his left side, with the lower leg straight and the upper leg drawn up towards the chest.

iv) Lift the upper buttock to expose rectal area and carefully inert the tip of applicator into the anus.

v) Depress the ointment tube to release the medication.

vi) After administration is over, remove the applicator from anus. The buttock should be held closed for few seconds.

vii) Remove the applicator from the ointment tube. Replace with the original cap.

viii) After each use, wash the applicator with soap and warm water and dry it.

Proprietary preparations: For anal fissures and haemorrhoids.

- ANOVETE ointment (Glaxo Allenbury's): Betamethasone valerate 0.05 per cent.
- SHIELD ointment (Smith Kline): Lidocaine 3 per cent, hydrocortisone acetate 0.25 per cent, Zinc oxide 5 per cent allantoin 0.5 per cent.
- XYLOCAINE JELLY and ointment (Astra-Zeneca) : Lignocaine 2 per cent and 5 per cent respectively.

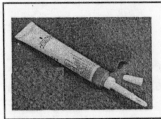
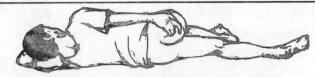

Lie on side with lower leg extended and upper leg bent, Lift buttock.

Insert applicator past rectal sphincter and squeeze tube

Figure 14.7 : Administration of Rectal Ointment

Vaginal creams or gels: The semisolid preparations containing anti-fungal, anti-infective agents are administered in the following way:

i) Remove the cap and pierce the protective seal.

ii) Attach the applicator to the nozzle of the tube.

iii) Squeeze the tube from the bottom to fill the product into the cylinder and push out the plunger as far out till the cylinder is filled.

iv) Always press the tube from the bottom permitting easy filling of the applicator and complete utilisation of the tube's tube's content.

v) Remove the filled applicator from the tube and close the tube with the cap.

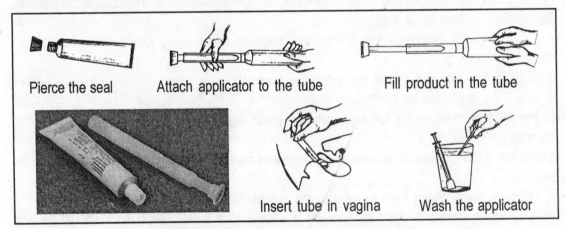

Pierce the seal   Attach applicator to the tube   Fill product in the tube

Insert tube in vagina   Wash the applicator

Figure 14.8 Administration of Vaginal Gels

vi) Lay on the back with the knees bent.

vii) Hold the filled applicator by the cylinder and gently insert the applicator into the vagina as deep as possible. Press the plunger completely to empty the contents of the applicator. With the plunger still depressed, remove the applicator from the vagina.

viii) After each use, the applicator should be taken apart for cleaning by holding the cylinder with one hand and pulling out the plunger with slight force. Wash with soap and warm water.

Semisolids

Proprietary preparations:

- CANDID–V GEL (Glenmark): Clotrimazole 2 per cent w/w. Fungicide and trichomonacide.
- GYNO-TERAZOL (Johnson and Johnson): Terconazole 0.8 per cent w/w. Fungicide
- CANTICID (Camlin): Miconazole 2 per cent. For treatment of Candidiasis.
- EVALON cream (Infar): Estriol 1 mg/g.

ADDITIONAL EXERCISE

Prescription No. 14.9

℞

Paraffin Ointment IP, BPC

White Beeswax	— 2.0 g
Hard paraffin	— 3.0 g
Cetostearyl alcohol	— 5.0 g
White/ Yellow soft paraffin	— 90.0 g

Melting Point

Principle:

Paraffin ointment is an example of oleaginous base prepared by fusion. White beeswax is a bleached product of yellow beeswax, the wax from honeycomb. It has a melting point of 62-65 °C. Hard paraffin is a mixture of solid hydrocarbons and has a melting point of 50-57 °C. Cetosteryl alcohol is mixture of solid aliphatic alcohols mainly stearyl and cetyl alcohol. It has melting point of 60-80 °C. The white soft paraffin is used for transparent to white coloured ointments and yellow soft paraffin is used when the ointment is coloured.

The product is a blend of stiffening agent, oil and water holding components and has occlusive and protective properties. Since all the ingredients are waxy and have the melting point closer to each other, they are mixed by fusion.

Apparatus: Porcelain dish, glass rod, ointment slab, spatula, water bath.

Compounding:

i) Grate solid waxy ingredients. Mix together and melt on water bath.

ii) Take away from heating source and stir continuously until solidification.

Container and storage: Store in well-closed, wide mouthed, bottles/jars in a cool place.

Category: Ointment base; emollient and protective.

Proprietary preparation:

- CETRABEN CREAM (Lyka): White soft paraffin 13.2 per cent w/w, liquid paraffin 10.2 per cent w/w for dry skin.

Prescription No. 14.10

℞

Simple Ointment, IP

Wool fat	—	5.0 g
Hard paraffin	—	5.0 g
Cetostearyl alcohol	—	5.0 g
White/Yellow soft paraffin	—	85.0 g

Principle:

Simple ointment is an example of anhydrous base having capacity to absorb water. This is a mixture of solid and semisolid bases compounded by fusion. Wool fat is pale yellow, tenacious, unctuous substance with melting point of 34-40 ℃. It absorbs about twice its weight of water, therefore is suitable for incorporate in the aqueous phase. But it is allergenic to some patients. For compounding, refer to prescription No.14.9.

Proprietary preparation:

• DERMADEW CREAM (HH Pharma): White soft paraffin. 7per cent, liquid paraffin 3 per cent in lanolin base, for dry skin.

Prescription No. 14.11

℞

Emulsifying ointment, I.P.

Emulsifying wax	—	30.0 g
White soft paraffin	—	50.0 g
Liquid paraffin	—	20.0 g

Principle:

Emulsifying ointment is an example of emulsifying ointment base prepared by fusion. The emulsifying wax is composed of mixed emulsifier, sodium lauryl sulphate (SLS) 1 part and cetostyl alcohol 9 parts. SLS is hydrophilic and an anionic surfactant having HLB 40 and cetostyl alcohol is non-ionic and oil soluble. The mixed emulsifier in optimum proportion produces emulsion of improved physical stability.

White soft paraffin and liquid paraffin give semisolid consistency. This base is water miscible and water-washable. It is suitable to incorporate oils, oil-soluble drugs, as well as water or water-soluble drugs. For compounding refer to prescription No. 14.9.

Proprietary preparation:

• HIMOST (Sigma): Light liquid paraffin 6 per cent w/w, white soft paraffin 15 per cent, Emulsifying wax 9 per cent for dry skin.

Prescription No. 14.12

℞

Macrogol Ointment, BPC

Macrogol 4000	—	35.0 g
Macrogol 300	—	65.0 g

Principle:

Macrogol (PEG) ointment is water-soluble ointment base prepared by fusion. Ointments of different consistencies can be produced by using different grades of PEG. The ointment is non-greasy, anhydrous and soluble in water. It is capable of solubilising water-soluble medicaments and is capable of increasing solubility, or dispersion of certain water-insoluble medicaments. Base has good skin penetration properties.

PEG 4000 is waxy solid with melting point of 50-56 ℃, it is soluble in 3 parts of water. PEG 300 is liquid macrogol completely miscible in water. PEG bases are hygroscopic.

Apparatus: Porcelain dish, glass rod, water bath.

Compounding:

i) Melt PEG 4000 on water bath.

ii) Take away from heating source. Add PEG 300 and stir continuously until solidification.

Container and storage: Store in well-closed wide-mouth bottles/ jar in cool and dry place.

Category: Ointment base.

Prescription No. 14.13

R

Iodine Ointment NFI 1979

Iodine	— 4.0 g
Potassium iodide	— 4.0 g
Purified water	— 4.0 ml
Simple ointment, Yellow	— 88.0 g

Principle:

Iodine is counter irritant. The higher local concentration of iodine is capable of producing excessive irritation and blistering; therefore, it should be uniformly distributed. The potassium iodide reacts with iodine to produce polyiodide, which is water-soluble and which in turn ensures uniform distribution. The simple ointment possesses water-holding capacity. Since iodine is coloured, simple ointment is made using yellow soft paraffin.

Apparatus: Porcelain dish, glass mortar, glass rod, water bath.

Compounding:

i) Crush the iodine in glass mortar. Mix it with potassium iodide and dissolve them in water.

ii) Melt simple ointment on water-bath. Add aqueous phase at 45°C. Stir continuously until solidification.

Container and storage: Store in well-closed iodine-resistant, wide mouth bottles/jar. Store in well closed in a cool place.

Handling precaution: Iodine is staining and sublimes; handle it with care.

Patient counselling: Ointment causes staining. Do not apply on broken skin.

Category: Counter irritant.

Prescription No. 14.14

R

Iodine Ointment, Non-staining BPC, BNF1952

Iodine	-5.0 g
Arachis oil	-15.0 ml
Yellow soft paraffin, to make	-100.0 g

Iodine Ointment, Non staining with Methyl Salicylate BPC, BNF1952

Methyl salicylate	-5.0 ml
Non-staining ointment of Iodine, to make	-100.0 g

Principle:

Iodine is counter irritant. The iodine ointment, due to their staining property, have poor cosmetic acceptability. The non-staining iodine ointment contains no free iodine, and therefore it does not stain. The unsaturated higher fatty acids or fixed oils containing unsaturated acids are allowed to react with iodine - producing non-staining product.

$$R\text{-}CH=CH\text{-}R\text{-}COOH + I_2 \longrightarrow R\text{-}CHI\text{-}CHI\text{-}R\text{-}COOH$$

These reactants are allowed to interact in closed vessels at temperature 50-60 °C, shaking the vessel occasionally. When the product turns greenish-black, it is tested for non-staining property. Iodine undergoes sublimation if reaction is carried put an in open vessel. It is insoluble hence, to ensure uniform mixing, the vessel should be shaken occasionally. Though the product is greenish-black, it is non-staining. The reaction usually requires not less than 1 hour for completion. Since iodine is coloured, yellow soft paraffin is used as base. Methyl salicylate is counter irritant, and since it is volatile, it should be added in non-staining iodine ointment during cooling at temperatures of 40-45 °C.

Apparatus: Porcelain dishs, glass mortar, glass rod, water bath.

Compounding:

i) Crush the iodine using glass morter. Heat the mixture of arachis oil-iodine in a closed vessel at temperatures of about 50-60°C with occasional shaking. When the product is greenish-black, take the vessel away from its heating source and check the product for non-staining property.

ii) Melt yellow soft paraffin on waterbath. Add it in a reaction mixture, stirring wells until it solidified.

iii) Add methyl salicylate in the above ointment during solidification at temperature of about 40-45°C. Stir until it solidifies.

Container and storage: Store in well-closed. iodine resistant, wide mouth, bottles/jars, in a cool place.

Handling precaution: Iodine causes staining and is sublime; handle it with care.

Patient counselling: Do not apply on broken skin.

Prescription No. 14.15
R
Resorcinol and Sulphur Paste BPC
Resorcinol, finely sifted — 5.0 g
Precipitated sulphur — 5.0 g
Zinc oxide, finely sifted — 40.0 g
Emulsifying ointment — 50.0 g

Category: Counter irritant.

Principle:

Resorcinol causes peeling of skin. Precipitated sulphur is mild antiseptic and keratolytic. Zinc oxide is mild astringent and antiseptic. Thick greasy preparation such as ointment should be avoided acne sure present. Most of the anti-acne drugs, are irritants and cause skin peeling, therefore, these must be applied only on the acne. These requirements are fulfilled by pastes. Emulsifying bases are less occlusive, water-miscible, washable, having skin cleansing properties and their mild oily nature ensures adhesion of product and allows drug penetration in acne. Prolonged application of resorcinol on the raw skin, may cause myxoedema and it also interferes with the thyroid function.

Apparatus: Porcelain dish, spatula, ointment slab, glass rod.

Compounding:

i) Sift the zinc oxide and resorcinol through mesh no. 85. Mix all powders by doubling up method.

ii) Melt emulsifying ointment on water bath. Allow it to cool by stirring continuously.

iii) Triturate the powder mixture gradually with equal amounts of soft base, each time using the ointment slab.

Container and storage: Store in well-closed, wide mouth bottles in a cool place.

Category and label: It is anti-acne. Apply on acne after washing and drying the area. For external use only.

Precaution during compounding: Sulphur and resorcinol are irritant, handle with care.

Patient counselling: Causes irritation if applied on broken or inflamed skin. Using it for a prolonged period of time may cause side effects. If irritation develops, discontinue its stet and contact a physician.

Prescription No. 14.16

℞

Magnesium Sulphate Paste NFI, BPC

Dried magnesium sulphate (Previously dried at 150°C for 90 min)	— 45.0 g
Phenol	— 0.5 g
Glycerine (Previously heated at 120°C for 90 min & cooled)	— 55.0 g

Principle:

Morison's Paste is its synonym. The paste is prepared by mixing anhydrous glycerine and magnesium sulphate. The higher osmotic pressure of the paste makes it useful to remove accumulated fluid in the treatment of carbuncles and boils. Phenol acts as antibacterial. Since it is hygroscopic, it should be stored in airtight containers.

Apparatus: Porcelain dish, glass rod, beaker,

Compounding:

i) Dry the excess of magnesium sulphate at 150°C for 90 min in oven.

ii) Dissolve phenol in glycerin. Mix dried magnesium sulphate in it using warm mortar.

Container and storage: Store in air tight, wide mouth glass bottles in dry place.

Category and label: Osmotic agent for carbuncles and boils. For external use only. Stir before use. Apply under dressing.

Patient Counselling: The effectiveness of paste is reduced if it absorbs moisture from the atmosphere. Shake the container before use.

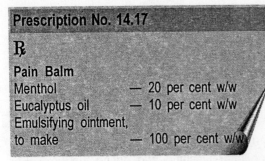

Prescription No. 14.17

℞

Pain Balm
Menthol — 20 per cent w/w
Eucalyptus oil — 10 per cent w/w
Emulsifying ointment,
to make — 100 per cent w/w

Principle:

Headache is common and is mainly due to tension and stress. Other reasons include hormonal factors, sensory stimulation due to bright light or loud sound and brain disease. Pain balm is first line symptomatic treatment for temporary relief. Menthol is obtained from peppermint oil. It is a crystalline powder with pleasant odour of peppermint. It is a freely soluble volatile oil. Eucalyptus oil is aromatic oil, soluble in fats and paraffin. It contains about 80 per cent eucalyptol. These are counter irritant and are used as ingredients in preparations for the nose and throat, to relieve decongestion and in treatment of common cold. These are formulated as inhalants, or as semisolid pain balm. The paraffin ointment, or emulsifying ointment, is used to formulate pain balm. The emulsifying property of an emulsifying ointment facilitates both skin penetration of volatile principles and ease of application, as well as removal.

Apparatus: Porcelain dish, water bath, glass rod.

Compounding:

i) Dissolve the menthol in eucalyptus oil.

ii) Compound the emulsifying ointment as per prescription 14.11.

iii) Cool the hot melt by continuous stirring. When the temperature of the mass is 40-45 °C, mix the volatile oil phase in it by stirring.

iv) Stir continuously until room temperature is attained.

Container and storage: Store in well-closed, wide mouth, jars/ bottles in a cool place.

Category: Remedy for headache, body pain and cold.

Label: For external use only. Ayurvedic medicine.

Patient counselling: Apply pain balm on and around the nose, throat, chest and back. Place 2-4 g pain balm in boiling water and inhale the vapours. Do not expose to direct heat. The use of pain balms as decongestants may be hazardous to infants.

In case of headaches, identify the factors that trigger off the headache, and take corrective measures. Pain balm is only for temporary relief. A patient should take a pain killer and complete rest. An ice pack may help relieve the pain. Drink plenty of water.

Proprietary preparations:

- VICKS VAPORUB (Procter & Gamble): Pudinah ke phool 2.82 g, kapoor 5.25 g, ajowan ke phool 0.10 g, turpin ka tel 5.57 ml, nilgiri tel 1.4 g, jaiphal tel 0.54 ml, ointment base to make 100 g.
- ZANDU BALM (Zandu) : Menthol 20 per cent w/w, Oil gaultheria 10 per cent w/w.
- IODEX RUB (Glaxo Smith Kline): Gandhapuro tel 2 g, turpine ka tel 400 mg, pudina ke phool 300 mg, nilgiri tel 400 mg, lavang ka tel 100 mg, in ointment base/20 g.

●●●●●

15 Suppositories

Suppositories are solid or stiffened semisolid dosage forms meant for insertion into body cavities, like rectum, vagina or urethral tract. They melt at body temperature, or soften, disintegrate, or dissolve in the body fluid of the body cavity, after insertion. Suppositories intended for vagina, urethra, ear or nasal cavity are also referred to as pessaries, urethral bougies, ear cones, nasal bougies respectively. These are either moulded in definite size and shape, or are compressed into tablets, or gelatin capsules.

Suppositories

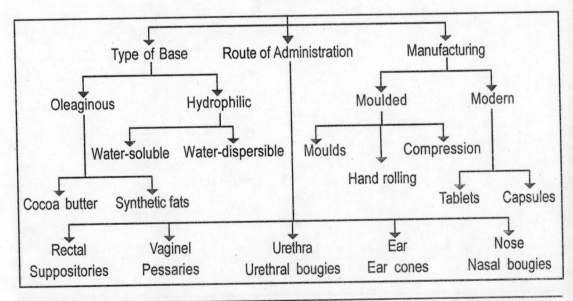

Types of Suppositories

Suppositories are compounded by moulding, either in moulds, by hand rolling or cold compression. The modern suppositories are either compressed tablets, gelatin capsules or liquids filled in plastic moulds.

1) Rectal suppositories: These may be either cone shaped with rounded apex, weighing about 1 gram, or torpedo shaped weighing about 2 grams. meant for infants cmlara Suppositories are usually half the weight and size of the adult suppositories. The torpedo shaped suppositories have their largest diameter up to about one fourth the distance from the top, the diameter then gradually decreases towards the base. Its advantage is that, when the widest part has been inserted, the sphincter muscle presses the suppository onwards into the rectum, minimising the possibility of expulsion. This shape of the suppositoies also allows incorporation of a larger amount of medicaments.

2) Pessaries (Vaginal suppositories): These are usually globular, oviform, cone-shaped or wedge-shaped. They vary in weight from 2-6 gms. Pessaries are generally prepared from glycero-gelatin or macrogol bases.

3) Urethral bougies: These are thin, pencil-shaped and pointed at one end to facilitate insertion into the male and female urethra. Male bougies are 4 g in weight and 100-150 mm in length, female bougies are of 2 g in weight and 60-75 mm in length.

4) Nasal bougies: Nowadays these are not much in use. They are similar in shape to urethral bougies, but about 9-10 mm long and weigh upto 1.2 gms. Nasal bougies are usually prepared from a glycero-gelatin base.

5) Ear cones: These are rare by use do; they are pencil-shaped cocoa butter products.

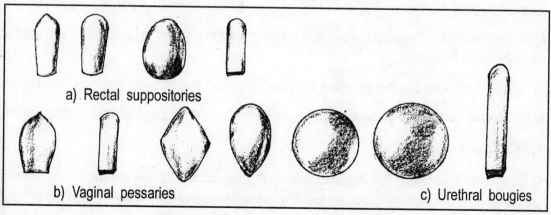

a) Rectal suppositories

b) Vaginal pessaries

c) Urethral bougies

Figure 15.1: Shapes of Suppositories

Merits of Suppositories

1) Local effects: Suppositories are frequently employed for local and systemic effects. The rectal suppositories intended for local action are employed to relieve constipation, pain, irritation and itching, associated with hemorrhoids and pruritus. Glycerin, bisacodyl and senna, which work as laxatives, by causing local irritation, are also examples of rectal suppositories for local effect.

Vaginitis and cervicitis as well as other vaginal infections, may be treated with vaginal suppositories. Urethral suppositories are only used to produce local effect, in the treatment of urethral infections.

2) Systemic effects: The rectum, as the site for systemic administration of drugs, is utilised quite frequently. An abundant blood supply at the site and rapid diffusion of drug through the rectal mucosa, permits rapid absorption of many drugs. Vagina, as the site for administration of drugs, is not generally used for systemic purpose.

3) First pass metabolism: The biotransformation of drugs in the liver can be avoided after its rectal absorption. However, the extent of drug being delivered to portal circulation increases as the depth of insertion of suppository from anus increases. Superior hemorrhoidal plexus vein drains the drug to the liver, where first pass metabolism of drugs occurs.

4) Alternative dosage forms: When a drug cannot be administered by oral route, either because of nausea, vomiting, or gastrointestinal disturbances, or in case of unconscious patients, or in infants and old patients, who find it difficult to swallow medications, suppositories serve as an alternate dosage form.

5) Unpleasant drugs: Body cavity is an alternate site for administering drugs having unpleasant taste and odour.

6) GI drug stability: To protect drugs that are degraded due to the pH of the GI tract and the enzymes present therein.

7) Gastric irritation: Drugs that irritate the gastrointestinal tract may be given by rectal route.

8) Prolonged drug release: Suppositories have been used for prolongation of drug action.

Limitations

1) Aesthetic objection: The main limitation of suppositories is the aesthetic objection of administering them into the body cavities. The administration of suppositories requires privacy.

2) Leakage: Sometimes melted suppositories leak from the body cavities, especially vaginal and urethral products.

3) Unpredictable absorption: Absorption from suppositories depends on the proper placement of the product in body cavities. The ability of retention of the product in body cavities, irritation, dehydration etc., affects drug absorption. Thus, the absorption of drug from suppositories is unpredictable.

4) Mucosal damage: Repeated administration of drugs, like local anaesthetics, dehydrating substances and irritants may cause mucosal damage.

Concept Clear : Suppositories

Suppositories: Suppositories are solid or stiffened semisolid dosage forms, meant for insertion into body cavities, such as rectum, vagina or urethral tract.
Local effects: To relieve constipation or pain, irritation, itching associated with hemorrhoids and infections of body cavities.
Systemic effects: Avoids first pass metabolism of drugs.
Alternative dosage forms: When a drug cannot be administered by oral route, suppositories serve as an alternative dosage form.
GI drug stability: To protect drugs from degradation in GIT.
Limitations: Poor aesthetic value, leakage from body cavities and mucosal damage.

FORMULATION OF SUPPOSITORIES

Drug

Suppositories are the alternative to oral route and sometimes as effective as parenteral route. By rectal route, drugs are administered for both local and systemic effects. Local anesthetics, laxatives and analgesics are employed for local treatment of the rectum and antibiotics are used for infections of the body cavities. Analgesics, antipyretics, sedatives, hypnotics have been formulated for systemic effect. The drug contained in suppositories may be in the form of dispersed insoluble powder, or it may be a solution in solvents like water, alcohol, glycerin or oil; or soft mass, oil, extracts, etc. The required properties of a drug used in suppositories, are as follows:

a) For systemic effect, drugs should have sufficient absorption from the particular body cavity for which it is meant.

b) Suppository is best suited route for drugs having first pass metabolism and drugs which degrade in GI fluid or irritate GI mucosa.

c) The drug should be soluble, or easily dispersible, in the suppository base. Drugs in solution state have better absorption and lipid soluble drugs possess high trans-mucosal penetration.

d) A reduced particle size, due to its increased surface area, increases bioavailability of the drug, but causes thickening of mass; whereas, coarse particles of the drug can cause irritation of mucosa.

e) The drug should be soluble in the base to achieve the desired homogeneity of a product, but should not have more affinity towards the base. The latter property may retard the easy release of drug from a formulation. A soluble drug should not lower the melting point of the base, e.g., camphor, phenol, chloral hydrate, etc., depress the melting point of cocoa butter, which can be corrected by addition of high melting point bases, such as beeswax.

f) Density and insolubility of a drug determines its distribution in the suppository and the amount of base required to mould it in the suppository. A minimum base should be required and a smaller and low weight suppository should be produced. The homogeneity of a product can be improved by reducing particle size of the drug, increasing viscosity of external base, or compounding close to solidification temperature of base.

g) The drug should be compatible and stable in the base and also at processing conditions.

Suppository Bases

The following are the ideal characteristics of suppository bases:

a) The base should produce a suppository that can retain its shape for insertion at room temperature, and preferably it should not soften below 30°C; but when administered ,it should melt at body temperature, or dissolve or disperse in body fluid, to release the medicament readily.

b) It should have a narrow and sharp melting point range (i.e., small difference between melting point and solidification point). At the same time, the base should permit easy incorporation of drug in it. Rapid solidification of melted mass minimises sedimentation of a suspended drug.

c) It should be easy to remove from the mould without sticking to it.

d) The base should be physicochemically stable on storage, and when heated above its melting point. Suppository should not soften/harden during storage.

e) It should have good manufacturing properties, such as wetting, emulsifying properties and high water number.

f) It should be compatible with a variety of drugs and should not interfere with release and absorption of drug substance.

g) It should be safe, non-irritant, and non-sensitising to mucous membrane.

Drug: For both local and systemic effects. Better for drugs that undergo first pass metabolism. It should be soluble in the base but should not affect the melting of base. It should be easy to disperse in the base with no sedimentation. Fine powder is good for improved absorption and for less irritation.

Base: It should retain the of the suppository shape during administration. It should melt, dissolve or disperse in body cavity. It should allow easy and uniform incorporation of the drug and easy removal

of suppository from the mould. Physicochemically stable and compatible.
Safe and economical.

Types of bases

1) Oleaginous bases

a) Cocoa butter   b) Cocoa butter substitutes or synthetic fats.

These bases melt at body temperature to release medicament.

2) Hydrophilic bases

a) Water-soluble Bases: Gelato-glycerin, soap-glycerin and macrogol bases.

b) Water dispersible bases   :   Emulsifying bases.

These bases are either soluble or dispersible in body cavities.

1) Oleaginous bases

a) Cocoa butter: Cocoa butter or theobroma oil is naturally occurring triglyceride with C_{12}-C_{18}. It is solid fat, which melts at 30-35 °C to form a thin, bland emollient oily liquid in the body cavities, allowing rapid drug release. It is most commonly used in rectal suppositories, but it has its limitations.

Limitations of cocoa butter:

a) As a natural material, there is considerable batch to batch variation in composition and physicochemical properties.

b) Being unsaturated, it becomes rancid on storage.

c) It exhibits temperature-dependant polymorphism. When the base is heated to about 33°C and slowly cooled, it produces stable beta (β) crystals, having melting point of 34-35°C. Overheating and rapid cooling causes complete destruction of the nuclei of beta form to produce least stable gamma (γ) crystals, which melt at about 15-18 °C. During solidification, there is a transition to the alpha (α) form (melting point 20-22°C) and beta prime (β°) form (m.p. 24-28°C). These metastable forms slowly revert to a stable beta form. This is the reason why freshly prepared suppositories melt at lower temperatures than aged suppositories. The lowering in melting point of bases allows settling of the suspended particles.

d) Cocoa butter is immiscible with body fluid and has poor water absorption capacity. The

Cocoa butter $\longrightarrow$ slow heating and slow cooling $\longrightarrow$ β (34-35 °C)

α (20-22°C) $\longrightarrow$ β⁰ (24-28°C) $\longrightarrow$ β (34-35 °C)

Cocoa butter $\longrightarrow$ over heating and rapid cooling $\longrightarrow$ γ (15-18 °C)

addition of water absorbent bases like lanolin, non-ionic emulsifying agents like tween, or fatty alcohols like stearyl and acetyl alcohol are various attempts to improve water holding capacity of cocoa butter. Higher lipophilicity of base can hinder release of lipophilic drug.

e) Certain soluble drugs, like volatile oil, camphor, menthol, phenol, chloral hydrate depress the melting point of cocoa butter. This effect can be minimised by addition of 4 per cent beeswax, or 20 per cent spermaceti. The use of 10 per cent lenete wax has been found to increase both, melting point as well as its water absorption capacity.

f) Because of its tendency to leak from the body cavities and its immiscibility with aqueous secretions, cocoa butter is not a good base for vaginal and urethral use.

g) Cocoa butter suppositories are liable to melt in warm climates. In such a case, the addition of beeswax (melting point 62-64 °C) increases the melting point by about 10-15 °C. Fractionated palm kernel oil (melting point 32-36 °C) is also recommended in such cases.

h) Low contractility during solidification causes suppositories to adhere to the moulds and hence necessitates the lubrication of moulds.

i) Cocoa butter has a low solidification point, which brings about sedimentation of insoluble drug at the apex of suppository formation. It therefore cannot be used for high speed production.

j) It has a disagreeable odour and its yellow to white colour that may get retained in the final product.

Concept Clear : Properties of Cocoa Butter

- Melts at body temperature
- Exhibits polymorphism
- Undergoes rancidification
- Soluble drugs depress melting point
- Melts in warm climates
- Leaks from the body cavity
- Low contractility
- Low solidification point
- Disagreeable odour

b) Synthetic fatty bases: Because of the shortcomings of the theobroma oil as suppository base, many combinations of fats and waxes have been suggested as substitutes. These include hydrogenated vegetable oils, such as coconut, palm kernel, cottonseed, peanut, fractionated palm kernel oil, witepsol, suppocire base, etc. Hydrogenation increases resistance to rancidification and increases chemical inertness. Witepsol bases are mixtures of triglycerides of natural saturated fatty acids having C_{12}-C_{18} and partial glycerides. On average, they have a melting point ranging from 33-35 °C, and are available in twelve grades. Suppocire bases are composed of a mixture of C_{10}-C_{18} saturated fatty acid mono-, di- and tri- glycerides obtained by hydrogenation and inter-esterification of vegetable oils. Suppositories made with synthetic bases like witepsol should not be cooled using ice, because they become brittle and fracture if cooled rapidly. As compared to the cocoa butter, these bases have following merits:

a) Due to their saturated nature, these bases are less prone to rancidity.

b) Do not exhibit polymorphism on heating.

c) Exhibit good water absorption and emulsifying properties.

d) They have very small melting range.

e) They solidify rapidly in the mould and shrink sufficiently, making lubrication of the mould unnecessary.

f) Melting points are not affected much by fat-soluble substances. Higher melting point bases can be mixed with low melting point bases to obtain desired melting range and have good drug release properties.

g) Suppositories of these bases are white, smooth and odourless.

2) Hydrophilic Bases:

Process of drug release from these bases is a function of dissolution of the base rather than its melting. Due to higher melting point of hydrophilic bases, problems of compounding, handling and storage can be effectively reduced. The hydrophilic nature also contributes to drug release and its absorption.

a) **Water-Soluble Bases:** These are of two types, gelled glycerin bases and macrogol bases.

i) **Gelled Glycerin Bases:** Glycerin is gelled either with soap or gelatin to produce base of desired viscosity, softness or stiffness. These bases are water-soluble and dissolve in the body fluids to release medicaments. Glycerin suppositoies consisting containing 91 per cent of glycerin gelled with 9 per cent sodium stearate soap, is official in U.S.P., which is used to evacuate the lower bowel. Gelato-glycerin suppositories are used exclusively for laxative purposes, or in vaginal therapy. The formula for gelato-glycerin suppositories I.P., contains 16per cent w/w gelatin and 70 per cent w/w glycerin. The U.S.P. formula recommends 20 per cent w/w of gelatin together with 70 per cent w/w glycerin. In order to use in hot climate or to make stiffer masses, amount of gelatin may be increased, e.g., B.P.C. formula contains 32.5 pcr ccnt of gclatin and 40 per cent of glycerin on weight basis. Desired properties of suppositories and thereby, drug release rate can be achieved by replacing glycerin partially or wholly by propylene glycol, or polyethylene glycol. In addition to their laxative effect, glycerin suppository bases have following limitations:

a) The hygroscopic nature of glycerin suppository bases may cause irritation to the rectal mucosa due to their dehydrating effect. Their hygroscopic nature also necessitates careful storage of suppositories.

b) Gelatin is incompatible with a large number of drug substances, like tannic acid, ferric chloride, etc. With ichthamol, suppository becomes insoluble and tannic acid may hydrolyse the gelatin.

c) Preparation of these bases is time consuming and they have a tendency to stick to the moulds, which necessitates mould lubrication.

d) Since they are liable to microbial growth, preservatives have to be added.

e) The mass cannot be processed by hand rolling.

ii) Macrogol bases: Macrogols, PEG or carbowaxes have been popularly used as water soluble bases, for preparation of both ointments and suppositories. These are polyethylene glycols which range from liquids, semisolids to waxy solids, as per molecular weight. The desired physical properties of these bases, like melting point, hardness and softness, can be achieved by using a suitable combination of high and low molecular weight polymers. Some typical formulas for water-soluble bases are as follows:

Formula- I

PEG 1000   96 per cent

PEG 4000   4 per cent

It is a low melting point soft base, dissolving more readily; it requires refrigeration during the summer.

Formula- II

PEG 6000   30 per cent

PEG 1540   70 per cent

It is harder, has higher melting point, and dissolves slowly.

Formula-III

PEG 4000   60 per cent

PEG 1000   30 per cent

PEG 400   10 per cent

It has intermediate characteristics, and can be used as a good general purpose, water-soluble, suppository base.

Due to their hygroscopic nature, PEG bases may dehydrate the mucosa and produce irritation. To reduce such discomfort, these suppositories are usually dipped in water before insertion. The incorporation of 10-20 per cent water in a base also overcomes mucosal irritation and facilitates addition of water-soluble drugs.

Merits of macrogol bases:

i) Macrogol bases, because of their high melting point, are especially suited for application in tropical climates.

ii) They have good solvent properties.

iii) In presence of even a little fluid in the rectum or vagina, PEG bases become soft and release medicament slowly for longer periods of time. Due to high viscosity, liquids are less liable to leak from the body cavities.

iv) Macrogol suppositories can be prepared satisfactorily by both moulding and by cold compression.

v) Macrogol suppositories are attractive, with a clean and smooth surface.

vi) They do not hydrolyse or deteriorate, or become rancid.

vii) They are physiologically inert.

viii) They do not support microbial growth.

Limitations of macrogol bases:

i) Because of their hygroscopic nature, they may cause irritation after insertion.

ii) Several drugs form complexes with macrogols, which results in slow rates of drug release. Due to complex formation, these have been reported to reduce preservative activity of parabens and quaternary ammonium compounds.

iii) Macrogol suppositories may produce fracture on storage, especially when they contain water. The formation of brittle and granular suppositories, due to crystallisation of dissolved material, after evaporation of water, has been reported.

iv) Macrogols are incompatible with number of drugs, including tannins and phenols and with plastic containers. The hydroxyl groups and water content cause hydrolysis of water-sensitive drugs.

b) **Water dispersible bases:** Water dispersible bases include several non-ionic surfactants, like tween, myrj and span. They act as self-emulsifying agents in water, forming soft, bulky and non-irritant emulsion, suitable for rectal treatment. They satisfy most of the criteria of an ideal suppository base such as:

i) Temperature stability

ii) Drug compatibility

iii) Non-toxicity, non-greasy

iv) Resistant to microbial growth

v) Good moulding ability

vi) Increased contact with mucus membrane

In order to promote the diffusion of drugs to the surrounding tissue, and their subsequent absorption, surfactants have been used with water immiscible bases like cocoa butter. They increase the contact of medicament with mucous membrane, and increase the interfacial area for release of drug by forming emulsion at the base-body fluid interface. Some surfactants are also reported to reduce drug release, and their subsequent absorption, due to complex formation.

Other Additives

The non-ionic surfactants, due to their non-toxicity, are used to improve dispersion of drugs. Surfactants also change permeability of the mucous membrane, improving drug absorption. The presence of soothing agents, such as glycerin, propylene glycol, castor oil minimises irritation of mucosa. Higher melting point waxes and fatty acid derivatives are used in combination with cocoa butter to overcome settling of insoluble drug during moulding and softening of suppository during storage; such additives include stearic acid, glyceryl monostearate cetyl, steryl alcohol, beeswax, paraffin wax, bentonite, etc. The oil-soluble antioxidants, such as BHT and BHA are suitable for oily bases. The blend of antioxidants with sequestering agents, such as citric acid and ascorbic acid, is more effective. Preservatives are more important in formulations containing water. The preservatives must not cause irritation of mucous membrane. Benzoic acid, sorbic acid and their salts, methyl and propyl paraben are common preservatives.

COMPOUNDING OF SUPPOSITORIES

Suppositories can be compounded by one of the following methods:
i) Moulding   ii) Hand rolling   iii) Compression.

i) Moulding

a) Cocoa Butter Suppositories:

In this method, medicament is dissolved, suspended or emulsified in a melted base and the mixture is poured into mould cavities to solidify.

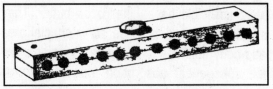

Figure 15.2 : Suppository Moulds

Suppository moulds: The suppository moulds are usually made of aluminium, brass or nickel-copper alloys and are available in various sizes having six to fifty cavities. Moulds with six to twelve cavities are more commonly used for compounding purposes. Teflon-coated moulds are available to prevent interactions of metals with medicaments, to make internal surface smooth and to prevent the suppositories from sticking to the mould. Suppository moulds are commonly made with a nominal capacity of 1 or 2 gram, moulds having 4 to 8 gram capacity are also available. Moulds of longitudinally split type can be opened by removing a screw.

Steps in moulding method

1) Cleaning of moulds: The opened plates are cleaned with detergent in hot water, wiped gently with a soft cloth and dried thoroughly.

2) Lubrication of moulds: To facilitate easy removal of suppository, mould lubricants are used. It is not necessary to lubricate the mould when synthetic fat or PEG bases are used, because they contract sufficiently on cooling within the mould to allow their easy removal. The best lubricant is one which is immiscible with the base, and which is able to provide a buffer film between the suppository mass and the mould surface. For cocoa butter suppositories, a thin film of mineral oil is applied. The lubricant composed of soft soap (1 part), glycerin (1 part) in 90 % alcohol 90 per cent (5 parts), is also used for cocoa butter suppositories. Such lubricants are unsuitable for suppositories containing metallic salts and for soap glycerin and gelato-glycerin suppositories. Arachis oil, almond oil or liquid paraffin may be used for glycerin suppositories. After lubrication, the mould is closed and placed inverted so as to drain off excess of lubricant.

3) Calibration of moulds: Suppositories are formulated on weight basis but the mould filling is based on capacity of cavity to hold specific volume of base. Although, the volume of base remains the same, the weight of the final suppository prepared, using the same mould varies from base to base, according to their specific gravity. For example, specific gravity of cocoa butter and gelato-glycerin is 1 and 1.5 respectively and therefore the weight of the suppository prepared using the same mould will not be the same. The capacity of mould should be determined by preparing blank suppository using base, weighing the product and taking the mean weight. If the calibration value of a particular mould for cocoa butter base is available, the calibration value for glycerol-gelatin base can be calculated by simply multiplying with 1.15 and with 1.25 for soap glycerin suppository.

4) Calculation of working formula: When the drug and base have the same specific gravity the actual weight of the drug is subtracted from the weight of the base, to produce a suppository using particular calibrated mould; otherwise, depending upon specific gravity of the drug, the weight of the base displaced by the drug is different. The most convenient way to calculate the quantities is to use the displacement value or the density factor. It is defined as the weight of medicament that displaces one part of the base; eg. the displacement value of zinc oxide in relation to cocoa butter is 5, it means 5 g of zinc oxide displaces 1g of cocoa butter.

The displacement values for some drugs are shown in Table 15.1. For liquids, displacement value is taken as 1, in this case, the weight of base required (B_R) is:

$$B_R = W_B - W_D$$

Where, W_B the total weight of base, W_D Total weight of drug. When the amount of medicament is very small, no deduction of drug quantity from the total weight of base is necessary, Hence, $B_R = W_B$.

For other drugs, the B_R is calculated by dividing the total amount of drug (W_D) by the displacement value (D_V); and subtracting the resulted value (Wi) from total weight of base (W_B).

i) $W_B = N \times C_V$ ii) $Wi = W_D / D_V$ iii) $B_R = W_B - W_i$

iv) $W_F = W_D + B_R$ v) $W_S = W_F / N$

Where, N the number of suppositories, C_V the calibration value of mould, W_F the

Table 15.1: Displacement Value of Drugs with reference to Cocoa Butter

Drugs	Displacement value	Drugs	Displacement value
Alum	2	Iodoform	4
Aminophylline	1.5	Ichthammol	1
Aspirin	1.1	Resorcinol	1.5
Bismuth subgallate	3	Zinc oxide	5
Boric acid	1.5	Zinc sulphate	2

working formula W_S the weight of suppository produced. W_S may slightly differ from the weight of suppository recommended for compounding. It is attributed to difference in specific gravity of drug and base. When the drug content is prescribed on the basis of weight of drug (g/mg) per suppository and when it is the percentage of drug in a suppository, it shows different working formula. But the intention of the prescriber should be interpreted. When the prescriber recommends 1 g suppository containing 40 per cent drug, it means his intention is to administer a dose of 400 mg.

During the preparation of a suppository, an excess of it (2 extra suppositories) must be made to minimise unavoidable losses.

Exercise No.15.1

Calibration of mould:

i) Type of mould: Metal mould with 6 cavities and 1 g capacity.

ii) Shred the cocoa butter. Weigh for 8 suppositories. Melt it.

iii) Fill it in lubricated moulds. Allow to solidify.

iv) Remove the overfilled base from the mould with a sharp knife.

v) Open the mould and eject the suppositories. Polish them.

vi) Take average weight of intact and undamaged suppositories.

vii) Calculation:

    a) Total weight of 6 suppositories   : 6.3 g L

    b) Average weight of suppository   : 1.05 g. Therefore, calibration value C_V of this particular mould is 1.05. (Use this value for further calculations).

Calculation of displacement value (D_V):

i) Weight of 6 cocoa butter suppositories (W_B)   = 6.3 g

ii) Weight of 6 medicated suppositories (suppose 40 per cent zinc oxide) (W_S)   = 9.2 g

iii) Calculate the amount of drug (W_D) = 9.2 x 40/100   = 3.68 g

iv) Calculate amount of suppository base (B_R)= (W_S - W_D)   = 5.52 g

v) Cocoa butter displaced by drug (B_D)= (W_B - B_R)   = 0.78 g

vi) Displacement value of drug is: W_D / B_D = 4.71 g

That is, D_V of zinc oxide is 5.

Calculations of working formula:

Calculate the working formula for 6 x 1 gm cocoa butter suppositories, each containing 200 mg zinc oxide when C_V w.r.t. cocoa butter is 1.05 g.

Calculations: 200 mg drug/suppository

W_B	=	$N \times C_V$	8.4 g	=	8 × 1.05 g
W_D	=		8 x 200 mg	=	1.6 g
Wi	=	W_D / D_V	0.34	=	1.6 / 4.7
B_R	=	W_B - Wi	8.06 g	=	8.4 - 0.34
W_F	=	$W_D + B_R$	9.66	=	1.6 + 8.06
W_S	=	W_F / N	1.21 g	=	9.66/8

5) Melting of cocoa butter base: Cocoa butter should be melted at a relatively low temperature in order to preserve stable β form. The calculated amount of grated base should be melted gradually at temperatures not above 40°C, using a small porcelain dish over a water bath. It is advisable to melt 2/3rd of cocoa butter, then remove the partially melted mass from the flame and stir to obtain melt.

6) Incorporation of Medicament in cocoa butter:

i) Insoluble medicaments: The powdered insoluble medicament is placed on slightly warm ointment slab and mixed with approximately equal weight of softened cocoa butter with the

---

help of a spatula. The uniform dispersion is then transferred back into the porcelain dish, heated slightly under agitation, till it is mixed with the remaining of the cocoa butter. It is immediately poured into moulds.

ii) Soluble medicaments: Soluble medicaments tend to lower the melting point of cocoa butter; the soft mass formed allows settling of suspended particles, if any, at the apex of the suppository. The soluble medicaments like chloral hydrate, phenol, camphor and volatile oils can be incorporated in cocoa butter upto 15 per cent without any significant effect; otherwise the melting point can be increased by adding beeswax, spermaceti or witepsol.

iii) If the formula contains semisolids like icthammol, soft extracts like belladonna extract, or viscous liquids like Balsam of Peru, they should first be softened by means of a little water or castor oil and then mixed with cocoa butter.

iv) Liquid upto 15-20 per cent can be incorporated in cocoa butter without softening effect; when the amount of liquid including volatile oils, is more than 20 per cent, the mass can be stiffened by addition of beeswax. When the non-volatile components are medicinally important, liquid can be evaporated to reduce the volume, eg. Belladonna liquid extract and hamamelidis liquid extract.

v) If permissible, the suppository of higher weight can be prepared to facilitate easy incorporation of solid or liquid drug.

vi) The volatile medicaments should be added at low temperatures, stirring continuously, during solidification of melted cocoa butter.

7) Pouring into mould cavities: Before pouring, it must be ensured that the mass is not too hot or too cool. Too hot a liquid mass, causes settling of suspended medicaments, whereas nearly solidified mass is difficult to pour. The pouring process should be conducted rapidly and uninterruptedly to avoid its solidification in the dish or formation of ridges on surface of suppositories. If solidification of mass does occur in the dish, it is warmed slightly. The cavities are overfilled to prevent the formation of depressions in the suppositories, which occur due to contraction of cocoa butter during cooling.

In case of insoluble drug, the powder per unit volume is a function of solid concentration and particle size. The reduced particle size thickens the mass, reducing the pouring ability.

8) Congealing: The well-filled moulds are cooled slowly. When mass has just solidified, the excess is trimmed off with a sharp knife or with a razor blade. After about half an hour, the moulds are opened longitudinally to remove the suppository. Whenever necessary, slight pressure is applied on broad ends of suppository for ejection.

9) Polishing: The excess lubricant is removed from the surface of suppositories by rolling them on filter paper or clean cloth.

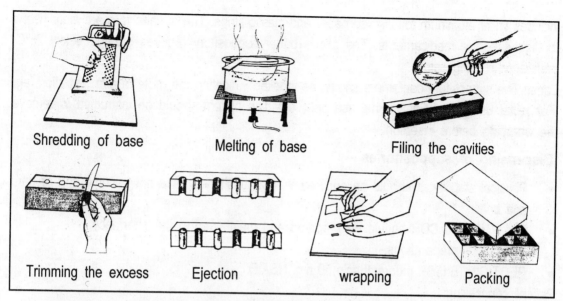

Shredding of base   Melting of base   Filing the cavities

Trimming the excess   Ejection   wrapping   Packing

Figure 15.3: Steps Involved In Compounding of Cocoa Butter Suppositories

A recent development in moulding involves the use of disposable plastic moulds. The warm liquid is directly poured in the pre-shaped packs made of plastic or aluminium and sealed. These do not need refrigeration during storage and transport. Refrigeration of such packs just before use causes solidification of the suppository in the desired shape.

Container and storage: Suppositories should be dispensed in shallow partitioned paperboard boxes, lined with impervious waxed paper. Partitioned boxes help to keep off the individual suppositories from touching and possibly sticking. In some cases, it is advisable to wrap each suppository before packaging in partitioned boxes. However, such packing offers little protection from air and moisture and plastic screw capped jars should be used. Wrapping material

---

Concept Clear :   **Compounding of Cocoa Butter Suppositories**

- Clean moulds using detergent in hot water and then dry.
- Lubricant should be immiscible with the base, and able to provide a buffer film. Mineral oil or mixture of soft soap and glycerin in alcohol, are suitable lubricants.
- The weight of suppository that could be produced by suppository base, using mould is called as mould calibration.
- Displacement value (D.V.) is the weight of medicament that displaces one part of the base.
- Cocoa butter should not be heated above 40°C.
- Incorporation of medicament: Soluble, insoluble, liquids, volatile ingredients.
- Moulding: Filling of mould in excess, slow congealing, trimming off of overfilled mass, removal and polishing by rolling onclean cloth.

includes tin or aluminum foil, waxed paper and plastic strips. The metallic foils are more useful for light-sensitive medicaments. The cocoa butter suppository requires storage below 25°C, preferably in refrigerator.

Label: The suppository containers should be labelled indicating the route of administration, eg. 'For rectal use only / For vaginal use only, etc. The patient should be instructed to remove the wrapping before insertion.

Dispensing of suppositories

- Physical stability: It should be ensured that suppositories have not become soft or hard and brittle.
- The PMR and CDR should be prepared and maintained in the pharmacy.
  Proprietary preparations.
- RECTICIN (BIISS): Indomethacin 50 mg. NSAID

Patient counselling:

Rectal suppositories: Unless otherwise indicated, a suppository is usually administered at night and morning after bowel movement.

i) Remove the wrapping. Bring the suppository to room temperature, ensure that it has softened or melted at this temperature.

ii) It is less discomforting for insertion if the suppository is lubricated with a water-soluble lubricant.

iii) Patient should lie on his left side, with the lower leg straight and the upper leg drawn up towards the chest. (Refer figure 14.7).

iv) Lift the upper buttock to expose rectal area and insert the tapered end of suppository past the rectal sphincter. A disposable finger coat or glove may be used.

v) After insertion the buttock should be held closed for few seconds. Patient should remain in bed for 5-10 minutes.

When suppository is in the form of liquid filled in plastic moulds, then it is refrigerated so as to solidify it. It is advisable that the suppositories are moistened with water just before administration.

Prescription No. 15.1

R

Bismuth Subgallate suppository, BPC
Bismuth Subgallate — 300 mg
Cocoa butter — q.s.
Dispense such 6 x 1 g suppositories

Principle:
Bismuth subgallate is an astringent used in hemorrhoids. Hemorrhoids or piles are due to swelling or enlargement of the veins in the rectal region. It is associated with pain and bleeding. Slight bleeding can be controlled by stool softening medicaments.

The soothing preparations containing mild astringents, such as bismuth subgallate and zinc oxide may give symptomatic relief.

Working formula: Calculate the amount for two extra suppositories. Consider C_v = 1 g

W_B	=	$N \times C_v$	8.0 g	=	8 × 1 g
W_D	=		2.4 g	=	300 × 8
Wi	=	W_D / D_v	0.89	=	2.4 / 3
B_R	=	W_B – Wi	7.2 g	=	8 - 0.8
W_F	=	$W_D + B_R$	9.6 g	=	2.4 + 7.2
W_S	=	W_F / N	1.2 g	=	9.6/8

The working formula for 8 suppositories each weighing 1 g is as follows:

Bismuth Subgallate — 2.4 g

Theobroma Oil — 7.2 g

Apparatus: Porcelain dish, beaker, knife, glass rod, suppository mould, water bath, ointment slab and spatula.

Compounding: Triturate the drug and pass the resultant powder through sieve no. 85. Shred and melt the cocoa butter. Triturate the drug with part of cocoa butter and melt it to produce a smooth paste. Transfer the smooth paste to a porcelain dish. Heat it, stirring continuously, to make a pourable mass. Fill the lubricated moulds as described under compounding.

Container and storage: Individually wrapped suppositories should be packed in glass or plastic screw capped jars. Keep in well-closed containers in a cool place. Protect from light.

Category and dose: For treatment of hemorrhoids. One at night and one in the morning, after bowel evacuation.

Label: For rectal use only. Remove the wrapping before insertion.

Patient counselling: Drink at least six to eight glasses of water. Take diet that is rich in fruits and vegetables. After a bowel movement wash around the anus gently with water, or it is better to pat the area with soft, slightly damped tissue. Follow the instructions given under dispensing of suppositories.

b) Glycero-gelatin Suppositories:

The basic moulding techniques remain the same as that of cocoa butter suppositories.

1) **Calibration of moulds:** Moulds are calibrated by preparing suppositories of plain base, or by multiplying cocoa butter calibration value by 1.15.

2) **Lubrication of mould:** The well-cleaned suppository mould is lubricated with liquid paraffin or arachis oil.

3) **Preparation of glycerol-gelatin mass:** Gelatin is soaked in purified water for about 10

minutes. Glycerin, previously heated to 100°C, is added and the mixture is heated on a water bath to effect a solution. If necessary, to adjust the weight, either hot purified water is added or the mass is heated to evaporate the water.

4) Incorporation of Medicament:

a) Soluble and thermostable medicaments are either mixed with a little amount of water or glycerin, before heating or can be dissolved in hot solution. The glycerin, or aqueous solutions, containing thermolabile drugs, are added in glycero-gelatin mass at low temperature just before pouring it in the mould cavities.

b) If insoluble, the medicament is first triturated in a warm mortar with sufficient glycerin and then mixed with glycero-gelatin mass just before pouring into moulds.

Continuous stirring is required during compounding to prevent 'skin' formation on the surface of glycero-gelatin mixture. As glycero-gelatin suppositories are often used for vaginal or uretheral administration, they should be free from pathogenic organisms. this can be achieved by heating the glycero-gelatin base at 100°C for an hour.

5) Pouring into mould cavities:
Skin formed on top of the mixture or entrapped air bubbles if present, should be removed by straining. The uniform mixture is poured at once into well lubricated mould cavities. Since glycero-gelatin mass does not contract appreciably upon cooling, the mould should not be over filled. The mass has to be poured rapidly, because if it solidifies, it is difficult to re-melt.

6) Congealing and Polishing:
The mass is allowed to cool in a refrigerator or on ice for about half an hour; and the moulds are opened to remove the suppositories. Ejected suppositories are rolled on a filter paper, or on a clean cloth, to remove excess lubricant.

c) Soap-glycerin Suppositories

1) Calibration of mould:
The suppository mould is calibrated by preparing the blank suppositories of the base, or by multiplying the value of cocoa butter base with 1.2.

2) Lubrication of mould:
Moulds are lubricated with liquid paraffin or arachis oil.

3) Preparation of soap glycerin base:
Glycerin is heated in a porcelain dish at 100°C. Sodium stearate is dissolved with gentle stirring and hot purified water is mixed in the mixture.

The weight is adjusted by evaporation or by addition of sufficient amount of water. The remaining stages are the same as that for glycero-gelatin suppository.

4) Incorporation of medicaments:
Soluble or insoluble medicaments can be incorporated in soap glycerin base. It is same as described under glycero-gelatin suppositories.

5) Pouring into mould cavities:
The hot mixture which is free from entrapped air is immediately

---

poured into a well lubricated mould.

6) Congealing and Polishing: The process is same as described under gelato-glycerin suppositories.

Container: The glycerin suppositories are highly hygroscopic. They require adequate wrapping with waxed paper and should be packed in a tightly closed containers to protect from moisture. They should be stored below 25°C, preferably in the refrigerator. The procedure is the same as the cocoa butter suppositories.

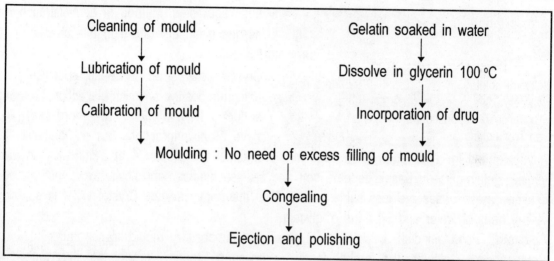

Figure 15.5: Steps Involved in Compounding of Glycero-Gelatin Suppositories

Prescription No. 15.2

℞

Glycerin Suppositories, IP
Gelatin	160 mg
Glycerin	700 mg
Purified water, to make,	1.00 g

Dispense 3 suppositories each weighing 1g

Principle:

Glycerin acts as laxative by stimulating the rectum, The stimulation is attributed to a mild irritant action of glycerin. Gelatin is a gelling agent used to impart semisolid consistency. Both of these also have water-holding properties, in turn softening and lubrication properties. Purified water is used for the softening of gelatin, so as to hasten its dissolution in glycerin. The presence of water also minimises dehydrating effects of glycero-gelatin suppository.

Apparatus: Porcelain dish, beaker, knife, glass rod, suppository mould, water bath.

Compounding: Calculate the formula for 1 extra suppository. Cut the gelatin in small pieces and soak Them in water for 5 min. Drain well. Heat the glycerin at 100°C. Add gelatin and heat on water bath to effect a solution. Adjust the weight. Pour it in a mould as described under compounding.

Container and storage: Wrap the individual suppository with wax paper and dispense in glass or plastic screw capped jars. Keep in cool and dry place.

Category and dose: As rectal evacuant. Infants 1 g, children 2 g, adults 4 g.

Label: 'For rectal use only'. 'Remove the wrapping before insertion'. 'Moisten the suppository with water just before administration'.

Patient counselling: Drink at least six to eight glasses of water. Take a diet that is rich in fruits and vegetables. Method of administration is as discussed elsewhere in this chapter.

Prescription No. 15.3

℞

Crystal Violet Pessaries, BPC
Crystal violet — 0.5per cent w/w
Glycerin Suppositories base — q.s.
Dispense 6 suppositories 2 g.
each weighing

Principle:

Crystal violet is an antiseptic; specifically it has gram-positive antimicrobial action. Women suffering from diabetes are more likely to have *Monilia* infection. But no longer is it recommended for application to mucous membranes. In the presence of a little fluid in the vagina, gelato-glycerin bases become soft and release medicament slowly for longer period of time. These bases are less liable to leak from the body cavities. Crystal violet is soluble in 200 parts of water and 30 parts of glycerin.

Apparatus: Porcelain dish, beaker, knife, glass rod, suppository mould, water bath.

Compounding: Calculate the formula for two extra suppositories. Prepare the glycero-gelatin mass as explained in Prescription No. 15.2. Sterilise the mass heating it at 100°C for an hour. Dissolve crystal violet in a minimum amount of glycerin and add this in the glycero-gelatin mass. Adjust the weight and pour in the mould as described under Compounding.

Container and storage: Wrap the individual suppository with wax paper and dispense in glass or plastic screw capped jars. Keep in a cool and dry place.

Category: For treatment of moniliasis.

Label: For vaginal use only. Remove the wrapping before insertion.

Patient counselling:

i) Clean the applicator using hot soapy water. The dry applicator should be stored in a clean area.

ii) Remove the foil wrapping and moisten the vaginal tablet by holding it under warm water for few seconds.

iii) Pull the plunger of the applicator and place a tablet in the cup of applicator.

iv) Patient should lie on her back with her knees elevated and slightly apart.

v) Hold the applicator at the bottom with her thumb and middle finger.

vi) Insert the applicator into vagina as easy as it goes. Press the plunger with index finger. Lie

Suppositories

for a few minutes to prevent expulsion.

vii) Take the applicator apart and clean it.

viii) When an applicator is not provided, the wide end of the pessary is inserted as deep in vagina as possible while the patient is in the lying position as in (iv) above.

Proprietary preparations:

- BETADINE Pessaries (Win-Medicare), POVID (Bliss): Povidone-Iodine 200 mg in water soluble base. Candidal, trichomonal or mixed infections.
- TODAY Vaginal contraceptive (Bliss chem. and Pharma): Nonoxynol-9. Spermicidal.
- KEMICETINE VAGINAL (Mac): Chloramphenicol 500 mg.

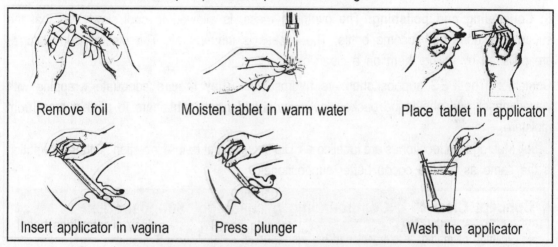

Remove foil   Moisten tablet in warm water   Place tablet in applicator

Insert applicator in vagina   Press plunger   Wash the applicator

Figure 15.6: Administration of Pessary

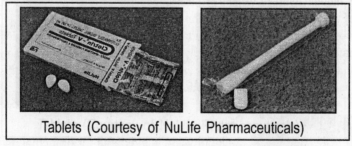

Tablets (Courtesy of NuLife Pharmaceuticals)

Figure 15.7: Vaginal tablets and Applicator

d) Macrogol Suppositories

1) Calibration of mould: The mould is calibrated by preparing and weighing the blank suppository.

2) Preparation of mould: The mould must be dry because the base is soluble in water. Lubrication of mould is unnecessary.

3) Preparation of macrogol base: The high melting point macrogol bases are melted first. Liquid macrogol and water, if present, are pre-warmed to the same temperature and these are added in hot melt and stirred well.

4) Incorporation of Medicaments: Water-soluble ingredients are dissolved in the water, which is added in macrogol mass. Insoluble medicaments are triturated with equal amount of melted base on warm ointment slab. The resultant drug dispersion is mixed with remainder of base just before pouring into a mould.

5) Pouring in mould cavities: Melted mass which has cooled almost up to congealing point, is poured to over-fill the cavities.

6) Congealing and polishing: The overfilled mass, is allowed to cool slowly, so that the suppository does not become brittle. The excess is trimmed off. The ejected suppositories are polished by rolling them on a clean cloth.

Container: The PEG suppositories are hygroscopic. They require adequate wrapping with waxed paper and should be packed in tightly closed glass containers to protect them from moisture.

Label: Macrogol suppositories are labelled as 'Dip in water just before insertion'. Other information is the same as for the cocoa butter suppositories.

Concept Clear : **Compounding of Macrogol Suppositories**

- Cleaning of moulds: Detergent and hot water. Dried.
- Lubrication of moulds: Unnecessary.
- Calibration of mould: Average weight of plain suppositories.
- Preparation of glycerol-gelatin mass: Fusion method.
- Incorporation of medicament: If soluble and heat stable, add during preparation of mass. Levigate insoluble drugs with liquid PEG/glycerin and then mix with the base.
- Moulding: Fill a mould in excess, congeal slowly, trim off excess medicament, remove & polish by rolling on a clean cloth.

Prescription No. 15.4

℞

Aminophylline Suppository, INF
Aminophylline — 500 mg
PEG 4000 1 part
PEG 1540 2 part q.s.

Principle:

Aminophylline is indicated for bronchial asthma. It is soluble in 1 in 5 parts of water. It undergoes hydrolysis with liberation of theophylline. The theophylline is also active, but is soluble in 120 ml of water, due to which, aminophylline precipitates in the presence of air, carbon dioxide or water. The oral and rectal absorption of aminophylline, therefore, is incomplete and variable. PEG base is a suitable base for aminophylline; it not only minimises the hydrolysis, but is also capable of dissolving the resultant precipitate. PEG, by its solvent action, contributes to effective absorption. To avoid use of water, one of the PEG components should be liquid or semisolid so as to dissolve the drug and to enable compounding at low temperature. In this formula PEG 1540 is a semisolid PEG.

      Use of aminophylline suppositories for more than a few days may cause proctitis, urticaria, erythema and exfoliative dermatitis. Taking into account the possible ill effects, these suppositories are no longer used.

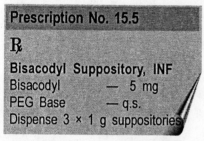

Prescription No. 15.5

R̲

Bisacodyl Suppository, INF
Bisacodyl   — 5 mg
PEG Base   — q.s.
Dispense 3 × 1 g suppositories

Principle:

Bisacodyl is a stimulant laxative. The adult dose by rectal route is 10 mg while the children dose is 5 mg. It stimulates the colon and produces faster action within 1 hour after the rectal administration, as compared to 5-6 hours after the oral route. A stimulant-laxative occasionally produces abdominal cramps. Prolonged use of bisacodyl may hamper normal process of defecation.

      Bisacodyl is white crystalline powder, very slightly soluble in water. The PEG base discussed under prescription No. 15.4 can be used. The final suppositories formed are white and have high aesthetic value.

Apparatus: Porcelain dish, beaker, knife, glass rod, suppository mould, water bath, ointment slab and spatula.

Compounding: Triturate the drug powder and pass through sieve no.85. Mix it with PEG 1540, to produce a smooth mass. Melt PEG 4000 in a porcelain dish. Transfer the smooth mass to a porcelain dish. Heat, stirring continuously, to make it a pourable mass. Fill the lubricated moulds as described under compounding.

Container and storage: Wrap the individual suppository and dispense in glass or plastic screw capped jars. Store in airtight containers in a cool place. Protect from light.

Category and dose: It is a stimulant laxative. One suppository in the morning.

Label: 'For rectal use only'. 'Remove the wrapping before insertion'. 'Moisten the suppository with water just before administration'.

Patient counselling: Drink at least six to eight glasses of water. Take a diet that is rich in fruits and vegetables. Method of administration is as discussed previously in this chapter.

Proprietary preparations:

- DULCOLAX (German Remdies); CONLAX (Bliss): Bisacodyl 10 mg.

ii) Hand Rolling

     This is the oldest and simplest method of preparing a suppository. No elaborate equipment, heating and determination of mould capacity is required. The soluble medicaments are dissolved in a small amount of water and, if necessary, mixed with a small amount of wool fat to facilitate easy incorporation into the suppository base. The powder of insoluble medicament is kneaded with the grated cocoa butter, using a mortar and pestle, until the resultant mass is plastic and thoroughly blended. If desired, fixed vegetable oil is added to make the mixture more cohesive and plastic. The mass is then rolled into a cylindrical rod of the desired length and diameter on a pill tile, which is pre-dusted with starch. The rod is cut into portions and then one end of each piece is made pointed.

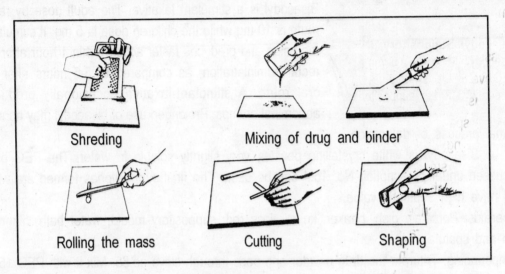

Shreding   Mixing of drug and binder

Rolling the mass   Cutting   Shaping

Figure 15.8: Preparation of Suppository by Hand Rolling

iii) Compression

More uniform and pharmaceutically elegant suppositories can be made by a cold compression process. The pharmacist should first calibrate the mould of the compression machine by preparing and weighing the blank suppositories. The suppository mass is prepared by mixing the powdered medicaments with the cold grated cocoa butter. The well-mixed mass is transferred to the hopper of a suppository machine. Pressure is applied by a hand-turned wheel, pushing a piston against the suppository mass, so that the mass is extruded into the mould. When the mould is filled, a movable retaining plate is removed and additional pressure is applied to eject the suppositories. The ejected suppositories have a small thread of mass (tail) which is easily clipped off. The retaining plate is returned and the processes are repeated.

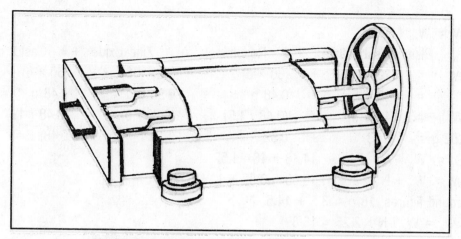

Figure 15.9: Suppository Compression Machine

Applicability of the compression process:

a) The compression process is most suitable for the preparation of cocoa butter suppository containing heat-labile and insoluble medicaments.

b) Avoids the possibility of settling of insoluble solids.

c) It avoids temperature related changes occurring, that is, polymorph of cocoa butter or degradation of the drug.

d) It increases the rate of production.

e) The major drawback of this process is, air entrapment occurs and it is unsuitable for suppositories that require heating, e.g. Gelato-glycerin and soap-glycerin suppository bases.

ADDITIONAL EXERCISE

Prescription No. 15.6

℞

Compound Bismuth Subgallate Suppository, BPC

Bismuth subgallate — 200 mg
Resorcinol — 60mg
Zinc oxide — 120 mg
Castor oil — 60mg
Theobroma oil — q.s.
Dispense 6 x 1g suppositories

Principle:

In addition to astringents, this preparation includes resorcinol. Castor oil is used for levigation and softening of powders. Prolonged application of resorcinol on raw skin may cause myxoedema and it also interferes with thyroid function.

Working formula: Since the solid content is high, double either the weight of suppository or number of suppositories. Prepare either 2 g suppository, or prepare 12 suppositories each of 1 g. Calculate the amount for two extra suppositories.

i) $W_B = N \times C_V$ $16 \text{ g} = 8 \times 2 \text{ g}$

---

ii) $W_i = W_D / D_V$

	Bismuth subgallate	+	Resorcinol	+	Zinc oxide	+	Castor oil
W_D =	(200×8)	+	(60×8)	+	(120×8)	+	(60×8)
=	1.6 g	+	0.48 g	+	0.96 g	+	0.48 g = 3.52 g
W_i =	(1.6 / 3)	+	(0.48 / 1.5)	+	(0.96 / 5)	+	(0.48 / 1).
1.52 g =	(0.53	+	0.32	+	0.19	+	0.48)

iii) $B_R = W_B - W_i$ 14.48 = 16 - 1.52

iv) $W_F = W_D + B_R$ 18.00 = 3.52 + 14.48

Taking round figures: 18 g = 3.5 + 14.5

$\qquad W_S = W_F / N$ 2.25 = 18/8

The working formula for 8 suppositories each weighing 2 g is as follows:

Bismuth Subgallate	—	1.5 g
Resorcinol	—	0.5 g
Zinc Oxide	—	1.0 g
Castor Oil	—	0.5 g
Theobroma Oil	—	14.5 g

Compounding: Triturate the powder drug separately and pass through sieve no. 85. Mix powders by the doubling-up method. Mix well with castor oil. Melt cocoa butter and triturate powder mixture with part of cocoa butter melt to produce a smooth paste. Rest of the producure is the same as for prescription No. 15.1.

Prescription No. 15.7

℞

Glycerin Suppositories, USP
Glycerin   —   91 mg
Sodium stearte   —   9 mg
Purified water   —   5 g
Dispense 3 suppositories each weighing 1g

Principle:
Glycerin is a stimulant. Sodium stearate is a gelling agent. The resultant soap also has stimulant effect. Water is added to minimise dehydration effect of anhydrous base.

Apparatus: Porcelain dish, beaker, knife, glass rod, suppository mould, water bath.

Compounding: Calculate the formula for 1 extra suppository. Heat the glycerin at 100°C. Dissolve sodium stearate with gentle heating. Add purified water. Adjust the weight. Pour in moulds as described in compounding.

Container and storage: Wrap the individual suppository with wax paper and dispense in glass or plastic screw capped jars. Keep in a cool and dry place.

Category: Rectal evacuant. Children up to 6 years 1 to 1.5 g; adults 3 g.

Label: 'For rectal use only'. 'Remove the wrapping before insertion'. 'Moisten the suppository with water just before administration'.

Patient counselling: Drink at least six to eight glasses of water. Take a diet that is rich in fruits and vegetables. Method of administration is as discussed elsewhere in this chapter. Proprietary preparation: Glycerin suppository (Apolo Pharma).

16 Pharmaceutical Powders

INTRODUCTION

Pharmaceutical powders are solid dosage forms consisting of a mixture of dry powder drugs intended for internal or external use.

Powders

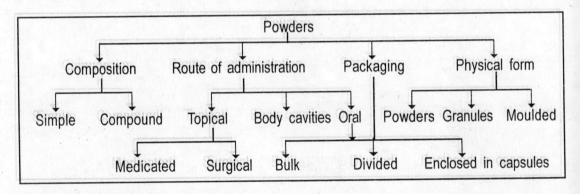

Types of powders:

According to composition: When a single active ingredient is dispensed as pharmaceutical powder, it is called as simple powder. Compound powder is mixture of two or more active ingredients.

According to route of administration: Oral powders and granules are taken orally either directly or after their dissolution in water. These are either bulk powders or divided powders. Powders for topical use are called dusting powders.

According to packing: Certain non-potent, large dose powders, dispensed in multi-dose bulk containers are called bulk powders. These are either effervescent or non-effervescent type.

When individual doses of powder are packed to supply potent drugs, where the accuracy of dose is extremely important, it is called divided powders. Unit dose of powder is also enclosed in hard gelatin capsules or cachets.

According to physical form: Powder can be agglomerated into granules or moulded into tablet triturates.

Advantages:

i) Divided powders provide means of administering accurate doses of insoluble drug.

ii) They provide flexibility in formulation; prescribers have choice of prescribing any suitable dose or drug combination.

iii) Powders are more chemically stable and less sensitive to microbial growth than the liquid dosage forms.

iv) Due to the high surface area, powders show fast dissolution and can produce rapid therapeutic effect than tablets do.

v) Provide alternative means to administer GI irritant drugs. Tablets and capsules containing irritant substances cause more GI irritation as compared to powders, where more rapid distribution of powders lessen local irritation.

vi) Convenient to dispense bulky or large dose drugs.

vii) Provide easier means of drug administration to pediatric and geriatric patients.

viii) Provide means of dispensing incompatible powders in the divided form.

Disadvantages:

i) Today, powders are administered very infrequently by oral route, because of the availability of dosage forms such as tablets and capsules, which are more convenient to handle and administer than powders.

ii) Inconvenient to administer. Usually it requires mixing with food or beverage.

iii) Compounding, especially of divided powders, is time consuming.

iv) Not very palatable way of drug administration.

v) Achieves less dose accuracy than that which can be achieved with tablets or capsules.

FORMULATION

1. Drug

i) Oral use: Active component in case of pharmaceutical powders is mostly solid and rarely liquid; the latter is usually adsorbed on the solid. Drug may be water-soluble or insoluble. It is reduced in size to ensure uniform distribution and their effectiveness. The smaller the particle size, the faster will be the rate of dissolution of drug. The effectiveness of oral insoluble powders, such as antacids and anti-diarrhoeal powders is high, if a drug has more surface area. Topical powders are less irritant in their fine form.

Active ingredient may be a low potent having small dose drug, which should be dispensed in the form of divided powders. It is difficult to attain uniform distribution of a low dose drug; and a specific method should be followed to ensure it.

High dose drugs are comparatively less potent drugs dispensed in the form of bulk powders. Bulk powders are appropriately used as antacids and laxatives. These include antacids (Magnesium trisilicate powder, chalk powder), anti-diarrhoeal (kaolin, pectin powder), or effervescent salts. In addition, powders contain some typical substances such as:

a) Hygroscopic substances, eg. ammonium citrate, sodium iodide, etc.
b) Efflorescent substances such as caffeine, citric acid, ferrous sulphate.
c) Eutectic substances such as menthol, thymol and camphor.
d) Oxidising agents such as potassium chlorate, potassium dichromate and reducing agents.
e) Liquids such as volatile flavour oils, tinctures or liquid extracts.
f) Dry powders of antibiotics for reconstitution.

ii) Not for oral use: The powders which are administered other than oral route include:
  i) Powders for external use: These are termed as dusting powders.
   a) Medicated dusting powders intended to be applied on intact skin have adsorption, astringent and protective properties. They are mainly composed of zinc oxide, boric acid, kaolin, talc, starch, etc.
   b) Surgical dusting powders are antibiotic powders used in treatment of wounds, burns and on broken skin and a the hence must be sterile.
   Eg. Barium sulphate powder, compound IP, is used as diagnostic agent to produce radio-opaque medium during X-ray diagnosis.
   c) The volatile substances are formulated as insufflations, which are blown into the
nasal cavity by means of insufflators for local effect.
   d) Douche powders are applied in vaginal cavity after dissolving in warm water as antiseptic or cleansing agent.
   e) Tooth powders composed of abrasive agents (insoluble calcium compounds) and surfactants. These are used to clean and polish teeth.

2. Additives

i) Diluents: The divided powder contains low dose drug and if needed, the dose should be made up to 120 mg by addition of suitable diluents. The common diluents include sucrose, lactose, glucose, starch, magnesium carbonate, etc. The topical powder formulations include talc due to their hydrophobic and high covering properties and starch for their absorptive nature.

ii) Processing aids: These include agents that facilitate easy compounding of powders, either minimising incompatibilities, or imparting specific functions; eg. glidants used to improve flow property, granulating agents used to produce granules and the hygroscopic and eutectic powders containing absorbents.

iii) Functional aids: Powders are converted into granules for various reasons. The granules are less hygroscopic, chemically more stable than powders and increase the bulk density of light powders. The effervescent granules minimise the violent generation of carbon dioxide. The evolution of gas causes deagglomeration of effervescent granules.

iv) Organoleptic additives: Owing to their solid state, powders are more palatable than liquid preparations, but are not too aesthetic a dosage form for oral administration. Coarse powders are unpleasant to take orally. Volatile oils or fruit juices are used along with sugars to give it palatability. The palatability of effervescent powders is attributed to the presence of citrus acids and generation of carbon dioxide.

Concept Clear : **Formulation of Powders**

Drug for oral use:
- High dose drugs are packed as bulk powders and low dose drugs are packed as divided powders. Typical types of drug compounded in powder are hygroscopic substances. Efflorescent substances. Eutectic substances. Oxidising and reducing agents and Liquids. Not for oral use:
- Dusting powders: Medicated dusting powders composed of zinc oxide, boric acid, kaolin, talc, starch, etc.; and surgical dusting powders containing antibiotics.
- Barium sulphate powder, compound IP, is used as diagnostic agent.
- Powders introduced in body cavities are insufflations.
- Douche powders are applied in vaginal cavity as antiseptic or cleansing agent.
- Toothpowders composed of abrasive agents and surfactants.

Processing aids   : Glidants, granulating agents, absorbants.
Functional aids   : Effervescent salts, disintegrating agents.
Organoleptic additives : Generation of carbon dioxide, volatile oils or fruit juice with sugars, citrus acids.

COMPOUNDING OF POWDERS

The fundamental operations in the compounding of powders are weighing, size reduction,

---

size separation and mixing. The minimum quantity of powder to be dispensed is 120 mg. To compound divided powders, at least one powder should be calculated in excess to avoid losses.

i) Size Reduction

The oral powders should be passed through mesh no. 60, whereas, externally applied powders, to avoid irritation, should pass through mesh no. 85. Trituration and pulverisation by intervention are usual methods of size reduction.

- a) **Trituration:** The dry grinding of solid substances, using mortar and pestle occurs by the mechanism of compression and attrition.
- b) **Pulverisation by intervention:** Solids, that are difficult to be powdered in the dry state are triturated with suitable volatile solvents. The solvent added evaporates quickly leaving behind the finely subdivided particles. Camphor, IP, is readily pulverisable in presence of a little alcohol, chloroform or solvent ether.

ii) Mixing

The following methods are adopted to mix powders:

    a) Trituration in mortar   b) Spatulation on paper or tile   c) Sifting   d) Tumbling

a) Trituration: Trituration of powder in mortar is employed both to mill and mix the powders. Potent substances are to be mixed with diluents by doubling up method or geometric dilution method. The small dose of potent drug and approximately equal amount of diluents are thoroughly triturated. The rest of diluents are then added in small increments, each increment is equal to the powder concentrate in mortar, triturating thoroughly after each dilution. To detect uniform distribution of potent drug, inert coloured substance may be added as marker. It is used in an equal amount to that of the potent drug during mixing. A porcelain mortar with rough inner surface is more suitable for milling and mixing than a glass mortar. Trituration produces more compact powder, which is difficult to flow and diffuse in liquid.

b) Spatulation: It involves blending of powders with a spatula on paper or tile. This method is not suitable for mixing of potent drugs. The large quantities of powders and powders containing eutectic and explosive substances, are mixed by spatulation. The latter type of substances should be mixed lightly to avoid inter-particulate friction between interacting substances. Placing the heavy powder on the top of the lighter powder can hasten spatulation.

c) Sifting: It involves the passing of powders through sifters. The resulting powders are light and fluffy. It is used to break loosely-held agglomerates. Powders that are required to be free flowing, loosely packed and rapidly dispersible, are better mixed by sifting.

d) Tumbling: It is the process of mixing in which powders are enclosed in a large container, that rotates about an axis causing the particles to tumble over each other.

Mixing of special type of drugs:

a) Hygroscopic substances: They take moisture from the environment and some of these liquefy or become soft. Therefore, substances like ammonium citrate, sodium iodide, etc., are supplied in granular form. Addition of light magnesium oxide may reduce the tendency of powders to become damp. The divided powders, containing such ingredients, must be double wrapped.

b) Efflorescent substances: Substances, such as caffeine, citric acid, ferrous sulphate and sodium potassium tartarate, liberate water of hydration on trituration, as a result of the heat developed, or in warm condition. Furthermore, any occluded moisture in the interior cavities of crystals, is released as crystals are reduced to smaller size. These drugs should be handled like hygroscopic powders.

c) Eutectic substances: Menthol, thymol, and camphor liquefy when intermixed. This can be avoided by dispensing individual ingredients separately, or compounding powder using diluents. An individual eutectic substance is mixed with diluents, and finally these mixtures are mixed together. The effective diluents for this purpose are magnesium carbonate, light magnesium oxide and kaolin. Heavy magnesium oxide and starch are also used. Mixing with the diluents prevents physical contact between liquefiable substances. Since the diluents are required in equal weight to that of eutectic substances, the total weight, and in turn, dose of powder increases to double the amount. To minimise bulk, one of the eutectic substance is mixed with diluents and another is mixed with resulting mixture. Alternatively, the eutectic substances are allowed to liquefy and the resulting small amount of liquid is absorbed in a suitable absorbent; but more amount of absorbent is likely to be needed by this method.

d) Redox agents: Trituration of oxidising agents such as potassium chlorate and potassium dichromate with a reducing agent, such as tannic acid, may result in a violent explosion. Such interacting substances should be dispensed separately, or mixed lightly in the presence of diluents such as magnesium carbonate, liquid magnesium oxide, starch or lactose. The latter approach avoids physical contact between interacting substances. Mixing, using mortar-pestle is not advisable. To avoid friction, spatulation or tumbling are convenient methods of mixing.

e) Addition of liquid: Liquid component in powders is usually flavour-oils or spirits of volatile oils. The medicated liquid drug is available either as tincture or liquid extracts. A small volume of liquid may be triturated with equal volume of powder component and the remainder of the powder is added in it with further trituration. When no suitable powder component is present in the formula, an additional absorbant, such as magnesium carbonate, starch or lactose is incorporated to produce dry powder.

When non-volatile matter is therapeutically useful, liquids can be concentrated by evaporation. Lactose is mixed in such a concentrate before it is dried completely. Lactose acts as absorbant to the resultant precipitate and thus avoids formation of sticky residue. Alternatively pharmacists can replace the liquid extracts with corresponding dry extract.

g) Powders obtained from natural sources: Powders like kaolin and talc may be contaminated with pathogenic microbes, and these require sterilisation by dry heat at a temperature above 160ºC for at least an hour.

h) Small dose drug: It should be triturated with other bulky drug, or additive and then this product concentrate should be further mixed to produce the final product. In case of powders containing low dose drug, the drug should be diluted by doubling up method with diluents like lactose; the resulting powder mix is termed triturate. Triturate of each powder should weigh 2 grain or 100 mg.

Packaging and Labelling of Powders

Powders are packed taking into consideration criteria like the potency of drug, route of administration and action of powder. They are packed in the following ways:

- Bulk containers (bulk powders).
- Individual dose in folded papers (divided powders).
- Dusting powders (dispensed in sifter-top jars or boxes) and
- Powders enclosed in cachets and in hard gelatin capsules.

Though the bulk powders and divided powders have different packing techniques, great precaution should be taken to protect volatile and hygroscopic drugs. Screw capped glass or plastic jars are superior to paper boxes to pack bulk powders. White bond paper, though opaque, gives inadequate protection to volatile, hygroscopic, deliquescent and efflorescent substances. These are well protected by double wrapping, i.e., white bond paper is lined with waxed paper and powder is packed by folding both papers together. Double wrapped powders are not necessarily powders containing potent drugs. To maintain stability some large dose powders are also packed as divided powders, eg. Siedlitz powder. Coloured papers are used to distinguish two parts of siedlitz powder. Cellophane envelops or aluminium foils are less time consuming and they provide better protection.

Label: Oral powders should have directions, like 'Place below tongue' and 'Swallow with water' or 'Dissolve in glass of water and drink'. Powders for other than oral route should be labelled accordingly, for example, dusting powders are labelled as 'For External Use Only', douches are labelled as 'For Vaginal Use Only', etc.

Dispensing of powders:

Physical stability: It should be confirmed that powders do not form lumps, cake or show colour change.

Patient counselling: The patient should be counselled regarding the disease, its therapy and directions to use the medication. Documents such as PMR and CDR should be maintained.

Storage conditions: Powders should be stored in well closed containers. The powders containing volatile ingredients should be stored in a cool place and hygroscopic powders in a dry place.

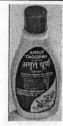 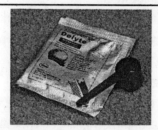 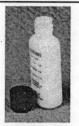

Jar (Courtesy Amrut Pharmaceuticals), Pouch (Courtesy of LiTaka Pharmaceuticals) Topical powder with perforated closure

Figure 16.1: Containers for Bulk Powders

Concept Clear : Compounding of Powder

- The minimum quantity of powder to be dispensed is 120 mg.
- One divided powder should be calculated in excess to avoid losses.
- Size reduction: Trituration by compression and attrition, using mortar and pestle. Pulverisation by intervention, using volatile solvent.
- Mixing: Trituration in mortar, spatulation on paper or tile, sifting and tumbling.
  Trituration: For potent substances. Produces compact powder.
  Spatulation: For eutectic, efflorescent and explosive substances.
  Sifting: Results in light and fluffy powders.
  Tumbling: Minimises environmental exposure.
- Hygroscopic and efflorescent components: Need absorbent components or are compounded into granules. Double wrapped.
- Eutectic substances: Liquefy after mixing. Dispense separately, add diluents or absorb the liquid in a suitable absorbent.
- Redox agent: Violent explosion. Dispense separately or mix lightly in presence of diluents.
- Liquid: Absorb in powder, concentrate by evaporation or replace with dry extract.
- Powders from natural sources require sterilisation.
- Small dose drug: Trituration. Triturate should weigh 2 grain or 100 mg.
- Size Separation: Oral powders # 60 and topical powders # 80 to 100.
- Packaging of Powders: Bulk containers (bulk powders), folded papers (divided powders), sifter-top jars (dusting powders) and powders enclosed in cachets.

POWDERS FOR ORAL USE

Bulk Powders: Non-potent drugs, where slight variation in accuracy of dose is tolerated are dispensed in bulk containers. Since glass is impermeable to moisture and atmospheric gases, wide-mouthed, plain, or amber, glass jars are used to dispense oral powders. A measuring spoon should be supplied with oral powders.

a) Non-effervescent type: These include large dose antacid powders (magnesium trisilicate powder, chalk powder), antidiarrhoea powders (kaolin, pectin powder) and electrolyte powders for rehydration. These powders are swallowed with water.

b) Effervescent powders: Effervescent salts are composed of citric acid, tartaric acid and sodium bicarbonate. Slightly acidic effervescent powders are more palatable. In presence of water, acid reacts with alkali to release carbon dioxide. The carbonated water masks the bitter and salty taste of medicaments.

Proprietary preparations:

- FYBOGEL ORANGE (Reckitt & Colman), NATUROLAX (Intercare): Isphaghula husk 3.5 g per 5.4 g. IGOL (Raptakos): Isphaghula husk 0.66 g per gram: Laxative.

- PEGLEC (Tablets India): Polyethylene glycol 118 g, sodium chloride 2.93 g, potassium chloride 1.48 g , sodium bicarbonate 3.37 g, anhydrous sodium sulphate 11.36 g. Bowel cleansing prior to X-ray examination.

- SPORLAC POWDER (Uni Sankyo): Lactic acid bacillus 150 million spores per 1.8 g. To normalise intestinal flora.

Prescription No. 16.1

R

Magnesium Trisilicate Powder, Compound NFI

Magnesium Trisilicate	- 25 g
Chalk powder	- 25 g
Heavy magnesium carbonate	- 25 g
Sodium bicarbonate	- 25 g

Principle:
This is an antacid powder. Refer Note 2, antacids.
Apparatus: Mortar and pestle, Sieves.
Compounding: Sieve the powders using sieve no. 60 and mix them by doubling up method, using mortar.
Container and storage: Packed in screw-capped glass or plastic jar. Store in well-closed containers in a dry place.

Category and dose: Antacid. 1-5 g.

Patient counselling: Take dose with water between meals or at bed time. Avoid administering to patients with hypophosphataemia and impairment of renal function. If diarrhoea occurs, discontinue the use and contact a physician. Do not co-administer with antidepressants, antiepileptic drugs and enteric coated dosage forms.

R

Compound Effervescent Powder, BPC
Powder No.1:
Sodium Bicarbonate — 2.5 g
Sodium Potassium Tartarate — 7.5 g
Powder No. 2:
Tartaric Acid — 2.5 g

Principle:

Synonym is Seidlitz powder. It is an effervescent type of laxative powder. Sodium potassium tartarate is a saline laxative. Sodium bicarbonate and tartaric acid are effervescent salts. In presence of water two molecules of sodium bicarbonate react with one molecule of tartaric acid to cause neutralisation. Carbon dioxide, which is evolved, makes the preparation more pleasant. Saline taste is covered by the acidic taste. 2.5 g sodium bicarbonate neutralises 2.23 g of tartaric acid. The 10-12 per cent unreacted tartaric acid contributes for slight acidic taste.

$$H_6C_4O_6 \quad + \quad 2NaHCO_3 \quad \rightarrow \quad Na_2C_4H_4O_6 \quad + \quad 2H_2O \quad + \quad 2CO_2$$

| Tartaric acid | Sodium bicarbonate | Sodium tartarate | Water | Carbon dioxide |

The neutralisation of tartaric acid by 2.5 g of sodium bicarbonate is:

$$\frac{2.5 \text{ g sodium bicarbonate}}{168.02 \text{ mol.wt. of sodium bicarbonate}} = \frac{x \text{ g of tartaric acid}}{15.09 \text{ g mol.wt. of tartaric acid}} = 2.23 \text{ g of tartaric acid}$$

The sodium potassium tartarate is tetrahydrate, i.e., has four molecules of water. It loses this water due to the heat produced during trituration. Furthermore, any accumulated moisture, in the interior cavities of crystals, is released as the crystals reduce in size. Sodium bicarbonate and tartaric acid are hygroscopic at high humidity; during compounding, or during storage, these powders may provide water required for effervescent reaction. To avoid reaction during storage, though it is bulk powder, it is divided so as to separate tartaric acid and sodium bicarbonate.

Apparatus: Mortar and pestle, sieve, wax paper and white bond paper and blue bond paper.
Method:

i)   Triturate the individual powder. Pass each through sieve no.60.

ii) Mix ingredient of Powder No. 1. Double wrap using blue paper.

iii) Mix ingredient of Powder No. 2. Double wrap using white paper.

Container and storage: Double wrapping. Store in dry place. Use within two weeks.

Category and dose: They are saline laxatives. Add one packet of each powder in a glassful of warm water and take the liquid while still effervescing.

Dispensing: These are hygroscopic powders. The swelling or moistening of powder indicates water uptake.

Patient counselling: Take fibrous food containing fruit pulp and excess water.

Modern Dispensing Pharmacy

Divided Powders (Chartulae): Potent drugs, for which accuracy of dose is extremely important are dispensed in the form of individual doses packed in folded paper. The minimum weight of divided powder is 120 mg. To compensate for the loss of material, the ingredients should be weighed in excess at least for one powder. After mixing, each dose of powder is weighed separately, or the powder bed of uniform thickness is divided into required number of blocks with a spatula. The division scale on pill tile serves as a guide to divide powders. Each division is then packed. The paper used for wrapping is either white bond paper, or moisture-resistant paper (glassine or vegetable parchment paper).

The method for fold packing of divided powders is as follows:

a) Cut paper 'chart' in appropriate size; the common paper sizes that have been used are 70 × 95 mm, 76 × 114 mm, 95 × 127 mm, 114 × 152 mm.

b) Fold over approximately ½ inch of the long edge of the paper (fold 1).

c) Place the weighed powder towards the folded edge of the paper. The reading of the balance must be adjusted on zero before each weighing.

d) Turn the unfolded long edge up and fit it into the crease of the top fold (fold 2).

e) Pull the top folds towards you until it divides the remainder of the paper approximately in half (fold 3).

f) Place the folded paper lengthwise on an open powder box and fold the ends so that the finished paper will just fit into the box.

g) The wrapped powders are dispensed in hinged cover cardboard boxes. The most common practice is to face all powder papers in the same direction with the top fold uppermost. Alternatively, the half of the powders is placed with the top folds upward and half with the top folds downwards.

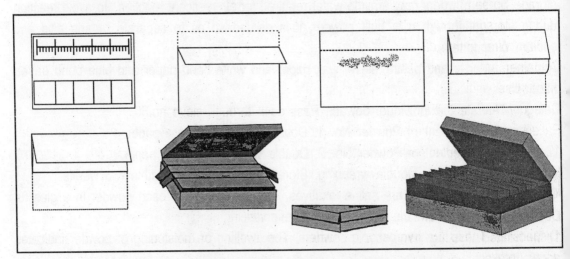

Figure 16.2: Paper Folding to Wrap Divided Powders

Pharmaceutical Powders

Cellophane, or plastic envelops, may be used instead of wrapping, for enclosing the divided powders. The cellophane envelops with built-in seal take less time than the traditional powder wrapping and secondly, they are best for hygroscopic drugs. Filling in the hard gelatin capsules proves a more suitable alternative to dispense divided powders.

Prescription No. 16.3

℞

Belladonna tincture — 0.6 ml

Aspirin — 0.3 g

Send 9 powders

Principle:

This is the example of powders containing liquid. Belladonna tincture and belladonna extract contains 0.03 g and 1.2 g of belladonna alkaloid per 100 ml respectively. Therefore 6ml of belladonna tincture can be replaced by 0.15 g of belladonna dry extract. The belladonna tincture can not be concentrated by evaporation because hyoscyamine gets readily converted by heat to less active atropine. Aspirin in presence of water readily undergoes hydrolysis to produce more irritant salicylic acid. The weight of each powder is above 120 mg, therefore, no diluents are required.

Working formula for 10 powders

Belladonna dry extract — 0.15 g

Aspirin — 3.0 g

Apparatus: Pill tile, spatula, beaker, sieves.

Compounding:

i) Sift powders through sieve no.60.

ii) Weigh the powders for one extra powder.

iii) Mix belladonna dry extract with equal amount of aspirin. Mix remaining aspirin by trituration.

iv) Spread powder mixture in the form of uniform layer on the pill tile, and with the help of spatula divide it in 10 equal portions.

v) Wrap individual portions and dispense.

Container and storage : Wrap in white demy paper or in cellophane envelop. Store in dry place. Use within two weeks.

Category: Antispasmodic; 1 powder three times a day for 3 days.

Patient counselling : Take after meals with plenty of water. Avoid administering to children under 12 years, and in breast feeding mothers, and to patients suffering from GI ulcer and in glucoma.

POWDERS FOR EXTERNAL USE

Dusting Powders: Powders for external use are termed as dusting powders.

1) Medicated dusting powders: These are intended to be applied on intact skin and have adsorptive, astringent, protective and lubricant properties. They are applied topically, where friction occurs between opposite skin surfaces. The additives in dusting powders are mainly included to facilitate easy application and to confirm skin residence. Zinc oxide and zinc sulphate are astringents, volatile oils are counter irritants, and starch and kaolin are absorbents. Aluminum stearate, magnesium stearate, zinc oxide and zinc stearate improve skin adherence of the   powders. Talc and zinc stearate impart slip property. Dusting powders are not applied on broken skin and areas that are very moist, otherwise the powder tends to cake and abrade the skin. Powder for external use can be dispensed in containers with perforated closure or in an aerosol containers for spraying.

2) Surgical dusting powders : These are used in the treatment of wounds, burns and on broken skin and these must be sterile. These should be packed in heat-resistant paper envelop, or in small sized glass, or plastic, bottles having nozzles.

Diagnostic Powders: Barium sulphate powder, Compound, IP, is used as diagnostic agent to produce radio-opaque medium during x-ray diagnosis. Though such powders are administered by oral route, these do not have medicinal value.

Insufflations: These are fine powders intended to be introduced into body cavities, such as ears, nose, vagina and throat. The volatile substances are formulated as insufflations, which are blown into the nasal cavity by means of insufflators for local effect. The powder is blown along with air current that is developed by pressing the bulb of insufflator. Now a days aerosols have replaced such techniques.

Douche Powders: These are applied in vaginal cavity, after dissolving in warm water, as antiseptic or cleansing agents. These powders mainly include antiseptics, astringents and deodorants, such as methyl salicylate, peppermint oil, thymol, menthol, eucalyptus oil, alum, tannic acid, zinc sulphate etc. The pH of resultant aqueous liquid should be in the range of 3.5-5. A special type of rubber syringe and nozzle is supplied with powder.

Toothpowders: Dentifrice powders composed of abrasive agents, such as insoluble calcium compounds and surfactants. These are used to clean and polish teeth.

Proprietary preparations:
- CANDID DUSTING POWDER (Glenmark): Clotrimazole 1 per cent w/w, talc. Antifungal.
- ABZORB Absorbable dusting powder (Croslands), MYCODERM-C (FDC): Clotrimazole 1per centw/w, talc and starch. Antifungal.
- MYCODERM (FDC): Salicylic acid 3 per cent, benzoic acid 6 per cent, menthol 0.08 per cent, starch 31 per cent, purified talc. Dermatitis.
- BETADINE (Win-Medicare), WOKADINE (Wockhardt): Povidone Iodine 5 per cent.Antiseptic.
- TANTUM VAG DOUCHE (Elder): Benzydamine 500 mg. Pre and post operative gynaecological surgery.

R

Zinc, Starch Dusting Powder, NFI

Zinc Oxide — 25 g
Starch Powder — 25 g

Principle:

This is medicated dusting powder. Zinc oxide is astringent and mild antiseptic and starch is absorbant.

Apparatus: Mortar and pestle, sieves.

Compounding:

i) Sieve the powders using sieve no 85.

ii) Mix them by doubling up method using mortar.

iii) Sift the powder.

Container and storage: Store in screw-capped coloured glass or plastic jars having a perforated seal; store in a cool place.

Category: Astringent, antiseptic and soothing powder.

Label: For external use only.

Patient counselling: Do not apply on broken skin and areas that are very moist, otherwise powder tends to cake and abrade the skin.

GRANULES

Granulation is the process of size enlargement, in which powders are made to adhere to form larger particles called granules. Granules can be used as dosage form, filled in hard gelatin capsules, or compressed in tablets.

Advantages:

The powders are converted into granules for the following reasons:

a) To increase bulk density, which that in turn reduces the volume and the size of container.
b) Suitable for large dose drugs, which have difficulty in compounding in the form of liquids.
c) To improve stability against humidity.
d) To ensure uniform distribution of added drugs.
e) To improve flowability.
f) To improve palatability.
g) To avoid violent effervescent reaction upon addition to water, the effervescent salts are converted into granules.

Disadvantages:

a) The multi-step process involves moistening and drying of powders.
b) Not suitable for water-sensitive and heat-sensitive drugs.
c) Requires more skill than it takes in making powders.
d) Slower drug action compared to powders.

Proprietary preparations :

- EVACUOL (Franco-Indian): Karaya gum 3.1 g, sennosides A & B calcium 15 mg per 5 g : Laxative.
- FROBEN-FR (Knoll Pharma): Flurbiprofen 100 mg. NSAID.
- HEPA-MERZ GRANULES (Win-medicare): L-ornithine-L- aspartate 3 g. Hyperammonaemia.
- Cap. OMEZOL (Megacares) E.C.Granules: Omeprazole 20 mg. Proton pump inhibitor
- ERYTHROCIN (Abbott): Erythromycin 400 mg. Antibiotic.

Non-Effervescent Granules

Granules, as dosage forms, are mainly compounded by wet granulation or are based on effervescent salts. Wet granulation is the process in which a granulating liquid is mixed with powder mixture to form a coherent mass, which is forced through a screen to yield wet granules, they are then dried. Typical granulating liquid includes water, ethanol and isopropyl alcohol, either alone or in combination or they may contain a dissolved or dispersed binding agent. The amount of granulating liquid that will produce a mass which is compactable and easily gripped in the hand, is usually sufficient. The resulting damp mass is then screened using 6 or 8 no. mesh screen, by hand. These granules are either air dried, or dried in the oven. After drying, they are again screened, using sieve no.16-22, to obtain the desired granule size.

Prescription No. 16.5

℞

Methylcellulose Granules, BPC

Methyl cellulose 2500	— 64.0 g
Amaranth colour	— 0.02 g
Saccharin sodium	— 0.1 g
Vanillin	— 0.2 g
Acacia powder	— 4.0 g
Lactose	— 31.86 g

Principle:

Methylcellulose swells in water, producing viscous colloidal solution. It is used as bulk laxative in the treatment of chronic constipation. When taken with water, it swells producing colloidal solution in upper GIT. After about 4-5 hours of administration, it enters the colon in the form of a gel, which increases the bulk and softens the stools. The dose of methylcellulose varies according to grade. In general, as laxative, 1 - 3.5 g of methyl cellulose should be taken with at least 300 ml of water. When it is taken with little amount of water, methylcellulose takes up water from GIT, restricting water loss and hence it also acts as an antidiarrhoeal and also controls colostomy.

The granules are prepared by wet granulation. Acacia acts as binder and lactose is diluent. Since methylcellulose swells in water, it is not needed to incorporate disintegrating agent. Vanillin and saccharin imparts palatability. The quantity of amaranth (20 mg) is not directly weighable; therefore, it is triturated with lactose.

100 mg amaranth + 900 mg lactose = 1000 mg triturate:

200 mg of triturate should be used for compounding. This technique also contributes to uniform distribution of amaranath colour.

Apparatus: Mortar and pestle, sieves.

Compounding: Mix methylcellulose, acacia, lactose (31.68 g) and amaranth triturate (200 mg) by doubling up method. Dissolve vanillin and sodium saccharin in minimum amount of water. Mix this solution with above powder mass. Continue mixing with sufficient water to form coherent mass and pass the coherent mass through a granulating sieve no.6 or 8. Dry these granules at temperature not exceeding 60^0C. Size these granules using sieve no.22.

Container and storage: Sachets containing unit dose, or bulk pack in plastic or glass jars. Keep in airtight containers.

Category and dose: Laxative: 1.5-6 g with at least 300 ml water.

Antidiarrhoeal: 1.5-6 g with little water.

Dispensing: If a product is moist and cohesive, or has formed a cake or shows colour change, it should not be dispensed.

Patient counselling: If constipated, take high fluid intake. In case of diarrhoea, minimise liquid intake for 30 minutes before and after the dose.

Effervescent Granules

The effervescent powders are converted into granules to avoid violent acid-base reactions upon addition to water and, in turn to minimise loss of solution due to uncontrollable effervescence. Secondly, granules, due to their reduced surface area, are less hygroscopic. The effervescent granules prepared by heating method should contain citric acid monohydrate, tartaric acid and sodium bicarbonate in the ratio of 1:1.55:2.94. Powdered sugar can be added in effervescent granules to improve palatability. Citric acid is used for duel purpose, to impart slightly acidic taste, which makes granules more palatable and to provide water of crystallisation as granulating liquid. The use of tartaric acid alone is not capable of producing granules of sufficient mechanical strength. One molecule of citric acid reacts with three molecules of sodium bicarbonate, releasing four molecules of water, whereas one molecule of tartaric acid reacts with two molecules of sodium bicarbonate, releasing two water molecules.

$$H_8C_6O_7.H_2O + 3NaHCO_3 \longrightarrow Na_3C_6H_5O_7 + 4H_2O + 3CO_2$$

Citric acid · · · · Sodium bicarbonate · · · · Sodium citrate · · · · Water · · · · Carbon dioxide

During heating of effervescent salts, acid releases water of crystallisation. In presence of this little water, partial interaction between acid and alkali occurs to produce more water. The water of crystallisation released by citric acid, plus water produced by reactions between acids and sodium bicarbonate, acts as granulating liquid. The 12-15 per cent loss of weight, which occurs during granulation, is attributed to partial reaction between acid and alkalis with formation of carbon dioxide and water.

Effervescent granules are prepared with the aid of heat, which is one of the method of dry granulation. The effervescent granules are also prepared by wet granulation using non-aqueous solvent, such as alcohol, as granulating liquid. In this method, it is not necessary to add citric acid.

Concept Clear : Granulation

- Granulation is the process of size enlargement in which powders are made to adhere to form larger particles.
- Non-effervescent granules are prepared by wet granulation method, which involves mixing the granulating liquid with powder, wet screening (# 6), drying and sizing (# 22).
- Effervescent granules are prepared from effervescent salt by heating method, or by using alcohol as granulating agent.
- Effervescent salts: Citric acid monohydrate, tartaric acid and sodium bicarbonate in ratio of 1:1.55:2.94.
- Citric acid imparts slightly acidic taste and provides water of crystallisation as granulating agent.
- 1 Citric acid + 3 sodium bicarbonate → 4 molecules of water.
  1 Tartaric acid + 2 sodium bicarbonate → 2 molecules of water.
- The water of crystallisation released by citric acid, plus water produced by partial reactions, act, as granulating liquid.
- The 12 -15 per cent loss of weight occurs during granulation.

Compounding: The 15 per cent extra quantities should be weighed to compensate the loss during compounding. The individual powder should be passed through sieve no. 60. Powders are mixed by the doubling up method and transfered to a hot porcelain dish. The powder mixture is heated further using water bath, pressing the powder with a spatula to form a damp coherent mass. The resultant mass is converted into granules of desired size. The water is allowed to liberate rapidly by placing effervescent salt in hot porcelain dish, otherwise slow heating increases loss of released water. For the same reason the powder mixture is not stirred, but pressed to make a coherent mass.

If any drug releases its water of hydration at or below $100^{0}C$, it should be removed by drying before its granulation. Otherwise, the excess moisture may produce moistened mass with chances of complete reaction between effervescent salts. Such formulations produce less evolution of gas when is placed in water. At the same time, a drug should not be exsiccated, or it should not be good absorbent, which would lead to absorption of water required for granulation. It makes the powder mixture dry and difficult to granulate.

Container and storage: Effervescent granules should be packed in wide-mouth glass jars and kept in a dry place.

Dispensing: The moist, cohesive or caked powder or generation of gas pressure inside the container, indicates moisture uptake and possibility of occurance of effervescent reaction. Add to a glass of water and take while effervescing.

Proprietary Preparations:

- CITRO-SODA (Abbot): Sodium bicarbonate 44.03per cent, sodium citrate (anhydrous) 15.75 per cent, tartaric acid 22.25 per cent, citric acid 17.88 per cent per 4 g. In indigestion, mild laxative.

Prescription No. 16.6	
R	
Effervescent sodium sulphate, Granules (BPC 1949)	
Sodium sulphate	50 g
Citric acid	21 g
Tartaric acid	24 g
Sodium bicarbonate	50 g

Principle:
Sodium sulphate is saline laxative and produces evacuation of bowel within 1 to 2 hours. It is poorly absorbed from GIT and retains water in the lumen. Sodium sulphate is decahydrate, which effloresces rapidly in dry air and liquefies in its water of hydration at about $33^0 C$. Therefore, it should be dried until it has lost about 55 per cent of its weight.

Apparatus: Porcelain dish, broad spatula, sieves.b

Compounding: Dry the sodium sulphate in a hot air oven to reduce its weight by 50-55 per cent. Weigh 15 per cent extra quantities. Pass the individual powder through sieve no. 60. Mix the powders by doubling up method and transfer to a hot porcelain dish. Heat the powder mixture using water bath, pressing the powder with spatula to form a damp coherent mass. Sieve the resultant mass into granules of 12-16 # size.

Container and storage: Pack in wide-mouthed, glass jars and keep in a dry place.

Category and dose: Saline purgative. 4-16 g.

Patient counselling: Add in water and take during evolution of carbon dioxide gas.

CACHETS

Cachets are used to enclose nauseous or disagreeable powders in tasteless concave pieces of wafers made of rice flour. When moistened with water, they become soft, elastic and slippery and these are easy to swallow. They vary in size from 3/4th to 1/8th in diameter and accommodate 0.2-2 g of powder.

Advantages:

i) It does not require complicated machinery like tablets/capsules.
ii) Cachets are useful for comparatively large doses of drugs, because, once they have been softened by immersion in water, even large size doses are easy to swallow as compared to hard capsules.
iii) Fast disintegration.

Limitations:

a) Poor mechanical strength and poor handling properties.
b) An attempt to increase fill-weight by compressing the powder may damage the wafer.
c) They provide less protection from environmental conditions than capsules do.
d) They are sensitive to moisture content.
e) They occupy more storage space than capsules.

Compounding: A mixture of rice flour and water is poured between two hot, polished, revolving cylinders. The sheet of wafer is formed after evaporation of water. One section of wafer is filled with the prescribed powder, and it is sealed by placing on the other section. The minimum weight of powder in a cachet should be not less than 200 mg. The cachets are of two types:

a) The wet seal-type of cachets consist of two halves both alike, concave in shape, having broad flanges. The empty half of the cachet is moistened with water and then turned over into position, so that the two halves of the cachet are joined by slight pressure.
b) The dry seal-type cachets have shallow body and cap. The cap, which is slightly larger in diameters, slips over the body.

ADDITIONAL EXERCISES

Prescription No. 16.7

℞
Oral Rehydration Salts, BP
Sodium chloride — 3.5 g
Potassium chloride — 1.5 g
Sodium citrate — 2.9 g
Anhydrous glucose — 20 g

Principle:
This formula is official in IP and BP as WHO-ORS citrate. The ORS formula is choice of treatment to treat water loss during diarrhoea. The ORS enhances the absorption of water and electrolytes. Glucose is absorbed in the small intestine, as in parts of nephron through transport carriers, coupled with sodium ions. Thus, increased glucose increases intestinal absorption of sodium and passive re-absorption of water; therefore, sodium chloride, potassium chloride and glucose are frequently used components of ORS. The palatability of powder is attributed to the presence of glucose and it is further built by the addition of citrates or fruit flavours. However, the higher concentration of glucose can cause osmotic diarrhoea and also aggravate existing diarrhoea. Therefore, the ORS should be

isotonic to body fluids. The osmolarity of body fluid is 286 + 4 mo sm/kg (280 m 05 ml). In this context, pharmacists should dispense the ORS formula of correct concentrations of salts and glucose and it should be reconstituted with 1 litre of water. Use of more powder and less water will not provide required osmolarity. The high salt concentration can lead to adverse reactions such as hypernatreaemia (exessive sodium in blood). The glucose: sodium ion molar ratio should be 1:1 to 2:1. The low sodium content ORS with 60mM/litre sodium ions is recommended for paediatric patients. The ORS also contains alkalising agents, such as sodium bicarbonate to counteract acidosis. However, the hygroscopic nature of sodium bicarbonate affects the storage stability of ORS formula.

Apparatus: White paper, spatula, sieves.

Compounding: Sieve the powders using sieve no. 60. Mix them lightly and pass through sieve no.60.

Container and storage: It is advisable to pack each dose in cellophane envelops and in air tight sachets. The bulk powders can be packed in screw-capped glass or plastic, jars. Store in well-closed containers.

Category and dose: Fluid and electrolyte replacement in diarrhoea. Reconstitute 1/4th quantity of the sachet with 250 ml of water. Dose varies according to fluid loss, usually 200–400 ml after every loose motion.

Label: Provides Na^+ 90 mmol, K^+ 20 mmol, Cl^- 80 mmol, citrate 10 mmol and glucose 111 mmol/litre.

- Patient counselling: Use within one hour after reconstitution. One sachet can be dissolved in 1 litre of water and stored in a refrigerator; it should be used within 24 hours. Drink extra water.

Proprietary preparations:

- ENERZAL (Mejda): Each 50 g contains carbohydrate 42.75 g, citric acid 1.19 g, sodium citrate dehydrate 0.88 g, sodium chloride 0.50 g, potassium chloride 0.45 g, sodium acid phosphate dihydrate 0.37 g, magnesium sulphate heptahydrate 0.30 g, calcium lactate pentahydrate 0.25 g.

- ELECTRAL (FDC) : Each 35 g contains sodium chloride 1.25 g, potassium chloride 1.5 g, sodium citrate 2.9 g, anhydrous dextrose 27 g, excipient q.s.

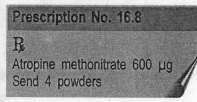

Prescription No. 16.8

℞

Atropine methonitrate 600 µg
Send 4 powders

Principle:

Atropine is obtained from natural sources but it rarely occurs in plants; and it is prepared by total synthesis. Atropine is antimuscarinic, tends to relax the oesophageal sphincter and dilates pupils. Atropine methonitrate is used in treatment of congential hypertrophic pyloric stenosis.

Atropine methonitrate should be given half an hour before food. Its dose is 0.6 mg. For small quantities of drug, weighing or measuring is done by the aliquot or by the triturating method. In latter case, an excess of the drug is weighed and diluted to a convenient weight. The part of the dilution that represents the desired quantity of drug is used in the prescription. Working formula: Calculate for 5 powders. Use lactose to make up each powder 120 mg.

Drug   : 600 µg × 5 = 3 mg

Total weight of powders   : 120 mg ×5 = 600 mg

The minimum weighable quantity is 100mg. Therefore take the minimum weighable quantity of drug and triturate it with lactose.

Trituration - I   Drug   : 100 mg
                   Lactose: 900 mg   Each 100 mg of Triturate - I contains 10 mg of drug.

Trituration - II   Triturate - I : 100 mg
                   Lactose: 900 mg   Each 100 mg of Triturate - II contains 1 mg of drug.

Trituration - III Triturate - II : 300 mg
                   Lactose: 300 mg   600 mg of Triturate - III contains 3 mg of drug.

Compounding: Sieve atropine methonitrate and lactose using sieve no.60. Mix these powders by doubling up method to produce triturates as above. Spread the powder on paper and divide it in 5 equal parts; weigh each aliquot 120 mg and wrap.

Container and storage: Wrap in bond paper. Store in dry place.

Category and dose: Antimuscarinic. 0.6mg half an hour before food.

Patient counselling: Avoid in paralytic ileus, ulcerative colitis, pregnancy and breast feeding. If it causes dryness of mouth, dilation of pupil, dry skin or palpitation, contact the physician.

Prescription No. 16.9

℞

Ispaghula Granules
Ispaghula 3.5 g
In effervescent base

Principle:

Ispaghula husk is mucilage containing drug obtained from dried seeds of plant. It relieves constipation by increasing faecal mass, which stimulates peristalsis. Because of its light and fibrous nature, there is difficultly in oral administration of ispaghula husk. The granulation is attempted to increase bulk density and to improve palatability. After contact with water, the husk swells and increases the faecal mass. If sufficient water is not taken along with these granules, swelling in presence of gastric fluid may cause intestinal obstruction, and therefore, adequate fluid intake should be maintained. This property provides dual action to ispaghula husk. At higher doses (3.5-9 g one to two times) with water, it acts as laxative and at lower doses (3.5 g 2-3 times), with no or little water, it acts as antidiarrhoeal.

The granules should contain above 90 per cent of ispaghula husk, otherwise; the dilute forms increase dose unnecessarily. The effervescent formula, or wet granulation formula, containing binders such as syrup can be employed for compounding of these granules. Effervescent granules are more palatable. The effervescent salts containing tartaric acid and sodium bicarbonate can be formulated using alcohol as granulating agent.

Working formula:
Ispaghula husk	: 3.50 g
Sodium Bicarbonate	: 1.25 g
Tartaric Acid	: 1.25 g

Compounding: Mix powders by doubling up method and add minimum alcohol to form a coherent mass. Screen it through sieve no. 6/22. Dry the granules that are retained on sieve no.22.

Container and storage: Granules are either packed in sachets (3.5 g husk/sachet) or as bulk pack (50 -90 per cent husk). The 5 ml teaspoonful should be provided with a bulk pack. Store in well-closed containers in a dry place.

Category and dose: Constipation, 1-2 sachets in 300 ml water 1-3 times daily.

Anti-diarrhoeal: 1 sachet 3 times daily.

Patient Counselling: maintain high fluid intake in constipation. In case of diarrhoea, minimise liquid intake for 30 minutes before and after the dose.

Proprietary preparations:

- HUSKY GRANULES (KAPL): Isphaghula husk powder 2.7 g, citric acid 0.66 g, sodium bicarbonate 0.62 g , excipients 1.42 g per 5.4 g. Laxative

Prescription No. 16.10

℞

Dry syrup
Amoxycillin trihydrate	— 5.5 g
Sodium Carboxy methyl cellulose	— 2.0 g
Sugar	— 90.0 g
Aerosil	— 0.8 g
Sodium benzoate	— 0.45 g
Tartrazine colour	— 20.0 mg
Pineapple flavour	— 1.0 g

Principle :

Amoxycillin is a broad-spectrum antibiotic with better absorption when given by oral route. It is effective for the treatment of chronic bronchitis, urinary tract infections, typhoid fever and dental prophylaxis. To overcome the problem of chemical degradation, it is better presented as dry powder, which has to be reconstituted with freshly boiled and cooled water. Sodium CMC is readily dispersible, viscosity enhancer. Sugar is diluent, sweetener and imparts body to the reconstituted liquid. Aerosil is used as glidant in 0.25-3 per cent concentration. Sodium benzoate is preservative. Tartrazine and pineapple are colour and flavour, respectively.

The 10 per cent overages should be calculated to compensate loss of amoxycillin trihydrate. The 20 g ± 100 mg powder has to be filled in amber glass bottles of 70 ml capacity with a mark at 40 ml. The reconstituted syrup contain 125 mg (137 mg on basis of averages) per 5 ml. Moisture content of powder should not be more than 1 per cent.

Compounding: All the processes should be conducted at a relative humidity of less than 40 per cent at 20^0C. Take dry sugar powder at 40^0C. Mix drug and other additives with sugar by the doubling up method for 30 minutes. Mix the remaining sugar. Fill 20 g of the resultant powder in a dry and clean bottle.

Container and Storage: Pack in amber glass bottles of 70 ml capacity with mark at 40 ml. 5 ml teaspoonful should be provided with pack. Store in a well-closed container in a dry place. The compounded dry syrup should be used within one month. The large scale manufactured products are stable up to 2 years. The reconstituted product should be used within two weeks.

Category and dose: Broad spectrum antibacterial. Up to 10 years, 125 mg every 8 hours. The dose may be doubled in case of severe infections.

Label: Shake well before use.

Patient counselling: Reconstitute the powder by pouring freshly boiled and cooled water up to the mark on the bottle. Shake the bottle for complete dispersion of the powder. Do not use boiled water for reconstitution. Use within two weeks after reconstitution. If diarrhoea occurs, contact the physician.

Proprietary preparations:

- ALLMOX (Lincoin), AMOXIVAN (Khandelwal), MOX (Rexcel): Amoxycillin 125 mg/5 ml.

Prescription No. 16.11

R

Compound Zinc Sulphate Powder, NF

Salicylic acid	— 0.5 g
Phenol	— 0.1 g
Eucalyptol	— 0.1 g
Menthol	— 0.1 g
Thymol	— 0.1 g
Zinc Sulphate	— 12.5 g
Boric acid	— 86.6 g

Principle:

This is medicated dusting powder containing eutectic and volatile substances. Salicylic acid, zinc sulphate and boric acid are applied topically for their antiseptic and astringent properties. Other aromatic ingredients are also antiseptic, and evaporation of these produce a cool feeling on the inflamed area. In the present formula, eutectic substances are more in number and it is complicated to triturate each separately to avoid liquefaction. Therefore, the eutectic substances are allowed to liquefy and the resultant liquid is adsorbed on solid components.

Apparatus: Pill tile, spatula, beaker and sieves.

Compounding: Mix phenol, eucalyptol, menthol and thymol and allow liquefying. Triturate salicylic acid and zinc sulphate to a very fine powder and mix the liquid of eutectic substances with powder. Add boric acid and continue triturating to get uniform mixture. Pass the powder through sieve no.85.

Container and Storage: Store in screw-capped, coloured glass, or plastic jars, fitted with a re-closable perforated lid; store in cool place.

Category: Antiseptic

Label: For external use only.

Handling precaution: Salicylic acid and boric acid are irritating.

Patient counselling: Do not apply on broken skin and areas that are very moist, otherwise powder tends to cake and abrade the skin.

Prescription No. 16.12

R

Body Powder

Zinc oxide	—	20 g
Menthol	—	0.25 g
Camphor	—	0.5 g
Zinc stearate	—	2.0 g
Talc	—	77.5 g

Send 40 g dusting powder

Principle:

This is medicated dusting powder containing eutectic and volatile substances. Zinc oxide is an astringent, menthol and camphor are antiseptics and when they evaporate, they produce a cool feeling on the inflamed area. Zinc strearate and talc imparts slip property and provides a covering. Talc is obtained from natural sources and before mixing with other ingredients, it should be sterilised by dry heat sterilisation. The formula contains menthol and camphor as eutectic substances and these can be mixed after trituration with other solids. Both, talc and zinc oxide, by virtue of their surface area, have capacity of adsorption. One eutectic substance should be triturated with one of the solid.

Apparatus: Pill tile, spatula, beaker and sieves.

Compounding: Mix separately, camphor and menthol, with equal amounts of zinc oxide and talc, respectively. Mix respective powders by doubling up method. Mix these two powders and add zinc stearate in it. Pass the powder through sieve no.85.

Container and Storage: Store in screw-capped coloured glass, or plastic, jars, fitted with a reclosable perforated lid; store in a cool place.

Category: Soothing on prickly heat.

Label : For external use only.

Handling precaution: Avoid unnecessary exposure of volatile substances.

Patient counselling: sprinkle powder liberally all over the body. Protect eyes.

Proprietary Preparation:

PERMICIL (Cipla): chlorophensin 1%, zinc oxide 16%, starch 51% in talc(w/w): prickly heat powder.

Prescription No. 16.13

Rx

Dentifrice, NF

Hard soap, fine powder	— 5.0 g
Precipitated calcium carbonate	— 9.35 g
Soluble saccharin	— 2.0 g
Peppermint oil	— 0.4 ml
Cinnamon oil	— 0.2 ml
Methyl salicylate	— 0.8 ml

Principle:
Precipitated calcium carbonate is an abrasive agent. It loosens the dirt adhering to the teeth. Hard soap is a detergent and by reducing surface tension, it hastens teeth cleansing. Foam produced during brushing holds debris in suspension. Methyl salicylate is antiseptic and analgesic. Peppermint oil and cinnamon oil are flavours. Saccharin is artificial sweetener.

Apparatus: Mortar and pestle, sieves, measuring cylinder.

Compounding: Pass the hard soap and precipitated calcium carbonate through sieve no.85. Triturate the soluble saccharin, oils and methyl salicylate with about ½ of the precipitated calcium carbonate. Mix hard soap with the remaining precipitated calcium carbonate, then mix the two powders thoroughly and sift through sieve no.85.

Container and storage: Pack in metal or plastic jars fitted with a perforated lid; store in well-closed containers in a cool place.

Category: Dentifrice.

Proprietary preparations:

- COLGATE Tooth Powder (Colgate-Palmolive).

●●●●●

17 Unit Dosage Forms

INTRODUCTION

The pharmaceutical dosage form, which contains a unit amount of drug, mostly a single dose, is termed as unit dosage form; such dosage forms guarantee accurate dosing. Solid dosage forms account for major portion of unit dosage forms.

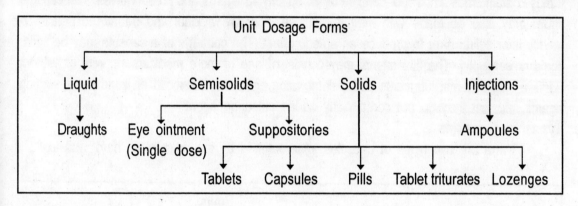

Advantages:

i) Greater accuracy and precision of dose.

ii) Portable, convenient to handle, identify and administer.

iii) Suitable alternative to powders, unless the powder mixture is too bulky or unless the patient cannot swallow a solid dosage form.

iv) More stable than multidose dosage forms, ensuring longer shelf-life periods.

v) Can be designed to make a medicament available to the body at pre-determined rates.

Disadvantages:

i) Drugs having high dose, or low bulk density, cannot be formulated into compact dosage form.

ii) Disintegration and dissolution of solid unit dosage form delays its effectiveness.

iii) Requires additional steps to present a particular dosage form, eg. conversion of powder into tablets.

CAPSULES

Definition and Types

Capsules are solid unit dosage forms intended for oral administration, usually containing a drug or mixture of drugs, enclosed in a hard or soft water-soluble 'shell' of gelatin or any other suitable material, which dissolves or disintegrates in water to release the medicament completely.

The capsule shell is basically made up of gelatin, the strength and flexibility of gelatin capsule shell is adjusted by addition of plasticizers, such as glycerin and sorbitol. Additionally, it may contain small amount of certified dyes, opacifying agents and preservatives. The capsule shells may also be made with methyl cellulose, polyvinyl alcohol and denatured gelatin to modify their solubility or to produce an enteric effect. The contents of a capsule may be solid, liquid or semisolid. The fill material may consist of one or more medicament, with or without additive, like diluents, lubricants and disintegrating agents or semisolid or liquid base, wetting agents, etc, but they do not contain any added colouring agent.

Types of Capsules

There are two types of capsules, differentiated by the adjectives, 'hard' and 'soft'.

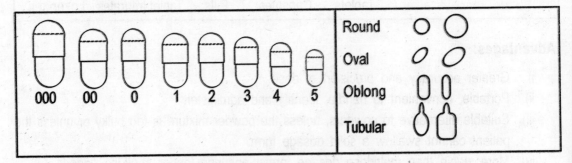

Figure 17.1 : Shapes and Sizes of Capsules

Table 17.1 : Difference between Hard Gelatin and Soft Gelatin Capsules		
No.	Hard Gelatin Capsules (HGC)	Soft Gelatin Capsules (SGC)
1	The hard gelatin capsule shell consists of two parts : cap and body.	Soft gelatin capsules are one piece, hermetically sealed shells.
2	HGCs are cylindrical in shape.	SGCs are round, oval, oblong and tubular in shape.
3	Eight sizes (000 to 5) are available for human use. 000 is the largest and 5 is the smallest size.	Content of capsule varies from 0.1 to 30 ml.
4	HGCs are used mostly for encapsulation of solids in the form of powder, beads, pellets or granules, small tablets and capsules, called as dry filled capsules (DFC).	SGCs consist of liquids or solids dissolved or dispersed in suitable base to give a paste-like consistancy, but may also consist of powders and granules. The sterile ophthalmic ointments are also dispensed for single use.
5	May show high weight variation if powder flow and mixing is poor.	The weight and drug content uniformity is more because dissolved or dispersed drug is volumetrically filled into capsules.
6	The encapsulated solid material has to disintegrate or dissolve before absorption of drug.	The drug is dissolved or dispersed in water miscible, or oily liquid, and show better bio-availability than solids.
7	The capsule shells are thiner and less flexible than soft gelatin shells. They contain plasticisers up to 5% by weight.	They contain 20-40% by weight of plasticisers. The shells are more thicker and more flexible than hard gelatin shells.
8	The filling of hard gelatin capsules is a multi-step operation. The content is filled into the body, which is then closed by slipping the cap over it.	Soft gelatin shells are formed, filled and sealed in a combined operation.

Advantages:

i)   Drugs having an unpleasant taste are enclosed in practically tasteless shell.

ii) Provide a smooth, slippery and easy-to-swallow capsule shell. If a patient experiences difficulty in swallowing a solid dosage form, the use of HGC is still an accepted alternative. This can be done by emptying the contents of the capsule into a beverage and administered.

iii) In contrast to tablets, capsules provide rapid bio-availability.

iv) The fill material requires minimum or no excipients.

v) Ready solubility of gelatin in gastric pH allows rapid release of medicament.

vi) The HGC is the only suitable dosage form to enclose coated beads for sustained release action. Formulation of such beads in a tablet form disrupts the coating.

vii) The tightly sealed capsule shell protects the enclosed drug from environmental degradation.

viii) Due to their elegance, ease of use and portability, capsules have become a popular dosage form.

ix) Capsules can be economically produced in large quantities and in a wide range of attractive colours.

Disadvantages:

i) Capsules are not suitable to fill liquid materials such as water, glycerin, or hydroalcoholic solutions, in which the shell dissolves.

ii) Capsules are also not suitable for low molecular weight, water-soluble or volatile organic compounds, which may migrate out or evaporate from the capsule shell.

iii) Rapid release of water-soluble salts, such as potassium chloride, potassium bromide and ammonium chloride, may cause gastric irritation.

iv) Capsules are also not suitable for very acidic or alkaline drugs, because acidic drug may hydrolyse the gelatin; whereas, alkaline drugs, due to their tanning effect, reduce solubility of gelatin.

v) Highly efflorescent or deliquescent powders may affect the capsule shell by their moisture-extracting effect, or making the capsule shells moist.

vi) The capsule shell contains 10-15 per cent water, which serves as plasticiser to maintain capsule elasticity. However, these undergo dehydration when stored in an atmosphere of low relative humidity, making the capsule brittle and hence crack easily. On exposure to high humidity gelatin shell becomes soft and, at times, capsules can stick to each other.

Formulation of HGC

Hard gelatin capsules are used for encapsulation of powder drug formulations. The beads, pellets or granules as conventional, or sustained release forms of medication, are also filled in it. In selecting a capsule size, the amount of powder that represents a dose should be weighed and the smallest capsule size that will accomodate the dose should be selected. The dry-filled formulations may necessitate the following additives :

1) Diluents : If the amount of drug powder representing a single dose of medication is not sufficiently bulky to fill the capsule, then a suitable powder diluent should be added. 60- 120 mg is the minimum weight of drug that can be filled in a smallest capsule and, generally, the minimum weight of a capsule should be 100 mg. Most common capsule diluents are starch, lactose and dicalcium phosphate.

2) Glidants : Powder used for capsule filling should have good flow properties. Glidants added to improve the flow properties are colloidal silicon dioxide, corn starch, talc, and magnesium stearate; usually up to 1 per cent concentration.

3) Surfactants : Surfactants like sodium lauryl sulphate, may be added in capsule formulation, to enhance drug dissolution by increasing the wetting of the powder mass.

4) Absorbants : Absorbants, such as oxides and carbonates of magnesium and calcium, may be used in formulation, particularly to prevent moisture absorption by hygroscopic substances.

5) Disintegrating agents : Disintegrating agents are particularly used as component of granules or pellets to be encapsulated in hard shells. Most common example includes sodium starch glycolate.

6) Antidust agents : Small amounts of edible oil can be mixed to impart cohesiveness to the powder, and to minimise dust generation.

Concept Clear : Hard v/s Soft Capsule

- Capsules, the solid unit dosage form, are of two types, hard gelatin capsules and soft gelatin capsules.
- Capsule shell is made up of gelatin, plasticisers, certified colours and preservatives.
- HGC formulation : Powders/granules; drug(s), diluents, lubricants and disintegrating agents.
- SGC formulation : Semisolid or liquid base, wetting agents, etc.
- HGC have two parts: Body and Cap; eight sizes, 000 (largest) - 5 (smallest).
- Capsules are tasteless, easy to swallow, but sensitive to moisture.

Filling of HGC

There are eight capsule sizes used for oral drug administration in human medicine. They are designated by numbers from 000 (the largest) to 5 (the smallest). The exact capacity of any capsule varies according to the density and compressibility of the formulation. The usual range of powder capacity for each size is summarised in Table 17.2. The fill weight is determined by bulkiness, or volume, occupied by the powder. Smaller capsules (Capsule No.5) usually accomodate 60-120 mg of powder and larger capsules can be filled with 600-1000 mg of powder.

Hard gelatin capsules are mainly used to fill dry powders. Hard capsules can be filled manually, or by use of hand-operated machines, semiautomatic or fully automatic machines.

The basic process of capsule filling involves rectification, separation, filling and joining.

Table 17.2: Different sizes of Hard Gelatin Capsules

No.	Capsule No.	Volume (ml)	Content (mg)
1	000	1.36	650-1000
2	00	0.95	390-1300
3	0	0.67	325-910
4	1	0.48	225-650
5	2	0.37	195-520
6	3	0.27	130-390
7	4	0.20	95-260
8	5	0.13	60-120

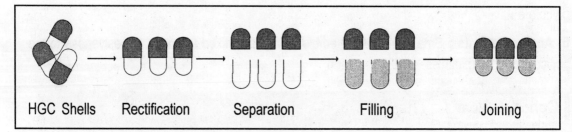

HGC Shells   Rectification   Separation   Filling   Joining

Figure 17.2: Basic steps in Filling of Hard Gelatin Capsules

Manual Methods: For capsule-filling by manual method, the working formula should be calculated to 10 per cent extra than actually required:

i)   For extemporaneous purposes capsules are generally filled by the punching method. In this method, well-formulated powder blends of desired particle size, is spread uniformly on a sheet of clean paper. Then, the open end of the empty capsule body is repeatedly pressed into the powder, firmly and uniformly, until it is filled. This method is unsuitable for powders that do not pack readily and tend to drop out of the body during filling (Fig.17.3a).

ii) In the other method, the body of the capsule is held horizontally facing the open end towards the heap of powder. Powder is filled and pressed with the help of spatula (Fig.17.3b).

iii) Filling of capsules by funnels is superior to the methods discussed above. In this method a measured quantity of powder is filled in bodies using funnels. If necessary the powder is pressed in the body by inserting the punch or glass rod, in bodies. After filling the bodies, the cap may be fitted loosely. These capsules are checked for fill weight. To ensure accuracy of dosage, each filled capsule should be weighed using an empty capsule of the same size as a tare. Rotating the well-filled and sealed capsule between the thumb and fingers gives completely and uniformly filled capsules.

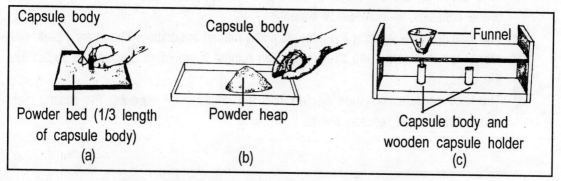

Figure 17.3: Manual Filling of Hard Gelatin Capsules

Hand-operated capsule filling machine:

A hand-operated, hard gelatin, capsule filling machine, consists of the following parts:
i)   A capsule loading plate having 24-300 holes to hold capsules of different diameters.
ii) A filling plate has corresponding number of holes to that of capsule-loading plate.
iii) A powder tray to prevent loss of material during filling.
iv) A pin plate having pins corresponding to the number of holes.
v)   A closure and ejection handle to raise or drop pegs into the corresponding holes of the filling plate.
vi) A locking handle to lock the body.
vii) A sealing plate with rubber top.

These machines are generally supplied with additional loading plates with various diameters of holes, so as to fill the desired size of capsules. Depending upon the filling capacity, one can prepare capsules at a productivity rate of 2000 capsules per day.
Working of hand operated machine:
i)   The carefully sorted empty capsules are filled into the loading plate, and the latter is placed over the filling plate.
ii) The bodies of the capsules are locked by operating the locking handle. It enables the separation of the two parts, holding bodies in filling plate and retaining the caps in the loading plate. The loading plate is lifted for separation.
iii) The locking handle is now released so that the body falls below the surface of the filling plate.
iv) The powder tray is placed on the filling plate to prevent any loss of the filling material.

v) The powder to be filled in the capsules is placed in a powder tray and spread with the help of a powder spreader, so as to fill the bodies of the capsule uniformly.

vi) The pin plate is lowered, if required, so as to press the powder into the bodies.

vii) After pressing, the pin plate is raised and more powder is filled into the bodies of the capsules to increase fill weight.

viii) The loading plate, holding the caps, is again placed in position. The sealing plate with rubber top is lowered; the closure ejection handle is activated, forcing the bodies into the caps.

ix) The filled capsules are then ejected from the machine by releasing the sealing plate and activating the ejection handle.

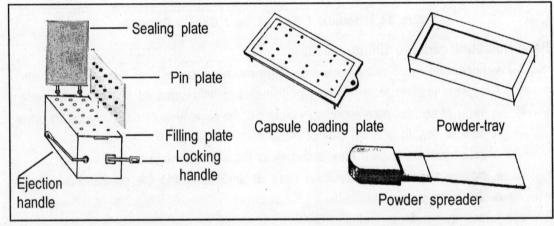

Figure 17.4: Hand Operated Capsule Filling Machine

The well-filled capsules are cleaned by wiping each capsule with a clean cloth, or by shaking the capsules gently with granular sodium chloride in a container. Then these capsules are rolled on a clean cloth to remove adhered sodium chloride. Clean capsules may be polished by rolling them in a towel, which has been previously sprinkled lightly with liquid paraffin. This gives very good shine to the capsules.

Container and Storage: Capsules are dispensed in bulk in amber glass, or plastic jars, preferably with child resistant closures. Capsules are protected from atmospheric moisture by keeping a desiccant bag on top of the capsules.

Dispensing: Hard, soft or sticky capsules or capsules with changed dimensions, should not be dispensed.

Patient counselling: Take with water. Unless otherwise directed, do not open the capsule. Store the capsules in a dry place.

Proprietary preparations:

- LANPRO (Unichem), LANZAP (Dr. Reddy's) : Lansoprazole 15 mg and 30 mg. ACICHEK (Boehringer Mannheim), OMECID (Saga Labs) : Omeprazole 20 mg. For treating gastric ulcers.
- DURASAL-CR (Raptakos) : Salbutamol 4 and 8 mg. THEO-ASTHALIN SR (Cipla) : Salbutamol 4 mg, Theophylline anhydrous 300 mg. For treating asthma.
- IMODIUM (Ethnor), PELOPEM (Mercury) : Loperamide 2 mg. Opioid antidiarrhoreal

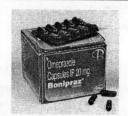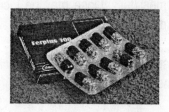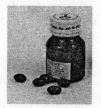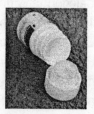

Blister pack (Courtesy LiTaka pharmaceuticals), Glass Jar and plastic jar with closures

Figure 17.5: Containers for Capsules

| Concept Clear | HGC Filling |

- Methods: Manual, hand operated machine, semiautomatic and fully automatic machines.
- Basic steps of capsule filling: Rectification, separation, filling and joining.
- Extemporaneous filling: Punching method, horizontal facing and funnel method.
- Hand-operated machine: Capsule loading plate, filling plate, powder tray, pin plate, closure and ejection handle, locking handle, sealing plate and powder spreader.
- Minimum capsule weight 100 mg.

Prescription No. 17.1

℞

Chlordiazepoxide HCl 10mg
Send 9 capsules
One capsule 3 times a day

Principle :

Chlordiazepoxide HCl is a sedative; it is available commercially in capsules containing 5, 10, and 25 mg. The working formula should be calculated for 10 capsules. In the given prescription the amount of the drug required is 10 × 10 = 100 mg. It should be apparent that 10 mg of chlordiazepoxide HCl powder would be insufficient to fill even the smallest capsule, generally available, and it necessitates inclusion of diluents such as lactose. Suppose the smallest capsule available in the laboratory is a No.4 capsule, Pharmacists should determine the weight required to fill a capsule. Supposing it is 150 mg,

Then, 150 mg - 10 mg = 140 mg lactose is required per capsule 140 × 10 = 1.4 g lactose for 10 capsules. The pharmacists should weigh 100 mg of chlordiazepoxide HCl and 1.4 g of lactose, followed by mixing by geometric dilution.

Apparatus: Mortar and pestle, funnel, spatula.

Compounding: Sieve chlordiazepoxide HCl and lactose through sieve no. 60 and mix it by doubling up method. Fill the powder mixture in the body of the capsule. Replace the cap loosely and weigh the capsules. If necessary, adjust the weight. Seal the capsules and make them dust-free.

Container and storage: Screw-capped glass jars. Store in well-closed containers.

Category and dose: Anxiety. 10 mg 3 times daily. Dose may be increased if necessary to 60-100 mg daily, in divided doses. For elderly patients, half of the adult dose.

Label: Keep away from children.

Patient counselling: Avoid prolonged use. Administer with caution if suffering with renal and hepatic impairment. May cause drowsiness, avoid driving. Effect of alcohol enhances, hence avoid taking with alcohol.

Prescription No. 17.2

R

Multivitamin Capsules

Vitamin B$_1$	— 10 mg
Vitamin B$_2$	— 10 mg
Vitamin B$_6$	— 3 mg
Vitamin B$_{12}$	— 15 mcg
Niacinamide	— 100 mg
Calcium pantothenate	— 20 mg
Send 30 capsules.	

Principle:

Vitamins are of great importance in body metabolism as co-enzymes. A balanced diet is the best source of vitamin; but no natural source contains all the water soluble vitamins. The regular vitamin supplements are not indicated in healthy individuals. However, their requirement increases during acute illness, fever, oral antibiotic therapy and other hypermetabolic states. The multiple deficiencies of water-soluble vitamins often co-exist and the repair of one vitamin deficiency may increase the need for another. Most megaloblastic anaemias are due to lack of either vitamin B$_{12}$ or folate. The other vitamins of vitamin B group include thiamine (Vit. B$_1$), riboflavin (Vit. B$_2$), pyridoxine HCl (Vit. B$_6$), pantothenic acid, para-aminobenzoic acid, biotin, choline. Vitamin B$_6$ is indicated in isoniazid-induced peripheral neuritis. These are also called as antiberiberi vitamins.

To compensate the loss of vitamins, overages are allowed during formulation, these include vitamin B$_1$ (15 per cent), Vitamin B$_2$ (15 per cent), Vitamin B$_6$ (20 per cent), Vitamin B$_{12}$ (100 per cent), Niacinamide (10 per cent). Since the amount of vitamin B$_{12}$ is very less, it is either dissolved in alcohol and the resultant solution mixed uniformly with sufficient diluents, such as lactose or starch; or vitamin B$_{12}$ is diluted with diluents to produce a triturate. For large scale manufacturing the overages must be calculated. The working formula, considering the overages, is given below.

Apparatus: Sieves, mortar and pestle, spatula.

Compounding: Calculate the formula considering overages. Prepare a triturate of vitamin B_{12} using diluents. Mix all the ingredients by doubling up method and sift the powder through sieve no.60. Fill in the capsule and check its weight.

Formula for 32 capsules

Vitamin B_1	:	368 mg
Vitamin B_2	:	368 mg
Vitamin B_6	:	115 mg
Vitamin B_{12}	:	960 mcg
Niacinamide	:	3.520 g
Calcium pantothenate	:	768 mg
Aerosil	:	70 mg
Thiourea	:	100 mg
Lactose	:	4.0 g
The total weight	:	9.31
Weight of each capsule	:	290 mg

Container and storage: Store in well-closed screw-capped glass jars.

Category and dose: Vitamin B deficiency. 1 capsule per day.

Patient counselling: Take balanced diet. Store capsules in airtight containers in a dry place.

Proprietary preparations:

B-LACT (Prem Pharma), BIOSTAR (Brown & Burk), BIOVITAL (Micro Labs), VITARAL (Glenmark).

TABLETS

Pharmaceutical tablets are unit solid dosage forms, prepared by compressing or moulding a drug(s) powder, with or without additives. They vary in shape and differ greatly in size, shape and weight, depending on the amount of medicinal substance and the intended mode of administration. Tablets can be swallowed whole, chewed or placed under the tongue (sublingual) or in the cheek pouch (buccal tablet).

Advantages:

a) Portable, convenient to handle, identify and administer.

b) More stable than liquid dosage forms, ensuring longer shelf-life periods.

c) Better accuracy and precision of dose.

d) Easy to modify drug release rate i.e. either to make fast dissolving tablets or to make medicament available to body fluids, in a controlled way, for prolonged periods of time.

e) Coated tablets can be prepared either to protect medicament from destructive influence of moisture and atmospheric gases, to mask bitter or unpleasant taste of medicament or to provide protection of medicament from destructive influence of gastric acid.

f) Tablets can be produced on mass scale for economy.

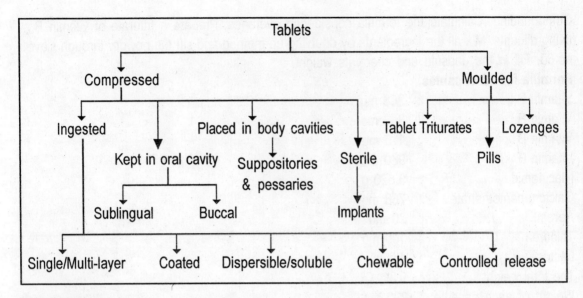

Disadvantages:
a) Drugs having low bulk density, cannot be formulated into dense compact tablets.
b) Some patients, particularly children, geriatric and those seriously ill, find it difficult to swallow solid dosage forms.
c) Disintegration and dissolution of tablet are the rate determining factors for drug absorption and in general, tablets show slow onset of action.
d) Not economical to produce compressed tablets on lab scale, requires machinaries, manpower and space.

Formulation of Tablets

Tablet formulation contains active ingredient and number of additives like diluents, binders and lubricants, which affect compressional characteristics of a tablet. Another group of additives helps to provide physicochemical stability, drug bio-availability as well as product acceptance. It includes disintegrants, colours, flavours and sweeteners.

Diluents are added when the quantity of medicament in each tablet is very small, e.g. lactose, mannitol, calcium phosphate, calcium sulphate, etc. Binders provide adhesiveness to powder blends during granulation and compression stages. Common binders include starch paste, polyvinyl pyrrolidone, tragacanth, etc. Lubricants are mixed with granules before compression. The glidants are employed to improve flow characteristic of granules, e.g. colloidal silica, purified talc. The antiadhesives prevents adhesion of material to the faces of punches and die walls, eg. Talc, sodium lauryl sulphate. Lubricant is third group, which reduces friction between die wall surface and powder mass, thereby allowing easy compression and ejection of the compressed tablet. Magnesium stearate is the most effective lubricant.

Disintegrating agents are added to tablets to promote break up (disintegration) of the tablet after ingestion, thus ensuring drug release. Common disintegrants include starch, microcrystalline cellulose, effervescent salts, ion exchange resins etc. Organoleptic additives like colours are incorporated into tablets to improve appearance or provide identity. When flavoured tablet is desired, it is usually done by spraying an alcoholic solution of volatile oils or other flavoring agents, onto the dry granules prior to compression.

Types of Tablets

Classification of tablets is usually based on the method of manufacture and on the intended usage. Broadly, they are classified into two classes, viz., Compressed tablets and Moulded tablets.

1) Compressed tablets: The conventional compressed tablet is meant for oral administration, which should disintegrate in water within 15 minutes and should dissolve specified drug as per the monograph. These are either single layer tablets or multilayer tablets. The single layer tablets are prepared by single compression cycle and usually composed of medicinal substances(s), with number of pharmaceutical additives. Multiple compressed tablets are compressed tablets prepared by more than a single compression cycle. Several different granulations are compressed on top of the other, to form a single tablet composed of two or more layers. Multilayer tablets are mainly used to separate incompatible substances, or get bimodal drug release.

Patient counselling: Swallow with water. For ease of administration, it can be broken or crushed. Proprietary preparations:

- CEMETIN (PCI), LOCK-2 (Cadila Healthcare): Cimetidine 200 mg; FAMOCID (Sun Pharma): Famotidine 20 mg & 40 mg; ZINETAC (Glaxo): Ranitidine 150 mg & 300 mg Treats hyperacidity.
- BETNESOL (Glaxo), CORTIL (Micro Labs): Betamethasone 0.5 mg. Treats inflammatory & allergic disorders in bronchial asthma.
- AMLODAC (Alidac), AMLOPRES (Cipla): Amlodipine 2.5, 5 & 10mg; ATELOL (Themis Pharma), BETACARD (Torrent): Atenolol 25, 50 &100mg. Antihypertension.

2) Coated tablets: Some compressed tablets are coated with various materials, including sugar and polymers. The reasons for coating includes i) Protection of the medicament from the environment, particularly light and moisture, ii) Masking unpleasant taste or iii) To improve ease of swallowing. Enteric coating technique is used to prevent the tablet from disintegrating in the stomach.

a) Enteric coating: Tablets coated with polymers like cellulose acetate phthalate and shellac, resist dissolution or disintegration in the stomach, but not in the intestine. Enteric coating is done to prevent the gastric content (acid and enzymes) attacking the drug and thus to protect the stomach from the irritant effect of certain drugs or when the drug absorption is enhanced in the intestine, which is preferable, to a significant extent. These tablets should not disintegrate in the acidic medium within two hours, but should disintegrate within one hour in the similated intestinal medium.

Patient counselling: Swallow the intact tablet with water. Take on empty stomach. Do not take with antacid.

Proprietary preparations:

- CANNACT (Astra-IDL): Diclofenac sodium 50 mg. NSAID
- ENSERA (Bombay Tablets): Serratiopeptidase 10 mg. Anti-inflammatory enzyme.
- PANTOCID (Sun): Pantoprazole 40 mg. Proton pump inhibitor.
- A.S.A. (German Remedies): ESCOPRIN (USV): Aspirin 50 mg and 75 mg respectively.

b) **Non-enteric coated tablets:** These include sugar and film coated tablet. Sugar coated tablets involves the successive application of coloured, or non-coloured, sucrose-based solutions to the tablets' core. The coating is water-soluble and is quickly dissolved after swallowing. Sugar coating is mainly done to improve palatability and appeal of the product.

Film-coating involves the deposition of coloured or uncoloured thin film of a polymer on the tablet core. Film-coating has the advantage over sugar-coating in that, that it is more durable, less bulky and a less time consuming coating operation. These tablets should disintegrate in water, or in simulated gastric medium, within an hour.

Patient counselling: Swallow the intact tablet with water.

Proprietary preparations:

- FORMET (Chemech): Metformin HCl, F.C. Tabs. 500 mg . Antidiabetic.
- WINCAP (RPG): Ciprofloxacin 250 mg, Tinidazole 300 mg. Antidiarrhoeals.
- CEBECT-TZ (Plethico), WINCAP (RPG): Ciprofloxacin 500 mg, tinidazole 300 mg. Antidiarrhoeals.
- FOURTUS B (Fourrts) : Multivitamin sugar-coated tablet.

3) **Dispersible and Soluble tablets:** These tablets disintegrate within 3 minutes in water to produce uniform dispersion or solution. Unlike conventional tablets these show faster action. These contain super disintegranting agents.

Patient counselling: Disperse in glass of water and drink.

Proprietary preparations:

- GASTROPEN (Morepen), CISATEN (Kamron): Cisapride 5 mg . For relief in constipation.
- GASTROGYL (Biological E): Ciprofloxacin 500 mg, tinidazole 600 mg. Antidiarrhoeals.

- NIMOTAS–CD (Intas): Nimesulide 100 mg. ROXICAP-DT (Seagull): Piroxicam 20 mg.NSAID.
- AMOTID (Dolphin), BIOMOX (Biochem): Amoxycillin 250 mg. Antibacterial.

4) Effervescent tablets: These are compressed tablets containing effervescent salts, which liberate carbon dioxide when in contact with water. The effervescence of carbon dioxide acts as a disintegrator. This also helps in masking unpleasant tastes of medicaments. Carbon dioxide is released due to chemical reaction between sodium bicarbonate and citric acid,or tartaric acid, in presence of water. Making effervescent tablets is one of the ways to produce dispersible or soluble tablets. When placed in water, these tablets should disperse or dissolve, with the evolution of gas, within 5 minutes.

Patient counselling: Dissolve or disperse in water and swallow.

Proprietary preparations:

- HISTAC-EVT (Ranbaxy): Ranitidine 150 mg. Treats hyperacidity.

5) Chewable tablets: These are compressed tablets designed to be chewed prior to swallowing. The antacids tablets are chewed as fine as possible and swallowed. Some antihypertensive drugs are also formulated in chewable form. Such tablets are chewed and swallowed after 2 minutes. The drug gets absorbed from the oral mucosa directly into the blood circulation. A disintegrating agent is not required in chewable tablets. Bad tasting drugs and drugs having extremely high dose are difficult to formulate in chewable tablets.

Proprietary preparations:

- CISADE MPS (Unichem) : Cisapride 10 mg, simethicone 125 mg; SYSPRIDE MPS (Systopic): Cisapride 10 mg, methyl polysiloxane 125 mg. Relives constipation.
- MOX (Rexcel) : Amoxycillin 250 mg. Antibacterial.
- ACIDIN–MPS (East India) Dried aluminium hydroxide gel 250 mg, magnesium hydroxide 200 mg, activated dimethicone 75 mg; GELUCIL PLUS (Parke-Davis), DIOVOL MINT TABS (Wallace). Antacid.
- SET cal (Indoco) : Calcium carbonate and vitamin D_3

6) Buccal and Sublingual tablets: Buccal or sublingual tablets are generally flat, oval tablets, intended to provide systemic effect by placing them in the buccal pouch (buccal tablets), or beneath the tongue (sublingual tablets), and allowing them to dissolve there. Absorption of drugs through the highly vascular mucosal lining of the mouth moves the drug through the sublingual or buccal capillaries and enters into general circulation from the oral venous drainage system to the right heart, by-passing the stomach and liver, i.e., first pass metabolism. Ideally the drug for sublingual, or buccal, use should be small in dose, usually not more than 10-15 mg and should not have an undesirable taste. Drugs administered by the sublingual or buccal route are either not absorbed from the gastrointestinal tract, or are rapidly metabolised by the first pass effect in liver.

Patient counselling: Sublingual and buccal tablets should not be chewed, crushed, or swallowed, but should only be placed under the tongue. Place the buccal tablet between the lip and gum, or between the cheek and gum. Allow the tablet to dissolve. Do not eat, drink, smoke, or use chewing tobacco, while a tablet is dissolving. Avoid touching the tablet with the tongue, it may cause the tablet to dissolve faster. Do not go to sleep while a tablet is dissolving, because it could slip down the throat and cause choking. If accidentally swallowed, replace it with another one.

Proprietary preparations:
- ISORDIL SUBLINGUAL (Wyeth Lederle): Isosorbide dinitrate 5 mg.Vasodilator.

7) Controlled release tablets: Most of the solid dosage forms are designed to release their medication into the body for rapid absorption, whereas, some products are designed to release the drug slowly for sustained drug action. The latter types of dosage forms are commonly referred to as controlled release, delayed release, sustained release, prolonged release, timed release or non-immediate action dosage forms. Controlled release tablets are designed in such a way that, the administration, of a single dosage unit provides the immediate release of some amount of drug that promptly produces the desired therapeutic effect and gradual and continuous release of remaining amounts of drug to maintain this level of effect over an extended period, usually 12 to 24 hours. (For detailed information refer Chapter 19).

8) Rectal tablets: For patients who have difficulty in swallowing tablets, rectal route can be used as an alternative. Tablets have some distinct advantages over semisolid suppositories which do not require refrigeration, as well as demonstrate better product stability. However, tablets are not very attractive for rectal administration, because they cannot disintegrate rapidly in the very small volume of fluid present in the rectum (Refer chapter 15).

9) Vaginal tablets: They are oval or pear-shaped, conventionally compressed, tablets, intended for insertion into the vagina, where tablets dissolve to release medicament. These are used in the treatment of local infections, as well as for systemic absorption. Vaginal tablets disintegrate in very small volumes of vaginal fluid. These are administered usually by means of a plastic inserter (Refer Chapter 15).

Proprietary preparations:
- GYNO–TERAZOL Ovules (Johnson & Johnson) : Terconazole 80 mg. Fungicidal.
- CANDID–V6 (Glenmark) vaginal tablets : Clotrimazole 100 mg. Fungicide and trichomonacide
- LOTRIL (Gufic), SURFAZ (Franco-India) : Ciclopiroxolamine 100 mg. For treating Candidiasis

10) Implants: Implants are small, rod-shaped or ovoid-shaped, sterile pellets composed o the highly purified drug alone, or in rate controlling system, intended for insertion into body tissue by surgical procedures, where the drug is slowly released, over a prolonged period of time, ranging from 3 to 6 months or longer.

11) Moulded tablets: These include tablet triturates, lozenges, pastilles.

- ALEX COUGH LOZENGE (Lyca), CHERICOF LOZENGES : Dextromethorphan HBr 5 mg. Treats dry cough.
- CHERANA COUGH LOZENGES (Knoll Pharma): Noscapine 10 mg. Treats dry cough.

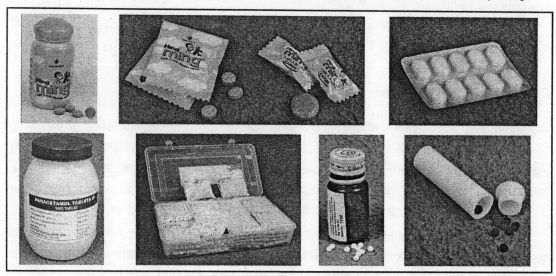

Figure 17.6: Containers for Tablets

Dispensing of tablets:

The tablets are mainly packed in strips or jars. Strips contain tablets in even number mostly, four, six, ten, etc. For b.i.d. and q.i.d. dosing, there are perfect packs. But when dose is t.i.d., the number of tablets for three days dosing are nine or for five days there are fifteen, and cutting of strips is inconvenient. After dispensing, nine tablets from a strip of ten units, it is very difficult to keep account of a single tablet, which bears no information about the batch number and expiry date. The general guidelines for dispensing of tablets are as follows:

- Do not dispense crushed/broken tablets or worn/torn strips.
- Cut the strips carefully without opening the pouch/blister of other tablets in strip.
- Always keep the cut portion of strip bearing the batch number in the pharmacy.
- Demonstrate the method to remove tablets from strip/blister backs.
- When a whole jar of tablets is dispensed, demonstrate the methods to remove the tablets. In form that minimum exposure to environment is necessary and that the desiccant bag has to be kept in bottle.

- The method for dispensing of units from bulk containers is given in Chapter 4.
Tablet Triturates

Definition and Uses: Tablet triturates, the term comes from the early practice of preparing moulded tablets from powder triturates of drug with diluents. These are prepared by moulding a moistened blend of potent drug and diluents with dilute alcohol as moistening agent. Unlike compressed tablets, tablet triturates are especially used for sublingual or for oral administration or to prepare other dosage forms such as hypodermic tablets, or dispensing tablets.

In the early days tablet triturates were used by the physician to prepare extemporaneous injections by dissolving a tablet in sterile water for injection. These were termed as hypodermic tablets. The current standards of sterility have made this concept outdated. Dispensing or compounding, tablets are used to compound other solid or liquid dosage forms, for example, liquid preparations for internal or external use can be compounded by dissolving the appropriate number of tablet triturates in water.

Formulation: Tablet triturates contain little or no binder, which otherwise have a retarding effect on disintegration or dissolution. Since these are designed mainly for administration of small doses of potent drugs, diluents are more useful additives among all the additives. Diluents which are used commonly include lactose, sucrose, mannitol or other soluble materials. Lactose is the standard diluent for tablet triturates, due to their fine particle size, inertness and whiteness. Due to high solubility, β-lactose is usually preferred over α-lactose. Tablet triturates made from lactose tend to crumble easily during handling; whereas, sucrose yields harder tablets. For this reason, mixture of lactose and sucrose is frequently used. In addition to diluents, the quality of tablet triturates depends upon the moistening agent, which is most commonly 50 per cent alcohol. Absolute alcohol is used to avoid decomposition of moisture sensitive drugs. However, alcohol alone tends to produce more friable tablets.

Compounding: Tablet triturates are compounded by moulding or, on large scale, by using tablet compression machine. Hand mould consists of two plates made from metal, hard rubber or plastic. The mould plate contains any number of die holds from fifty to several hundred. The lower plate has corresponding number of pegs, which fit into the holes of mould plate to eject tablet triturates.

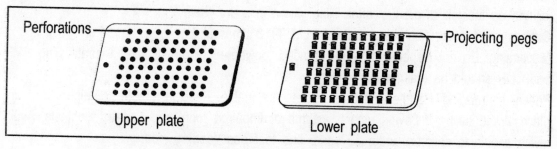

Figure 17.7: Tablet Triturate Moulds

The capacity of each mould cavity (holes) is determined by calibration, taking average weight of dried tablet triturates made up of only base. The well triturated powder is moistened with 50 per cent alcohol. The workable mass should be moist enough to have inter-particular adhesion, but should not be over wetted. An over wetted mass is likely to stick to the moulds, as well as it may produce hard products. Generally, 0.8 ml of 50 per cent alcohol is sufficient to moisten 4 grams of lactose. The mould plate is placed on a clean tile and the mass is pressed into the holes with a broad spatula. If the mass is sticky, both surfaces of the mould plate should be dusted with a little amount of starch, talc or lactose. The well filled moulds are allowed to stand to evaporate moistening liquid. The mould plate is then placed over the peg plate and gently pressed down to eject tablet triturates. The ejected tablet triturates are spread evenly, in single layer, on a sieve, or on a thin cloth stretched upon a frame and dried in a chamber with warm circulating air. Plastic or glass jar is used as container. Since tablet triturates are friable, cotton is placed at the bottom of the jar and on the top of the product after filling.

Prescription No. 17.3

R

Paracetamol	125 mg
Aspirin	300 mg
Tablet triturate base q.s.	

Principle:

Tablet triturates are rapidly dispersible. The kid tablets of paracetamol, or dispersible tablets of aspirin, can be formulated in the form of tablet triturates. The use of alcoholic moistening agent also preserves the chemical stability of aspirin. The TT base mostly contains sucrose 20 parts and lactose 100 parts.

(Refer paracetamol elixir, chapter 4).

Apparatus: TT mould, spatula and pill tile.

Compounding: Calibrate the mould cavities preparing tablet triturates of the base. Calculate the formula. Calculate for some extra tablet triturates, then mix drug with TT base by doubling up method. Moisten paracetamol-containing mass with 50 per cent alcohol (note: Use absolute alcohol, for aspirin). Press the wet mass in cavities. Allow it to dry. Place on lower plate for ejection.

Container and storage: Pack in well-closed plastic or glass jars. Place cotton at the bottom of jar and on the top of product after filling. Store in a dry place.

Category and dose: Analgesic, antipyretic. 1 TT 3 times a day.

Dispensing: Do not dispense broken, abraded, powdered or moist tablet triturate. The PMR and CDR should be maintained.

Patient counselling: Handle with care, tablets are friable. Keep in airtight containers in a dry place. Avoid taking if having ulcers, asthma or impaired renal and hepatic functions. Avoid giving aspirin to children under 12 years and to breast feeding mothers.

Prescription No. 17. 4

℞

Diazepam 2.5 mg

Send 3 TTs

Principle:

Diazepam is anxiolytic. Adult dose is 2.5 -10 mg 2-4 times a day. For children upto 3 years 1-6 mg daily in divided doses.

Working Formula: Calculate for 4 TTs. Use lactose as diluent.

Drug: 2.5 mg × 4 = 10 mg

Weigh the minimum quantity of drug and triturate it with lactose. Mix the triturate containing 10 mg drug with TT base.

Apparatus: TT mould, spatula, pill tile.

Compounding: Calibrate the mould cavities preparing tablet triturates of TT base. Calculate the base required, then mix the drug with TT base by doubling up method. Moisten the mass with 50 per cent alcohol. Press the wet mass in cavities and allow to dry. Place on lower plate for ejection.

Container and storage: Pack in plastic or glass jars. Place cotton at the bottom of the jar and on the top of the product after filling. Store in well-closed containers, in a dry place.

Category and dose: Anxiolytic. 1 TT at bed time.

Patient counselling: Avoid taking it with alcohol. Take it with caution during cimetidine therapy. Avoid giving to children under six months.

LOZENGES

Definition and uses: Lozenges are round disc, oblong, triangular or rectangular shaped solid dosage forms, intended to be sucked. The viscous liquid produced in the mouth retains the medicament in contact with the affected area for a prolonged period of time. These are mainly used for treatment of local infections of the mouth and throat and are occasionally used as means of slow release of drugs for systemic action. The drugs routinely incorporated into lozenges include antiseptics, local anesthetics, antitussives, decongestants, vitamins, etc. Lozenges containing fluoride are used for the prevention of dental caries. Lozenges stimulate the mouth secretions and thus provide a demulcent and comforting effect in minor throat or oral cavity irritations.

Formulation: The lozenge base should ensure that there is no disintegration and should help slow dissolution of lozenge. The base mostly includes sugar, glycerin, liquid glucose and adhesives, like acacia, tragacanth, gelatin, methyl cellulose, or similar materials. Moulded glycero-gelatin lozenges are referred to as pastilles, while compressed lozenges are often referred as trouches.

Compounding: Extemporaneously, lozenges are prepared by moulding method and on large scale by compression method. Blend of medicament with base containing sucrose, acacia, is converted into pliable mass by adding water, syrup or tragacanth mucilage. Usually 6-7per cent acacia or 1-3 per cent tragacanth gives sufficient adhesion to the mass. The lozenge mass is rolled out on a board, with a roller, to form a sheet of uniform thickness. The sheet of required dimension is cut into round discs, rectangular shaped by means of a sharp knife, or lozenge cutter. Like pill making, cylindrical pipe is also made and cut to form lozenges. The lozenges are usually one gram in weight. The resultant lozenges are dried in a hot air chamber at moderate temperatures.

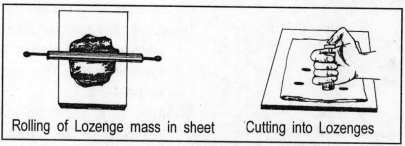

Rolling of Lozenge mass in sheet   Cutting into Lozenges

Figure 17.8: Compounding of Lozenges

The method of preparation of lozenges (pastille), using glycero-gelatin, is based on the principle of gelling of glycerin with gelatin. The most commonly used base contains one part of gelatin, two and half parts each of glycerin and water on weight basis. Gelatin is softened in water with the aid of heat. Mixture of softened gelatin and glycerin is heated below 120°C to form a clear solution. The medicament is added in gel just before stiffening of the mass with continuous stirring. The mass is poured at once in tray to form a sheet of uniform thickness. When cooled, the sheet is sized into squares with a sharp knife. Alternately, the liquid mass is allowed to solidify in cavities of metal mould or starch mould. Starch mould is made by forcing a peg plate into the bed of starch to produce cavities of required shape and size.

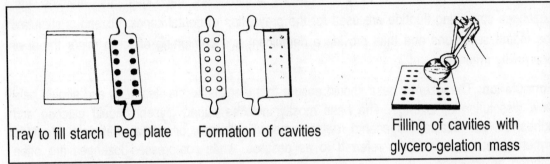

Tray to fill starch | Peg plate | Formation of cavities | Filling of cavities with glycero-gelation mass

Figure 17.9: Compounding of Glycero-Gelatin Pastilles using Starch Mould

Container and storage: Airtight containers like screw-capped glass or plastic jars or tubes are mostly used. Lozenges may be individually wrapped in wax paper or aluminum foils. They are stored in a cool and dry place.

Dispensing: The moist, sticky, soft or broken lozenges should not be dispensed. The PMR and CDR should be maintained.

Patient counselling: Remove the wrapper and suck one at a time whenever necessary. Do not drink water immediately after taking lozenge.

Prescription No. 17.5

℞

Benzalkonium Lozenges, BPC

Each ten lozenges contains,

Benzalkonium chloride solution	— 0.01 ml
Menthol	— 6.0 mg
Thymol	— 6.0 mg
Eucalyptus oil	— 0.02 ml
Lemon oil	— 0.02 ml
Lozenge base for 10 lozenges	— 10 g
Sucrose	
Powdered acacia	— 0.7 g

Principle:

Benzalkonium chloride is an antimicrobial agent and along with volatile substances, it is used in treatment of throat infections. A lozenge usually weighs 1-2 g.

Apparatus: Lozenge board, roller, lozenge cutter and spatula.

Compounding: Triturate an individual ingredient with mixture of sucrose and acacia powder. Mix the base by doubling up method. Add sufficient quantity of water to produce coherent mass and roll the mass into a sheet of uniform thickness and cut it into lozenges.

Containers and storage: Wrap each lozenge in wax paper and pack in a tube. Store in a well closed container.

Category and dose: Throat inflammation. Suck whenever necessary.

Label: Do not swallow. Suck it slowly.

Unit Dosage Forms

Prescription No. 17.6

℞

Bismuth Lozenges, Compound BPC
Each ten lozenges contain,

Bismuth Carbonate	— 1.5 g
Heavy Magnesium Carbonate	— 1.5 g
Calcium Carbonate	— 3.0 ml
Rose Oil	— 0.0006ml
Lozenge base for 10 lozenges	
Sucrose	— 10 g
Powdered acacia	— 0.7 g

Principle:

It is used as antacid in treatment of dyspepsia.

Apparatus: Lozenge board, roller, lozenge cutter, spatula.

Compounding: Triturate an individual ingredient with a mixture of sucrose and acacia powder. Mix the base by doubling up method. Add sufficient quantity of water to produce a coherent mass. Roll the mass into a sheet of uniform thickness and cut it into lozenges.

Containers and storage: Wrap each lozenge in wax paper and pack into jars or tubes. Store in a well-closed containers. Protect from light.

Category and dose: Antacid. Suck whenever necessary.

Label: Do not swallow. Suck it slowly.

PILLS

Definition and Uses: Pills are small spherical or oval shaped solid dosage forms intended for internal use. Most of the pills weighing between 60 and 300 mg and larger pills upto 2 gm are used for veterinary purposes. The latter are known as bolus. The smaller pills are superseeded by compressed tablets and capsules. Pills due to their smallness and spherical shape are easy to swallow and are also suitable for administration of the medicaments in concentrated form. Medicaments with bitter taste can be administered in the form of coated pills. Pills are not suitable to be administered in case of large dose drugs, drugs which irritate are corrosive or deliquescent and when fast action is required.

Formulation: The excipients required in compounding of pills are diluents and adhesives. The excipient used in pills gives essential characteristics to the pill, such as size, adhesiveness, firmness, disintegration and solubility. The best excipient is that, which quickly and easily makes a good pill mass, to produce pill of small size. Commonly used pill excpients can be classified as follows:

a) Adhesive excipients: Acacia mucilage, tragacanth mucilage, liquid glucose, syrup, honey, etc.

b) Liquid excipients: Water, alcohol, glycerin.

c) Absorbant excipient: Powdered liquorice root, acacia, tragacanth, kaolin, calcium phosphate, etc.

Adhesive excipients are required for substances that are insoluble in common solvents, or those that form solutions of not enough viscosity to produce a pasty pill mass. Acacia has been used in the form of 10-25 per cent solution. Tragacanth, when used alone, does not produce pills as hard as when acacia is used. Though, syrup possesses good excipient properties, honey is more adhesive due to presence of waxy and gummy material in it. Due to its low viscosity, it is easier to mix with powders than syrups. Liquid excipients interact with pill ingredient such as acacia, tragacanth or sugars, to produce an adhesive mixture. Alcohol or alcoholic tinctures are preferred over water when the formula contains a resinous matter and when rapid drying is required.

The surface of a pill often acquires dampness due to the presence of glycerin. Absorbant excipients are used to convert liquid, or soft ingredients, into semisolid mass. Powdered liquorice root has stiffening effect and it is useful in pill-containing oils. Animal soap (curd soap), like sodium stearate is usually combined with powdered liquorice root. Wool fat is a suitable pill excipient for oily ingredients. Petrolatum and Canada balsam are very useful for oxidisable substances or where aqueous or alcoholic liquids have to be avoided.

Conspergents are dusting powders used to prevent pill mass from sticking during compounding and to prevent the pills from adhering to each other. The most commonly used powders for this purpose are starch, talc, lycopodium and liquorice root powder.

Compounding: Considerable skill and care is required to produce pills of uniform weight and to maintain high level of hygiene. Pill tile and roller must be covered with white paper. A circular piece of white paper must fit exactly inside the pill rounder and hands must be spotlessly clean. The medicaments are thoroughly mixed with solid and liquid excipients to form a pill mass. When the weight of the mass indicates that a pill is exceeding 300 mg, the mass must be divided to prepare twice the number of pills and the direction is changed to take two pills at a time. The pill mass is rolled on the pill tile using a broad spatula to form a rope of uniform diameter and of exact length. The length of rope is determined by number of pills required. The pill tile or pill machine is lightly dusted. The rope made from pill mass with blunt ends is placed on the division line scale and cut into desired number of pills. The cut pieces are rolled into globular shape in the palm of one hand with finger of the other hand, or on pill rounder using a flat spatula. The slightly dusted pills are air dried. Sometimes, pills are coated to improve the finish, to mask unpleasant taste, to improve stability, or to change solubility. The coating material includes varnish (resins), sugar, gold, silver, enteric polymers, etc.

Container and storage: Pills are dispensed in screw capped glass or plastic jars. A thin layer of cotton is placed at the bottom and on the top of pills to prevent ratting and breaking of pills. Pills should be stored in airtight containers in a cool and dry place.

Unit Dosage Forms

Dispensing: Pills that are moist, sticky, broken or powdered, must not be dispensed. PMR and CDR must be maintained.

Patient counselling: The pills should be swallowed with water, or sucked in mouth, as per directions of the physician.

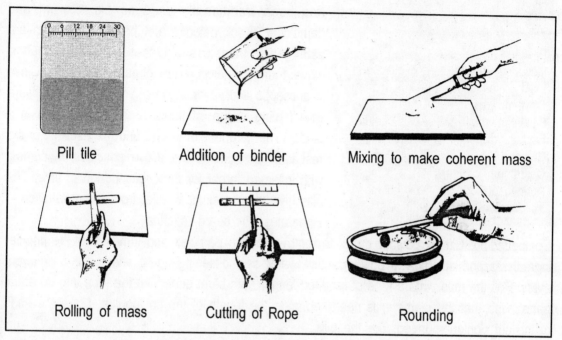

Pill tile   Addition of binder   Mixing to make coherent mass

Rolling of mass   Cutting of Rope   Rounding

Figure 17.10: Compounding of Pills

Prescription No. 17. 7

℞

Compound Phenolphthalein, Pills, BPC
Each 10 pills contains
Phenolphthalein — 0.3 g
Belladonna Dry Extract — 50.0 mg
Aloin — 0.15 g
Liquid Glucose Syrup — q.s.

Principle:

Aloin is extracted from aloes and in dose of 15-60 mg. It is used as purgative. It is an irritant purgative. It contains anthraquinones, which act on, the bowel in eight to twelve hours. Phenolphthalein is also an irritant purgative, and produces prolonged effect. Belladonna is an antispasmodic drug.

Apparatus: Pill tile, knife, spatula.

Compounding: Mix fine powders of phenolphthalein, belladonna dry extract and aloin. Add liquid glucose and knead to form pill mass. Roll the mass in to a rope of required length and of uniform diameter.

iii) Cut the rope in 10 equal parts and round them into pills. Dry in air.

Container and storage: Pack in screw capped glass, or plastic jars. A thin layer of cotton is placed at the bottom and on the top of pills. Store in airtight containers in a cool and dry place. Category and dose: Laxative. Dose: 1 to 2 pills.

Prescription No. 17. 8

℞

Throat Pills

Each pill contains

Liquorice powder	—	4.0 mg
Black catechu	—	30.0 mg
Clove powder	—	1.5 mg
Beleric myrobalan	—	5.0 mg
Fennel powder	—	5.0 mg
Camphor	—	1.0 mg
Cardamom powder	—	1.5 mg
Nutmeg powder	—	1.5 mg

Acacia gum q.s. Send 20 pills.

Principle:

Liquorice is a sweet saponin containing drug, which has been traditionally used as expectorant and demulcent. Black catechu and beleric myrobalan are astringents. Volatile substances such as camphor, clove, fennel, nutmeg are respiratory stimulants. Clove is antiseptic and vaporisation of volatile oil produces a cool feeling in the inflamed throat. Acacia gum is a binder. The hardness of the pill and the viscosity of the resultant liquid keeps the active principles in contact with inflamed throat for prolonged period of time. The pills give temporary local relief from throat irritation.

Apparatus: Pill board, spatula.

Compounding: Sift all powder drugs to remove foreign particles and lumps. Mix the powder ingredients and add acacia powder. Use water as moistening agent and make a coherent mass. Roll the mass into a rope of required length, with blunt ends. Cut the rope into 20 equal parts, such that the diameter is nearly equal to the length of the cut portion. Make the ends of the cut portion rounded. Dry the pills.

Container and storage: Plastic jars. Store in a well-closed plastic jars in a cool place.

Category and dose: Throat pills. Hold 1-2 pills in the mouth for slow dissolution whenever there is discomfort in the throat.

Label: Suck the pills slowly.

Patient counselling: Do not swallow the pills with water or do not chew them. Avoid smoke, dust. Avoid oily food. Drink plenty of water. Additionally use gargles.

Proprietary preparations:

- YOGI KANTHIKA (Yogi Ayurvedic, M.S.) : Mulethi 42per cent, Sunth 10per cent, Jaiphal 4.75 per cent, Ajwan ka satva 0.25 per cent, Sheetcichini 2.55, Tulsi 2.5 per cent, Lavang tel 2 per cent, Pudina tel 2 per cent, Kapoor 2 per cent, Mulithi satva 30 per cent, Babool ki goond q.s.

- KHO-GO (Ahilya Ayurvedic, Mumbai) : Acacia catechu 32.5, Areca catechu 10.4, Glycyrrhiza glabra 3.9, *Terminalia bellerica* 5.2, *Foeniculum vulgare* 5.2, *Piper cubeba* 2.6, *Elettaria cardamomum* 1.3, *Myristica fragrans* 1.3, *Caryophyllous aromatica* 1.3, Borniol 1.3.

Unit Dosage Forms

Prescription No. 17. 9

℞

Digestive Pills

Each pill contains:

Ginger	40 mg
Shankha bhasma	40 mg
Sajji Kshar	35 mg
Caraway	10 mg
Black pepper	8 mg
Amla	50 mg
Sucrose	50 mg
Lemon juice	q.s.
Starch paste	q.s.

Principle:

The volatile substances are carminative, stomachic and digestive. These increase salivary and gastric secretions. Shankha bhasma and sajji kshar are antacids. The pills should be held in the mouth for some time, so as to stimulate saliva and then swallowed.

Compunding: Use starch paste as binder and proceed with same as Prescription No.10.8.

Category and dose: Digestive and carminative. 1-2 pills after food.

Patient counselling: Do not take fatty food. Avoid alcohol and coffee. Walk after taking food. Drink plenty of water.

Proprietary preparations:

- HING-MING (Sanjivani): Hing 4.3mg, Sunthi 8.6 mg, Mire 6.9 mg, Pimpli 2.6 mg, Saindhav 60.1 mg, Jire 25.7 mg, Krishna lavan 51.5 mg, Imali kshar 34.3 mg, Nimbu Satva 10.3 mg.

- HAJMOLA (Dabur): Samudra Lavan 96 mg, Imli sarr 61 mg, Sharkara 341 mg, Kshudhvardak imli churna 100 mg consisting of imli sarr 25 mg, Jeeraka 20 mg, Krishna lavan 15 mg, Kali mirch 12 mg, Nimbu sarr 12 mg, Sunthi 6 mg.

- PACHAK VATI (Sharandhar Pharma, Pune): Sunthi, Chitrak, Hing, Sajii kshar, Shanka bhasma, Shuddha Gandhak, each 45 mg, Sauvarchal 60 mg, Amalaki 120 mg.

●●●●●

18 Sterile Products

Sterile dosage forms are completely free from microorganisms. These include injections, eye preparations, irrigating fluids, dialysis solutions, vaccines, blood products, etc. The term parenterals is derived from the Greek word *para* (besides) and *enteron* (the gut); the medicines applied topically to the skin, eye or ear, or those that are inhaled can be called as parenterals, but generally, the term parenteral refers to injections. A parenteral can be defined as a sterile fluid that does not utilise the GIT for entry into the body tissue. It gains entry into the body by routes other than the alimentary canal; and is packed in a manner suitable for administration by hypodermic injection.

Injections and eye preparations are mainly manufactured on a large scale. However, a dispensing pharmacist should be familiar with the types of injections and how they differ from non-sterile products. Hospital pharmacists have to operate different sterilisation equipments and work in aseptic areas. This chapter briefs about the important aspects of sterile products.

Advantages:

i) An immediate physiological action must be achieved in emergencies like cardiac arrest, asthma and severe imbalance of fluids and electrolytes, due to certain diseases.

ii) Prolonged drug action is possible, i.e., intramuscular injection of penicillin.

iii) Provides local effect thus avoiding systemic toxicity, as in local anesthetics, used in dentistry and anticancer drug injected in the cancer tissue.

iv) Convenient when oral route is not suitable:
    a) As in case of unconscious or unco-operative patients.

b) To avoid absorption or degradation of drugs in alimentary canal, e.g. Insulin and hormones.

v) Dose accuracy is greater.

vi) Direct control over pharmacological parameters is possible, such as onset of action, plasma levels, etc.

Disadvantages:

i) Must be administered by a trained person.

ii) Requires frequent visits of the patient.

iii) Requires asepsis during manufacturing and administration.

iv) Painful process.

v) Difficulty in correcting errors once administered.

vi) High manufacturing and packaging cost.

Types of Injections

Injections are sterile, pyrogen-free preparations intended to be administered in the skin layers, muscles, veins, or in particular organs, for rapid drug action.

1) Dosage forms:

a) Solution or suspension ready for injection.

b) Dry soluble/insoluble powders ready for reconstitution with sterile water for injection, before administration.

c) Emulsions.

2) Package:

a) Single dose units: Ampoules, pre-filled disposable syringes or infusion solutions.

b) Multiple dose units: Multiple dose vials.

c) Parenterals having volume less than 100 ml are called small volume parenterals (SVP) and those having volume greater than 100 ml are termed as large volume parenterals (LVP).

3) Route of administration:

a) Intradermal (Intracutaneous): Only small volume of fluids, up to 0.1 ml, is injected Into the superficial layer of the skin. Its use is generally restricted to diagnostic tests and certain vaccines.

b) Subcutaneous route: Subcutaneous (S.C.), is one of the primary routes of injections. These, administrations refer to injecting up to 2 ml into the loose connective and adipose tissues beneath the skin, usually of the arm or thigh, i.e., insulin injection.

c) IM administration, also a primary route, means injecting into the muscle mass in the upper arm (2 ml) or in the buttock (maximum up to 5 ml), which provides means for prolonged release of drugs formulated as aqueous, or oily, solution or suspension.

d) IV. route, another primary route, is used when an immediate systemic response is required. Injection is directly given into a vein. It is the main route for large volume parenterals. Injections above 10 ml are given by IV route. This route has the ability to restore rapid fluid and electrolyte balance, immediate response in emergencies and to provide continuous nutrition. Substances that are comparatively irritant, can be given by this route because of their rapid dilution. Suspensions should not be administered by IV route, because of the danger of possible blockage of the capillaries by the insoluble particles. In such cases, IM or SC route is preferred.

e) The other route includes intracardiac injection, i.e., injecting into the heart, usually in emergency situations such as cardiac arrest. Intraarticular route is injecting in to the joints in conditions such as rheumatoid arthritis. Hypodermoclysis is infusion of large volumes of solution into SC tissue, mainly for prolonged drug release. Intraspinal refers to injection into the spinal column.

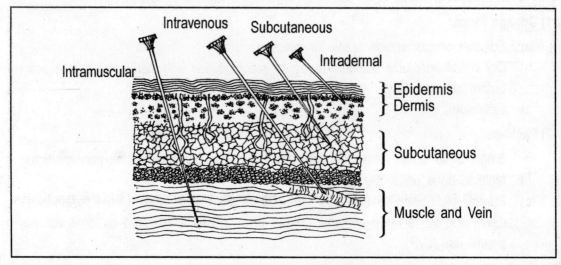

Figure 18.1: Routes for Injection

Requirements

1) Sterility: Sterile is an absolute term, which means free from all living microorganisms. The products which directly come in contact with tissues, bypassing natural barriers, such as injections, products for inflamed and infected eye, surgical powders and medical devices must be sterile.

Sterile Products

2) Free from particulate matter: Presence of extraneous, unintended foreign and insoluble substances in parenterals is the main cause of irritation and may lead to capillary blockage. Limits are set for the presence of particulate matter in injections (clarity).

3) Freedom from pyrogen: Pyrogens are chemically lipopolysaccharides and are metabolic products of living microorganisms, especially Gram-negative bacteria. When injected, they raise body temperature (pyretic). Water, container and chemicals used for preparations of injections are the main sources of pyrogens.

4) Isotonicity: Injections must be isotonic, i.e., have same osmotic pressure as that of the body fluid. 0.9 per cent w/v sodium chloride aqueous solution has same osmotic pressure as blood and it is isotonic. Paratonic solution (non-isotonic) may cause irritation and pain after injection. The solution having greater osmotic pressure than blood are hypertonic, which may cause shrinkage of blood cells. Hypotonic solutions have lower osmotic pressure than blood and can cause swelling of cells followed by haemolysis.

5) Stability: Parenterals, like other dosage forms, should remain physicochemically stable in the final container, throughout its shelf life. The product should not be dispensed if it shows any sign of leakage, if the content is not clear, contains visible particles, or shows any colour change.

Concept Clear : **Sterile Dosage Forms**

- Sterile means completely free from microorganisms.
- Parenterals means administration by other than oral route; but generally it refers to injections.
- Injections: Immediate effect in emergency. Suitable for unconscious, uncooperative patients and for administering drugs that are not absorb, or those that degrade, in the GIT.
- Requirements: Sterile, free from particulate matter, freedom from pyrogen, isotonic.

FORMULATION OF INJECTIONS

1) Vehicle: The majority of parenteral products are aqueous in nature because of their physiological compatibility; high dielectric constant and hydrogen bonding capacity, which makes water a good solvent for ionisable electrolytes, and substances such as alcohols, aldehydes, ketones, etc. Absorption of drugs normally occurs rapidly and completely when it is administered in the form of an aqueous solution.

a) Water for Injection (WFI): WFI is clear, colourless, odourless, pyrogen-free water, prepared freshly by distillations or by reverse osmosis and contains no added substances. It has pH within the range of 5-7 and it is used for preparation of parenteral products which are to be sterilised. The total dissolved solid content should not be more than 10 ppm and ionic

---

contaminants must not be more than 0.1 ppm. When WFI cannot be used immediately after its production, it is stored either at 5°C or 60-80 °C, to prevent production of pyrogens by inhibiting the growth of microorganisms.

b) Sterile Water for Injection (SWFI): SWFI is sterilised WFI, suitably packed in single dose containers, not larger than 1liter. These are used for preparation of injection by admixing with other sterile ingredients under aseptic conditions and which are not terminally sterilised. The SWFI is used as sterile vehicles for reconstitution of sterile dry powders just before injections. A higher solid content is allowed in SWFI as there are chances of leaching of material from glass containers during its sterilisation. Secondly, when packed in 30 ml or smaller containers, SWFI may contain bacteriostatic agents. The limit for dissolved solid is upto 40 ppm. Containers of larger quantities of SWFI should contain low levels of solids, so as to avoid toxicity due to injection of larger quantity of a bacteriostatic agent.

c) Non-aqueous vehicles: Though an aqueous vehicle is generally used for an injection, it has limitations if the drug is insoluble in the aqueous phase and if it hydrolyses. The non-aqueous vehicles presently employed for injections are fixed vegetable oils, glycerin, propylene glycol, PEG and, to a lesser extent, ethyl oleate, isopropyl myristate. In addition to all required properties, these should allow thermal sterilisation and should remain clear when cooled. Oils must be absorbed by body tissues, this precludes use of mineral oil.

2) Added substances: Added substances are selected either to improve solubility, physicochemical stability, maintain sterility or to improve safety of the parenteral formulation. Colours are never added to parenteral formulations.

a) Solubilising agents: To enhance the solubility of drugs, parenteral formulation contains co-solvents, some chemical additives and surfactants. Co-solvents, such as alcohol and liquid PEG (polyethylene glycol), not only improve the solubility of drugs in water but also reduce hydrolysis of drugs, for example, sodium benzoate to solubilise caffeine, ethylenediamine is used in aminophyllin injection. The non-ionic surfactants have been used to solubilise drugs such as vitamins, hormones and volatile oils.

b) Buffers: Changes in pH of parenteral preparation may occur because of chemical degradation, interaction with container and dissolution of gases. The ideal pH of injection should be 7.4, which is the pH of the blood. pH of parenterals administered other than I.V. route is generally adjusted to a pH between 4 and 9. Blood is an excellent buffer that can tolerate an injection with pH 3 to 10.5. To achieve the greatest buffer capacity, buffer which has a pKa within ± 1 of desired pH is selected. Buffer systems commonly used for injectables are acetates, citrates, phosphates and glutamate. Effect of ionic strength of buffers on isotonicity should be considered while selecting buffers. Buffers should not be used in intracardiac and intraocular injections.

c) Antioxidants: The commonly used antioxidants for aqueous parenterals are sodium and potassium salts of the metasulfite and sulfite ions. Chelating agents, such as EDTA, citric acid and tartaric acid, are used to improve the effectiveness of antioxidants. Protection from oxidation can be achieved by bubbling nitrogen or carbon dioxide through the solution prior to filling and maintaining the solution under a blanket of these inert gases.

d) Preservatives: The IP recommends the use of anti-microbial agents in preparations packed in multi-dose containers. Preservatives should not be added when the volume to be injected as a single dose exceeds 15 ml. The most frequently used preservatives include benzethonium chloride, benzalkonium chloride and phenyl mercuric nitrate upto 0.01 per cent; phenol, cresol and chlorobutanol upto 0.5 per cent and combination of methyl paraben upto 0.18 per cent with propyl paraben upto 0.02 per cent.

e) Tonicity modifiers: Injections have to be made isotonic with blood first, by adding sodium chloride or dextrose. The slightly hypertonic injections can be tolerated if given by I.V. route, owing to fast dilution of injections after administration. To facilitate absorption of drug from tissues, the SC and IM injections can be made hypertonic. If a preparation is hypertonic, either it is injected by a suitable route, or it is injected slowly allowing sufficient time for dilution.

f) Wetting and Suspending agents: The improper formulation of suspensions not only affects the dose uniformity, but also determines its syringeability and injectability. The sedimentation of insoluble drug makes it difficult to take an accurate dose in the syringe (syringeability) and to inject with an even flow, without clogging, under given pressure (injectability). Wetting agents, such as polysorbate 80, pluronic and sorbitan trioleate and suspending agents such as sodium CMC, PVP and gelatin, are used to maintain physical stability of parenteral suspensions.

g) Dry powders for injections: Drug, which is unstable in liquid form is filled in vials, which is reconstituted using sterile water for injection. To enhance reconstitution, the powder may be aseptically crystallised or lyophilised. When the same injection is to be given by two different routes, the required volume of SWFI varies; e.g. Ceftriaxone sodium injection USP, 1g of which is reconstituted using 9.6 ml of SWFI for IV administration, and using 3.6 ml of SWFI for an IM injection.

h) Containers: For parenterals, the commonly used containers are glass ampoules sealed by fusion of glass or plastic vials closed with a rubber stopper and sealed with an aluminium crimp. Ampoules are made of Type I glass and the medicaments filled in it are for single use. Since ampoules are opened by breaking the glass, there are chances of glass particles entering the solution. Vials with rubber stoppers are used for multidose products. However, rubber particles generated from closures may contaminate the product and multiple withdrawals may result in microbial contamination. Drugs administered in an emergency are available in pre-filled syringes.

Large volume parenterals (LVP) are packed in glass bottles, PVC collapsible bags or semi-rigid infusion bags. Glass bottles are made of Type I or Type II glass. The PVC and semi-rigid bags have two ports, one for attachment of infusion set and other for addition of small volume parenterals. Nowadays, PVC bags employed for Form-Fill-Seal (FFS) technique is the most accepted container. LVP containers have a graduated scale, which can be read either in an inverted or upright position. The sterile container containing LVP are further wrapped with moisture barrier polythene.

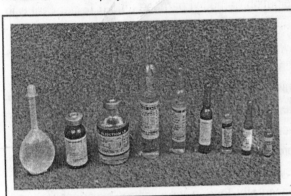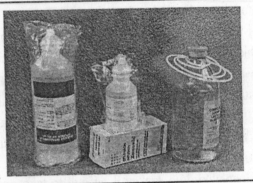

Figure 18.2: Containers for Injectable Products

Concept Clear : Formulation of Injections

- Water for Injection (WFI): WFI is pyrogen free, but non-sterile water, prepared freshly by distillation, or by reverse osmosis and contains no added substances. It is used for preparation of parenteral products that have to be sterilised.
- Sterile Water for Injection (SWFI): SWFI is sterilised WFI suitably packed in single dose containers, not larger than one litre. These are aseptically mixed with sterile ingredients or for reconstitution of sterile dry powders just before injections. Contain preservatives.
- Other additives: Solubilising agents, buffers, antioxidants, preservatives, tonicity modifiers and suspending agents.
- Containers: Glass ampoules sealed by fusion of glass, or plastic vial, closed with a rubber stopper and sealed with an aluminium crimp, or pre-filled syringes, are for single dose injections. The vials are used for multidose products. Large volume parenterals are packed in glass bottle, PVC collapsible bags or semi-rigid infusion bags.

STERILE FACILITY

Sterilisation

The most popular sterilisation method is thermal sterilisation, either by dry or moist heat. A hot air oven is used for dry heat sterilisation. The equipments are sterilised for 2 hours at 180°C, which normally kills microorganisms by oxidation. This process is used for sterilisation of glassware and metal equipments. In moist heat sterilisation, the steam generated in an autoclave causes coagulation of cellular proteins of microorganisms and sterilisation occurs within 10 minutes at 121°C and 15 pounds pressure. Rubber closures, gloves, uniforms, filters of various types, etc., can be sterilised by this technique. Non-thermal methods of sterilisation include filtration, ionising radiation and chemical sterilisation. Heat-labile substances like penicillin, vitamins, catgut, disposable needles and syringes are routinely sterilised by ionising radiation or chemical sterilisation. The former is based on lethal mutations in microorganisms by electromagnetic or particulate radiation. Chemical sterilisation using ethylene oxide gas, is used extensively to sterilise plastics, medical instruments and hospital bedding. Ethylene oxide acts by alkylating those bacterial proteins, which are needed for reproductive processes. A material containing little moisture is more susceptible to gaseous sterilisation. However, residual gas must be allowed to dissipate after sterilisation. Heat-labile solutions are clarified and sterilised using membrane filters of porosity ranging from 0.45 - 5 mm and then filled aseptically into the sterile containers and sealed.

Aseptic Processing

The environment for preparing and handling of sterile products should be aseptic, instruments should have a high standard of cleanliness and absolute control on microbial contamination should be maintained. Sterile preparations are processed either by aseptic filling in which sterilised material is filled and sealed in sterile containers; or the product is filled in clean containers, and the sealed container is terminally sterilised.

In general, ingredients, containers and equipment flow from the supply room either to the clean-up area, or to the compounding area. Clean-up area is mainly used for cleaning and assembling equipment and containers. This area is specially constructed and cleaned so as to prevent deposition of particles or other contaminants inside the area, as well as on the equipment. Clean-up area does not need to be aseptic. Compounding area is used for compounding of preparations. Its construction is same as clean-up area with more control maintained on the microbial load.

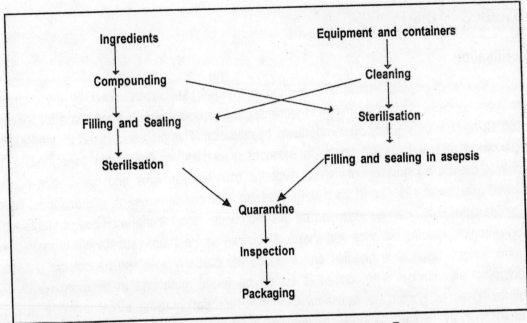

Figure 18.3: Preparation of Parenteral Dosage Forms

Aseptic area is a specially constructed area, where the ceiling, walls and floor must be sealed; all counters should be of stainless steel so that they can be washed and sanitised. The area should not have any such places where accumulation of dirt can occur. Personnel should have entry into this area through an airlock. The environmental control of an aseptic area can be maintained in following ways:

Air cleaning: An aseptic area must be maintained as free as possible from particulate matter. The air supplied must be thoroughly filtered. HEPA (High efficiency particulate air) filters are used to cleanse the air. These filters are capable of removing particles of 0.3 mm and above, with an efficiency of 99.97 per cent. This clean air is introduced into the aseptic area to maintain a positive pressure, which prevents the outside air from rushing into that area.

Laminar flow: It distributes filtered air with a uniform velocity along parallel lines resulting in total sweep of a confined area. The velocity of the airflow is 100 ± 20 feet per minute. Laminar airflow units can be placed above filling machines, such that vertical airflow or horizontal airflow takes place across the surface of working area. The laminar airflow can be arranged so as to cover the entire room or be limited to the working area only. The laminar hoods are used for covering only the work area.

Clean room: It is generally classified as, class 100. It means that it does not contain more than 100 particles, sized 0.5 mm, or larger, per cubic feet. The filtered rooms should be aseptic of class 100. On this basis, clean rooms are classified as class 10,000. The entire facility is irradiated with ultraviolet lamps to assure disinfection.

Personnel: The essential factors for working in sterile area is a properly motivated, neat, orderly and reliable staff. The personnel must be healthy. The uniforms, i.e., facemask, caps, gloves, disposable boots, apron, goggles, etc., should be freshly laundered and sterile. The flow of both personnel and goods should be in one direction only, i.e., from the cleanest to the sterile area with no crossover.

DISPENSING OF INJECTIONS

Checking of products: During manufacturing, the injections are checked for ensuring sterility, absence of pyrogens and the limit of presence of particulate matter. In addition, at the time of dispensing, the injections must be checked for the following criteria:

i) Damage to the container, as even minor damages may result in contamination.

ii) Presence of any suspended particles.

Patient counselling: Ask the patient to handover the injection to the medical practitioner immediately after purchase. Some injections have specific storage conditions, which must be followed diligently. Warn them not to open the pack including the outer wrapper.

Advice to the doctors:

i) Return the injection for replacement, if leakage is found on squeezing, or if the contents are not clear, or contain visible particles.

ii) Do not remove the inner container from the overwrap until ready for use.

iii) Injections should not be used if any suspended particle is visible.

iv) The reconstituted suspension should be used immediately. Shake vial vigorously before withdrawing the dose.

v) Discard any unused portion.

Proprietary preparations:

a) Single Dose injections:

Ampoules:

- NEUROBION FORTE (Merk): I.M., Multivitamin injection.
- PERINORM (IPCA) IM, IV, Metoclopramide HCl. Hyperacidity, GI sedative.
- PHENERGAN (Nicholas): IM, slow IV, Promethazine HCl. Antiemetic.
- FORTWIN (Ranbaxy): IV, IM, SC, Pentazocin lactate. Analgesic, antipyretic.
- ATROPINE SULPHATE INJ., IP (T. Walkers): IV, IM, SC, Antimuscarinic.

Dry Powders for reconstitution:

Dry powder is packed in vials and supplied with SWFI.

- PENIDURE LA 12 (Wyeth): IM, Benzathine Penicillin injection, IP. Antibacterial.
- C-TRI 250 (Zuventus): IM, IV, Ceftriaxone for injection, USP. Antibacterial.
- TAXIM Injection (Alkem): IM, IV, Cefotaxime for injection, USP. Antibacterial.
- NOVA CLOX-1000 (Okasa): IM, IV, Amoxicillin sodium and Cloxacillin. Antibacterial.

b) Multidose injections:

- PERINORM (IPCA) IM, IV, 5 ml vial. Metoclopramide HCl. Hyperacidity, GI sedative.
- AVIL-RC (Hoechest Marion Roussel): IM, slow IV, 10 ml; Pheniramine maleate. Classical antihistamine.
- G-MYCIN (BPL Pharma): IM. IV, 20 ml; Gentamycin. Antimicrobial.
- FEBRINIL (Sigma), IM, 15 ml; Paracetamol. Antipyretic.
  LVP 100 ml
- CIPLOX (Cipla): IV, Ciprofloxacin Injection, IP. Antibacterial.
- METROGYL (JB Chemical) Slow IV, Metronidazole Injection, IP. Antibacterial.
  LVP 500 ml,
- HAEMACEEL (Nicholas) Each 100 ml contains polymer from degraded gelatin (Equivalent to the nitrogen content of 0.63 g) 3.5 g, electrolyte in m.mol/lit Na^+ 145, K^+ 5.1,Ca^{++} 6.25, Cl^- 145 in WFI. Electrolyte.
- COMPOUND SODIUM LACTATE INJECTION, IP: (Denis Chem) Each 100 ml contains Sodium lactate solution USP equivalent to sodium lactate 0.32 g; Sodium chloride 0.6 g, Potassium chloride 0.4 g, Calcium chloride 0.027 g in WFI.
- SODIUM CHLORIDE AND DEXTROSE INJECTION, IP (Denis): Each 100 ml contains. Dextrose unhydrous 5 g, Sodium chloride 0.9 g, in WFI.

Insulin Injection

Insulin is choice of drug for Type-1 diabetes. According to onset and duration of action it is classified as follows:

Type	Examples	Onset (hr)	Duration (hr)
Short acting	Regular	0.5 to 1	3 to 8
Rapid acting	Lispro, Aspart	<0.25	6 to 12
Intermediate acting	Lente, NPH	1 to 2	18 to 24
Long acting.	Ultra lente, Glargine	4 to 6	24 to 36

Pre-mixed insulin containing 30:70 and 50:50 regular and NPH insulin, are also available. Insulin vials are available in two strengths, 40 IU and 100 IU with corresponding syringes.

Patient Counselling: Lead a healthy life style taking low sugar diet, high fiber vegetarian diet and regular exercise. Avoid alcohol and smoking. Take medicines regularly and at the scheduled time. Take care of the feet and avoid injury. Explain time for administration of oral hypoglycemic agents. Most of these are taken on full stomach. Take acarbose with the first few mouthfuls of food. Insulin should ideally be taken half an hour before a meal. Explain storage conditions and demonstrate method for insulin injection.

Self administration of insulin:

i)   Follow the directions given by the physician concerning the dose and time of injection.

ii) Make sure that the purchased product is of correct type and strength of insulin.

iii) Do not change the medicine except on doctors' advice.

iv) Use syringe that is marked according to the dose of insulin.

v)   Wash hands with soap and water before using the injection.

vi) Insulin injection is either a clear solution or a cloudy suspension. Suspension should be rolled between the palms until the content is uniformly distributed. Do not shake the insulin vials; it may produce air bubbles that can get into the syringe.

vii) Insulin is ideally given half an hour before a meal.

viii) Keep the vials out of refrigerator for 10-15 minutes before injecting.

Preparation of syringe: Use of disposable syringe is advisable; otherwise a sterilised syringe should be used. Sterilise the syringe as follows:

i)   Boil the syringe, plunger and needle for 5 minutes in water. When cooled, remove the articles from the water. Insert the plunger into the syringe and attach the needle. Move the plunger in the syringe several times to make it completely free of water.

ii) Avoid cleansing the needle with alcohol as it may dissolve the silicone coating and increase the pain at the site of injection.

Filling the syringe with insulin:

i)   Roll the vial between the palms until the liquid gets uniformly dispersed.

ii) Wipe the top of the vial with an alcohol swab.

iii) Pull the plunger back to draw air into the syringe. The volume of air should be equal to the dose. Introduce air in the vial.

iv) Turn the vial and syringe upside down and draw the correct dose of insulin into the syringe. Withdraw the needle and expel the air from the syringe and check that the dose is correct.

v)   Inject immediately.

vi) To take two types of insulin:

- Take regular insulin injection first.

Modern Dispensing Pharmacy

- Without moving the plunger, insert the needle in the second type of insulin bottle and withdraw the correct dose.
- Do not inject the extra insulin back into the bottle, but throw it away.

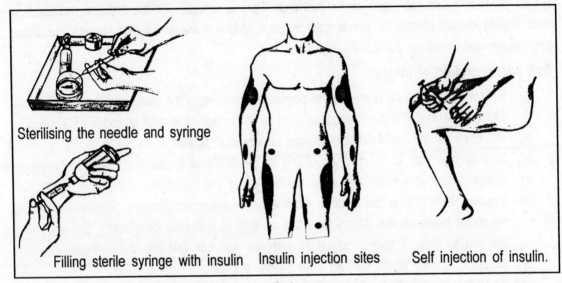

Sterilising the needle and syringe

Filling sterile syringe with insulin   Insulin injection sites   Self injection of insulin.

Figure 18.4: Administration of Insulin Injection

Method to inject insulin:

i) Insulin is administered as subcutaneous injection at different locations shown in Fig 18.4. SC injection into abdomen wall results in a faster absorption than from other sites.

ii) Insulin suspension should never be given intravenously.

iii) Choose the injection site. Clean the area using an alcohol swab. Pinch up the skin between fingers. Inject the needle at 90° angle into the skin.

iv) A different spot, at least a finger-width away, from the last shot should be selected for each consecutive injection. Repeated injection at a single site may cause hard fatty deposit (lipodystrophy) and delayed absorption of insulin.

v) After removing the needle, the area should be pressed or rotated within an anatomical region in order to avoid lipodystrophy, but should not be rubbed heavily.

Storage of insulin:

i) Insulin injection vials should be stored in the refrigerator between 2 and 8 °C; but never be kept in, or very close to, the freezer compartment. It should be kept in the door compartment, below and away from the freezer.

ii) Earthen pot (Refer Chapter 6) can be used to store insulin.

Sterile Products

iii) Insulin should ideally be stored horizontally.

iv) Do not store insulin on the top of a refrigerator or, T.V., near the stove, or in luggage bags, during air travel. It may heat the insulin.

v) When travelling, always carry one additional set of insulin, as there are chances of breakage of glass bottles.

Proprietary preparations:

- ACTRAPID (Novo Nordisk) Neutral highly purified (procaine) 40 IU per ml.
- HUMAN MIXTARD (Knoll): Highly purified biphasic insulin (monocomponent human) 40 IU per ml.
- MIXTARD-30 (Knoll): It contains a mixture of 30 per cent rapid acting, and 70 per cent intermediate acting, isophane insulin per 100 IU/ml.
- ACTRAPID MC (Knoll): Highly purified monocomponent pork neutral insulin, 40 IU per ml.

Note 4: Diabetes Mellitus

An elevated level of sugar in the blood is called as diabetes mellitus. It is a metabolic disorder characterised by chronic hyperglycaemia and disturbances of carbohydrate, fat and protein metabolism associated with absolute or relative deficiencies in insulin secretion and/or insulin action. Insulin is a hormone that helps the body use glucose for energy. The beta cells of the pancreas make insulin. When the body does not produce enough insulin and/or the cells ignore the insulin, it results in elevation of blood glucose level.

Blood sugar levels are estimated at different time intervals. Fasting plasma glucose (FPG) means estimation of blood glucose in patient fasting for 8-10 hours. FPG 70-100 mg/dl is considered as normal, 100-126 mg/dl is pre-diabetic signal and in diabetic if it is above 126 mg/dl. PPG (post-prandial glucose) is blood glucose estimated 4-6 hrs after eating a meal. It should be 180 mg/dl. Glycosylated hemoglobin test (HbA1c) indicates average blood sugar level over 8-12 weeks period and it should be below 6 per cent.

Accordingly, there are two major types of diabetes, viz., Type 1 diabetes when the body doesn't produce insulin and Type 2 diabetes, where either the body does not produce enough insulin to keep the blood glucose level normal, and/or the cells ignore the insulin. Type 1 diabetes mellitus treatment requires insulin injections. Type 2 diabetes is more common and can be treated by oral hypoglycaemic agents like Gliclazide, Glimepiride, Metformin, Pioglitazone, Rosiglitazone, Acarbose and Miglitol. The other types of diabetes include, gestational diabetes, which develops during pregnancy and may persist as Type 2 diabetes later in life. The secondary diabetes is drug-induced by certain drugs, or by pancreatic, hormonal, or other disorders.

Signs and symptoms of diabetes mellitus include polyphagia, polyurea, polydipsia, blurred vision, fatigue, weight loss, dry skin and frequent infections. Diabetic patients may suffer from hypoglycemia when blood glucose level falls too low. Mild conditions can be treated by immediate administration of sugar-based edibles like biscuits or chocolates. Hypoglycemia may be fatal and needs emergency hospitalisation. The symptoms of hypoglycemia are headache, fatigue, looking confused, looking pale, fast heartbeats and in severe cases, falling unconscious and going into coma.

OPHTHALMIC PREPARATIONS

Ophthalmic preparations are sterile preparations intended for application to the eye for a localised effect on the surface of the eye; these mainly include aqueous or non-aqueous solutions or suspensions and ointments.

Requirements

Most of the requirements of ophthalmic preparations are the same as that of injections. Some important points are as follows:

- Except for ophthalmic preparations used during eye surgery, preservatives should be added to ensure sterility. The former are usually packed in single dose containers. The preservative for ophthalmic preparations includes benzalkonium chloride, chlorbutanol, phenylmercuric acetate, phenylmercuric nitrate, etc.
- Ophthalmic preparations need not be pyrogen-free, as pyrogens-cannot cross the eye membrane.
- Ophthalmic solutions are preferred over suspensions and ointments. The later are useful to increase the corneal contact time.
- Lachrymal fluid has an osmotic pressure corresponding to that of a 0.9 per cent sodium chloride solution. The eye preparations should be isotonic.
- Lachrymal fluid has pH of about 7.4 and ideally ophthalmic solution should have the same pH. However, practically, the buffer should maintain a balance between comfort, solubility, stability and activity of drug.
- Viscosity of the eye drops determines its residence in the eye, which should be 15-25 cps. Viscosity enhancers include hypromellose, polyvinyl alcohol.
- Ointment base used should be non-irritating, have melting or softening point close to body temperature. Mixture of yellow soft paraffin, liquid paraffin, wool fat or lanolin is generally used as base.
- The commonly used container for ophthalmic solutions or suspension, is a multi-dose container (5 ml, 10 ml). Glass containers are supplied with sterile plastic droppers. Plastic bottles are produced by FFS technique with built-up nozzle. Eye ointments are packed in smaller plastic tubes fitted with a narrow gauge tip. (Fig. 18.5)
- Label: Not for injection. For external use only. Shake well before use (if it is a suspension).

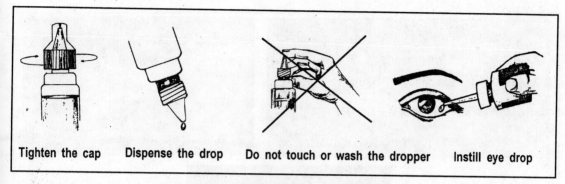

| Tighten the cap | Dispense the drop | Do not touch or wash the dropper | Instill eye drop |

Figure 18.5: Plastic Eye drop Container

Dispensing

Checking product: The product should not be dispensed if it leaks, contains foreign matter, is turbid or if the dropper is open.

Patient counselling: a) Fitting the dropper: Place the dropper on the vial as explained in Figure. 18.5. When the vial is a plastic bottle with built-in nozzle, tighten the cap on the nozzle. The spike in the cap will make a dispensing hole on the nozzle. Remove the cap and dispense drops applying gentle pressure. Replace the cap.

b) Mode of use: The patient should look upward for instillation of eye drops. The eyedropper should be held above the eye with the right hand and with the left hand, the patient should pull the lower eyelid down. Eye drops should be dropped quickly without touching the dropper to the eye. After instillation, the patient should keep the eyes open for 30 seconds. If more than one drop is to be administered, a three to five-minute interval between drops is recommended. This allows distribution of drug in the eye and minimises loss by drainage. Ointment should be placed onto the margin of the eyelid.

Warnings:

i) If irritation persists or increases, stop the use and consult the physician.

ii) Do not touch the tip of the dropper to any surface, or do not rinse it, since this may contaminate the product.

iii) Use it within one month after opening the vial.

iv) Remove contact lens before instillating the eye drops and do not wear them during eye infection.

v) Stay away from irritant factors such as dust, smoke, and swimming pool water. Wear goggles.

vi) Do not touch the eyes frequently to avoid re-infection. Rubbing causes redness of eyes.

vii) Do not share towels, goggles and glasses.

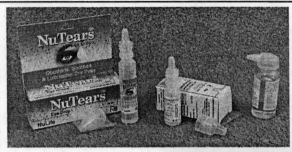
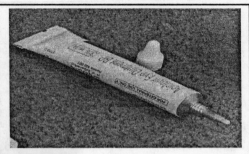
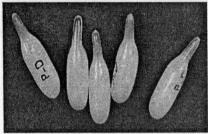

Plastic eye drops 10 ml and 5 ml (Courtesy of NuLife Pharmaceuticals and Miaami Pharma and Chemicals). Glass vial with dropper, Opthalmic ointment in collapsible and Soft capsules (applicaps).

Figure 18.6: Containers for Ophthalmic Preparations

Proprietary preparations:

Eye drops

- OCUCHLOR (Elder), CHLORMET (Milmet): Chloramphenicol 0.5%. Antibiotic.
- ALCIPRO (Alkem), CEBRAN (Blue Cross): Ciprofloxacin 3 mg/ml. Antibiotic.
- SOFRAMYCIN (Hoechest Marion Roussel): Framycetin 0.5%. Antibiotic.
- GARAMYCIN (Fulford), GENTICYN (Nicholas Piramal): Gentamicin 3 mg/ml.
- MILBETA (Milmet) Betamethasone 0.1%. Antiinflammatory.
- DICLORAN (Unique): Diclofenac 0.1%. OCUFLUR (FDC): Flurbiprofen 0.03%. NSAID.
- PILOCAR (FDC), PILOPRESS (Centaur): Pilocarpine 1,2,4%. Cholinergic.
- DILATE (Micro Vision), CYCLOGIK (FDC): Cyclopentolate 1%. Mydriatic.

Eye ointment

- ACIVIR (Cipla), HERPEX OPHTHACOPS (Torrent): Acyclovir 3%. For treating Herpes Simplex infection.
- CHLOROMYCETIN APLICAPS (Parke-Davis): Chloramphenicol 1%. Antibiotic.
- CIPLOX (Cipla), ZOXAN (FDC): Ciprofloxacin 0.3%. Antibiotic.
- BETNESOL (Glaxo), Betamethasone 0.1%. Antiinflammatory.

•••••

19 Novel Drug Delivery Systems

ORAL DRUG DELIVERY SYSTEMS

Novel Drug Delivery Systems (NDDS) is the extension of conventional dosage forms, developed on novel ideas to achieve improved patient compliance, modified drug release, delivery of drug to site of action, more efficient administration of drugs by various routes, and for better therapeutic effect. The examples of NDDS are as follows:

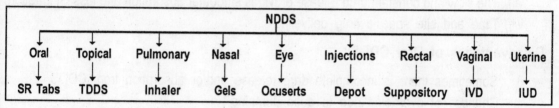

The conventional dosage forms are designed to provide drug rapidly to the body. For example, the disintegration time of conventional tablets is less than 15 minutes and a single dose of drug is provided by them. Drug dissolved in GI content enters in blood circulation to elicit its action. This type of dosage forms need frequent dosing to achieve therapeutic effect, hence shows fluctuation in systemic drug concentration. The Sustained Release Dosage Forms (SRDF) are based on slow drug release for extended period of time. Controlled Drug Delivery Systems (CDDS) provide constant release of contained drug at predetermined rate and for a predetermined time period.

Advantages of Oral CDDS:

i)   Deliver drug at a controlled rate over an extended period of time.

ii) More uniform blood concentration, in turn more consistent and prolonged therapeutic effect.

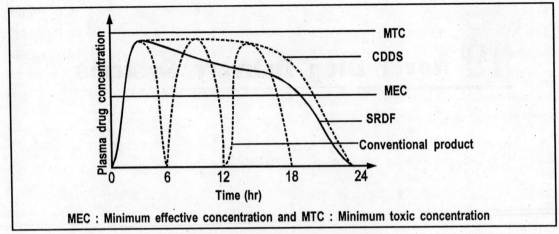

MEC : Minimum effective concentration and MTC : Minimum toxic concentration

Figure 19.1: Plasma Drug profile

iii) Improved patient compliance due to the reduced dosing frequency and avoidance of night time dosing.

iv) Less chances of missing of dose.

v) Reduce adverse effects associated with intermittant dosing.

vi) Reduce daily dose of drug.

vii) The slow and constant drug release provides smoother absorption and less GI irritation.

viii) Time and site specific drug delivery.

Disadvantages of Oral CDDS:

i) Sometimes there is incomplete drug release and/or absorption from CDDS.

ii) Chances of overdoing due to dose dumping.

iii) Increased cost.

iv) Unpredictable and poor *in vitro : in vivo* correlation.

v) Increased potential for first pass clearance.

vi) Reduce flexibility of dose adjustment.

vii) Need for additional patient education and counselling.

Techniques to Control Drug Release

CDDS works on principle of drug release in two portions. The initial dose should release immediately to achieve steady state plasma concentration that promptly produces the desired therapeutic effect. It is followed with a gradual and continuous release of remaining drug to extend the steady state level over prolonged period of time. Tremendous research has been taking place in this field and too many techniques are available to achieve controlled drug release. The most common techniques used are as follows:

1) Polymer coating: Tablets, capsules or granules can be coated with polymer to retard the drug release. These polymers may be hydrophobic, hydrophilic-swellable, or have pH dependent solubility. The insolubility, concentration and thickness of water-insoluble polymers govern the rate of drug release. The diffusion of drug from the cohesive gel formed by swellable polymer is another mechanism. Delayed release from enteric polymer is best example of pH-dependent drug release.

2) Matrix tablets: The physical mixture of drug and polymer is compressed into a tablet; the nature and concentration of polymers are rate determining factors.

3) Microcapsules or coated beads: To minimise 'all or non-effect' of the controlled release tablets or capsules, and to achieve controlled release of two drugs simultaneously, the coated beads or microcapsules are filled in hard gelatin capsules. After the disintegration of the capsule, the individual beads or microcapsules show desired controlled drug release.

Sometimes, the CDDS discussed above are bio-adhesive to GI mucosa, or float on the gastric content and have prolonged gastric residence.

4) Pro-drugs: The drug is chemically modified to alter pharmacokinetic properties. The bonding of drug with pharmacologically inactive moiety and site-specific breakdown of such bonds is common approach of pro-drug.

The other techniques include, increasing the particle size and reducing rate of dissolution of the drug, use of ion exchange resin, osmotic agents, etc.

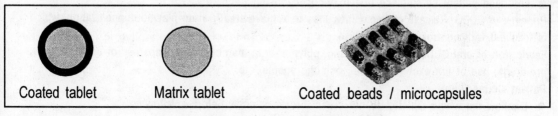

Coated tablet   Matrix tablet   Coated beads / microcapsules

Figure 19.2: Fabrication of Oral CDDS

Dispensing

SR Tablets and capsules should be observed for intactness. Broken/cracked or adhered dosage forms must not be dispensed.

Patient counselling: Swallow the whole tablet. Do not crush, break, or chew before swallowing. Do not open the capsule and sprinkle the beads onto the food unless told to do so by the physician. Take the medicine at about the same time each day. Some medicines are to be taken each morning after fasting overnight, or at least 1 hour before eating. However, majority of medicines are to be taken in the morning or evening after food. No two CDDS of drugs show the same super-imposable drug release profile, because of the difference in the technique used to control drug release. Therefor, do not change brands without the permission of the physician. Unless otherwise, directed do not refill the prescription.

Advise to the doctors: Physician should check the progress of the patients at regular visits; it helps the doctor to decide the dose of a particular medicine.

Proprietary preparations:

- DICARD (Intas), ICIDIL -CD (ICI): Diltiazem 90 mg. Antihypertensives
- FELOGARD ER (Cipla): Felodipine 2.5, 5 and 10 mg respectively. Antihypertensives
- CALCIGARD RETARD (Torrent), DEPICOR (Merck): Nifedipine 20 mg. Antianginal
- BRONCODRIL XL (USV), THEOBID SR: Theophylline 200 mg. Anti-asthma.
- DIC-SR (Dee Pharm): Diclofenac sodium 100 mg. NSAID.

Capsules:

- BETA NIFEDINE (SPPL), CALBETA (Torrent) : Atenolol 50 mg, Nifedipine SR 20 mg. Antihypertensive.
- DURASAL CR (Raptakos), VENTORLIN (Glaxo Allenburys) : Salbutamol 10 mg.

Concept Clear : **Oral CDDS**

- Deliver drug at a controlled rate over an extended period of time.
- More uniform blood concentration, in turn more consistent and prolonged therapeutic effect.
- Improved patient compliance due to reduced dosing frequency.

Principle of CDDS: Release of immediate dose to achieve steady state plasma concentration, which is followed with controlled drug release.

Fabrication of oral CDDS: Polymer coating, polymer-drug matrices, microcapsules or coated beads, pro-drugs, use of ion exchange resin, osmotic agents, etc.

Patient Counselling:

- Swallow the whole tablets. Do not crush, break, or chew before swallowing.
- Do not change brands without permission of the physician.
- Unless otherwise directed, do not refill the prescription.

INHALATION DRUG DELIVERY SYSTEM

Patient counselling in the administration of drug for the treatment of respiratory diseases is one of the prime areas where positive input can have significant bearing on success of the therapy. Bronchial asthma is a disease of airways where narrowing of the airways occurs causing symptoms of dyspnoea, wheezing and coughing. Asthma may be the result of multiple stimuli including allergy. These patients may have a family history of allergic diseases. The

Novel Drug Delivery Systems

airborne allergens, drugs like aspirin and NSAIDs, exposure to chemicals, infections, physical exertion and emotional stress are the different stimuli. Other reasons are chronic bronchitis (excessive mucus production), loss of elasticity of alveoli (emphysema) and smoking.

The present trend in NDDS is effective delivery of the drug to its site of action. Rapid action can be obtained even with a reduced dose. Due to the direct delivery of the drug to the large surface area of the tracheobronchial tree and alveoli, even a smaller inhaled dose can produce rapid action, with reduction in systemic side effects. Here drugs are administered for both local as well as systemic effects in to the respiratory tract. The pulmonary drug delivery is based on three types of aerosol generators:

      1) Inhalers   2) Rotahalers   3) Nebulisers.

1. Inhalers

i) Metered Dose Inhalers (MDI) :

Aerosol is a pressurised pack, where micronised drug is dissolved or suspended in a liquid propellant and packed in a sealed container. The pressure inside the container is created by vapour pressure of the propellant. The high velocity aerosols, which are generated by activation, are inhaled. The actuation of container is linked with a metering valve. On actuation, a metered dose is released, therefore it is called as MDI (Metered Dose Inhalers).

When not in use, the metering valve is open to the contents of the container. When inverted and pressed from above, the meter valve seals the content of the container, but is open to the atmosphere to generate an aerosol spray. The aerosol spray contains fine droplets or micropowders surrounded by the propellant. The vaporisation of propellant reduces particle size and these smaller particles are inhaled. Finer the aerosol particles, more effective is the targetting. For the dose to take effect, the actuation of inhaler must be synchronised with inspiration. MDI are small in size and handy to carry and use.

The limitations of MDI are as follows:

  i)   Almost 50 per cent of patients use the inhaler incorrectly.

  ii)   Children, arthritic patients and patients during an acute asthmatic attack, face the problem of synchronisation.

  iii) From conventional inhalers, though it is used correctly, only 10 per cent of the dose released from it reaches the lungs. Almost 80 per cent is deposited in the oropharyx and the remaining adheres to the device. The deposited drug is then swallowed, the systemic absorption of which leads to side effects.

  iv) Some patients may actuate the device more than once during single inspiration.

Patient Counselling:

- Remove the cap of the inhaler and shake the container before use. In case the inhaler is new, the first dose should not be inhaled. Point the nozzle into the air, away from the face and press the top of the canister, to spray the aerosol two times into the air. Always hold the canister upright while actuating. Breathe out gently, but not quite fully, just before placing the mouth piece in the mouth.
- Hold the mouthpiece about one to two inches in front of the widely opened mouth or place the mouthpiece in the mouth between the teeth and seal the lips around it. Make sure the tongue or teeth are not blocking the path of the spray or that the spray does not hit the roof of the mouth. Start slow inhalation and actuate the inhaler by pressing the canister. Coordinate inhalation and actuation. Continue slow and deep inspiration for some time after actuation to receive the complete dose. Avoid breathing through the nose after actuation.
- Remove the inhaler. Close the mouth and hold the breath for 10 sec. There should be an interval of one minute between two consecutive doses.
- Close the mouthpiece. Clean it at least once a week.
- Use the blue adapter for bronchodilator inhalers and brown adapter for steroid inhalers. Bronchodilators are taken whenever necessary, whereas, steroid inhalers are prophylactic and these are for regular use as per the physician's directions. Use the inhalation method recommended by a physician.

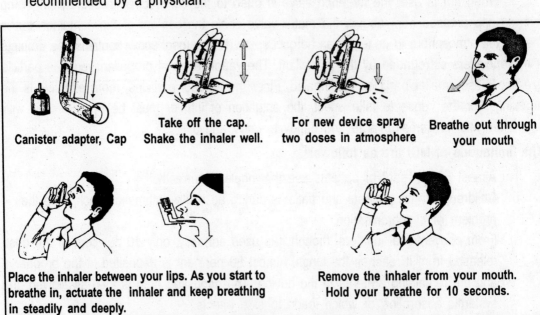

Figure 19.3: Administration of Drug using MDI

Novel Drug Delivery Systems

ii) Long Tube Inhalers (Spacehaler)

The limitations of MDI are mainly attributed to the use of a short mouth piece. The aerosol particles released from MDI are comparatively bigger in size, have high velocity and contain more propellant. The poor synchronisation of these, leads to deposition of more aerosols in the throat. The attachment of a long tube to the mouthpiece of MDI overcomes these problems. While covering the long distance in the tube, the resistance created by air reduces the velocity of aerosols, allows vaporisation of propellant, which causes the droplets to decrease in size. The mist of aerosol particles, which remain suspended in the tube (spacer), can be conveniently inhaled after a few seconds of actuation.

Advantages:

i)   Inhalation of aerosols using spacer increases lung deposition to 100 per cent and decreases throat deposition by 90 per cent.

ii) Reduction in velocity of aerosol particles allows synchronisation between actuation and inhalation.

iii) Evaporation of propellant in spacer tube, before inhalation, minimises side effects of the propellant.

iv) Due to the instant vaporisation of propellant and the associated chilling effect in the throat, many patients stop breathing, this is termed as the cold-freon effect. The transition stage further increases deposition of drug in the upper respiratory tract. The spacers minimise the spray hitting the throat.

v)   The smaller aerosol generated after vaporisation of propellant possesses good lung deposition.

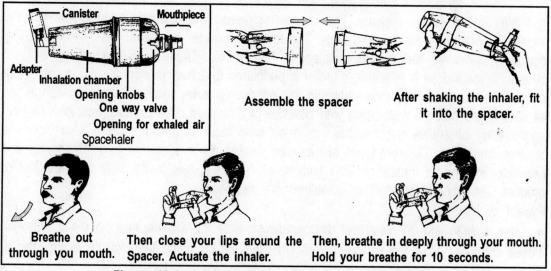

Figure 19.4: Administration of Drug using Spacehaler

vi) Unlike MDI or dry powder inhalers, spacers do not require deep inspiration.

vii) Arthritic patients can conveniently concentrate their attention first on actuation and then on inhalation.

Patient Counselling:

- Attach the spacer to the MDI according to instructions and gently shake the whole assembly three or four times. Breathe out gently, but not quite fully, just before placing the mouth piece in the mouth.

- Place the mouthpiece of the spacer into the mouth between teeth and over the tongue; seal it with the lips. Actuate the inhaler by pressing the canister and inhale the aerosol within one or two seconds, slowly for three to five seconds. Avoid breathing through the nose after actuation. Without removing the inhaler from the mouth, hold the breath for 10 sec. Breathe in and out slowly two to three times. Keep an interval of one minute between two consecutive doses. Do not put more than one dose into the spacer at the same time.

- When dosing is finished, remove the spacer from the inhaler. Close the mouthpiece and clean the spacer at least once a week.

Proprietory preparations:

- ASTHALIN (Cipla): Salbutamol 100 µg/md.
- BECLATE (Cipla): Beclomethasone dipropionate 50, 100 & 200 µg/md.
- FLOHALE(Cipla): Fluticasone propionate 25, 50 & 125 µg/md.
- PULMICORT (Astra-Zeneca): Budesonide 100,200 & 400 µg/md.
- BRICANYL MISTHALER (Astra-Zeneca): Terbutaline 250 µg/md.

2. Dry Powder System (Rotahaler)

In the dry powder system, the micronised drug is mixed with a carrier, such as lactose and filled into a gelatin capsule. The capsule is placed within a device, which pierces the capsule or separates its cap and body. The resultant powder is inhaled. Now multi-dose dry powder systems are also available instead of the capsule. These contain a number of small blisters. When a dose is required, a blister is punctured to deliver powder for inhalation. These are called as Diskhalers. During inhalation, the released powder passes through a mesh. It has all advantages that are associated with absence of propellant. The powder must be free from aggregates; otherwise the resultant irritation may lead to excess mucus secretion and bronchoconstriction. Different types of rotahaler devices are available to hold the capsule and generate powder for inhalation. The techniques for using the device vary from product to product. The general counselling guidelines are as follows:

Patient counselling:

- Use a clean and dry Rotahaler device. Always store the capsule in a dry place in a well-closed container. Hold the rotahaler vertically. Hygienically place the capsule in the device just before use. Hold the mouthpiece firmly with one hand and rotate the base. The fin separates the two halves of the rotacap.

- Breathe out gently, but not quite fully just before placing the mouthpiece into the mouth. Place the mouthpiece into the mouth between the teeth and over the tongue; seal it with the lips. Inhale the powder slowly for three to five seconds. Slowly breathe two to three times in and out in the device. Avoid breathing through the nose after actuation. Remove the inhaler from the mouth and hold the breath for 10 sec.
- When dosing is over, clean the Rotahaler as per instructions given by the manufacturer.

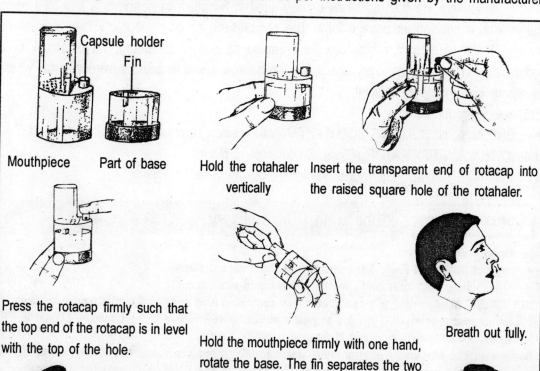

Capsule holder
Fin

Mouthpiece   Part of base

Hold the rotahaler vertically   Insert the transparent end of rotacap into the raised square hole of the rotahaler.

Press the rotacap firmly such that the top end of the rotacap is in level with the top of the hole.

Hold the mouthpiece firmly with one hand, rotate the base. The fin separates the two halves of the rotacap.

Breath out fully.

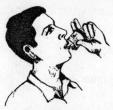

Grip the mouthpiece between teeth and seal lips around it. Tilt head slightly backwards. Breath in through mouth deeply.

Remove the rotahaler from mouth and hold breath for 10 seconds.

Figure 19.5: Administration of Drug using Rotahaler

- There should be an interval of one minute between two consecutive doses. Do not put more than one capsule into the rotahaler for a single dose.

Proprietory preparations:

- ASTHALIN Rotacaps (Cipla) : Salbutamol 200 µg.
- FORATEC (Protec) : Formoterol 12 µg.
- BECLATE (Cipla) : Beclomethasone dipropionate 100, 200 or 400 µg.

3. Nebulisers

Nebulisers are the machines usually used in hospitals to generate a fine mist using the inhalation solution as dosage form. The compressed air or ultrasonic waves are utilised for generation of aerosol, which can be breathed by normal breathing, via facemask or a mouthpiece. Nebulisers are very useful for giving large doses in acute severe asthma, where breathing becomes very difficult.

Proprietory preparations:

- BRIKANYL NEBULISING SOLUTION (Astra-Zeneca): Turbutaline sulphate 10 mg/ml.
- ASTHALIN RESPIRATOR (Cipla): Salbutamol 5 mg/ml.
- FLOHALE (Cipla): Fluticasone propionate 0.5 mg/2 ml, 2 mg/ml.

Concept Clear : **Inhalation Drug Delivery**

Inhalation Drug Delivery
- Targeted delivery of drug to the tracheobronchial tree and alveoli.
- Rapid action, small dose and reduction in systemic side effects.

MDI: Aerosol is pressurised in a sealed container containing drug and liquid propellant. On actuation, a metered dose is released. Finer the aerosol particles, more effective is the targeting. Limitation: Not synchronised in actuation and inspiration.

Spacehaler: The attachment of long mouth piece to MDI. It reduces velocity of aerosol, reduces particle size and improves synchronisation. Increases lung deposition, decreases throat deposition and related side effects.

Patient Counselling:
- Gently shake aerosol devise before use.
- Breathe out gently. Place the mouthpiece between teeth and over the tongue; seal it with the lips.
- Inhale slowly for 2-3 seconds. Hold breath for 10 seconds.
- Keep an interval of one minute between two consecutive doses.

Rotahaler: The gelatin capsule containing micronised drug is pierced or separated and the resultant powder is inhaled.

Nebulisers: The machines usually used in hospitals to generate fine mists using the inhalation solution as dosage form. Useful to give large doses in acute severe asthma.

TRANS-DERMAL DRUG DELIVERY SYSTEM

The adhesive patch containing dissolved or dispersed drug when applied on intact skin, delivers the drug at a controlled rate to the systemic circulation. The drug release may be upto 7 days.

Proprietary preparations:

- NITRODERM TTS (Novartis) : Glyceryl trinitrate 5 & 10 mg per 24 hrs.
- ESTRADERM MX (Novartis) : Estradiol releasing 0.025, 0.05 & 0.1 mg.

Advantages:

i) There is increased patient compliance, as problems such as GI irritation and frequent dosing are avoided.

ii) There is improved effectiveness of a drug as drug degradation in GIT and first pass metabolism are avoided.

iii) Constant plasma drug concentration is maintained without the peaks and troughs pattern.

iv) Easy to terminate drug therapy by removing transdermal patch.

Limitations:

i) Only suitable for small dose drugs with some amount of skin penetration properties.

ii) Skin irritation and sensitisation can occur.

iii) It is costly.

Patient Counselling: Clean and dry the area on the skin that has little or no hair and is free of cuts, or any irritation. Remove the previous patch if any, before applying a new one. Apply the new patch to a new area each time. Area should be protected from the environment and any disturbance from daily routine. The adhesive patch should not be trimmed or cut to adjust the dosage. If a patch becomes loose, press it properly or apply a new patch if there are chances of it falling off. Used patch must be disposed of properly.

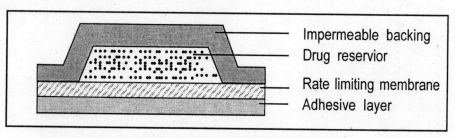

Figure 19.6: Transdermal Patch

Concept Clear : TDDS

TDDS: The adhesive patch when applied to the intact skin delivers the drug at a controlled rate.
- Avoid GI irritation and reduced dosing frequency.
- Avoid degradation in GIT and first pass metabolism.
- Easy to terminate drug therapy.
- Suitable for small dose drug with skin penetration properties

Patient counselling:
- Clean and dry the area on the skin which has little or no hair and is free of cuts, or irritation.
- Remove the previous patch. Apply a new patch to a new area.
- Do not trim or cut the patch.

20 Pharmaceutical Calculations

ALLIGATION METHOD

Alligation method is used for two types of calculations:

a) Calculation of resulting strength of product (X_n, P_c) produced by mixing two or more products or compositions (X_n) of different concentrations (P_c).

$$X_1P_1 + X_2P_2 = \Sigma X_nP_c$$

$$\frac{\Sigma X_nP_c}{\Sigma X_n} = X_nP_c$$

b) Calculations of the proportion (X_n) in which two or more products or compositions of different strength (P_c) should be mixed to get product of required strength ($X_n P_c$).

The first method is called alligation medial and the second method is called as alligation alternate.

Exercise 20.1 What is the percentage of zinc oxide in an ointment prepared by mixing 20g of 5% ointment, 10 g of 7% ointment and 30 g of 2% ointment ?

	$X_n \times P_0$	
	20 x 5 =	100
+	10 x 7 =	70
+	30 x 2 =	60
$\Sigma X_n = 60$	$\Sigma X_n P_c = 230$	

$$\therefore \quad \frac{\Sigma X_n P_c}{\Sigma X_n} = \frac{230}{60} = 3.83\%$$

Proprietary Preparations: Zinc oxide ointment: 7.5% w/w, lotion 5% w/v.

Exercise 20.2 In what proportion should 50% and 90% alcohol mixed so as to make 60% alcohol.

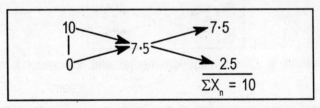

Thus, 30 parts of 50% alcohol and 10 parts of 90% alcohol are to be mixed to get 40 parts of 60% alcohol.

Exercise 20.3 What is the percentage (v/v) of alcohol in a Ammonium chloride mixture, BPC containing 5 ml of Aromatic solution of ammonia, BPC and 10 ml of Liquid extract of liquorice, IP and enough water to make 100 ml. Aromatic solution of ammonia, BCP contains 3% v/v alcohol and liquorice liquid extract, IP contains 20% v/v of alcohol?

$X_n \times P_c$		
05 x 03	=	15
+ 10 x 20	=	200
+ 85 x 00	=	0
$\Sigma X_n = 100$	$\Sigma X_n P_c = 215$	

$\therefore \quad \dfrac{215}{100} = 2.15\%$ v / v

Exercise 20.4 In what proportion should 10% w/w Povidone Iodine ointment be mixed with white petroleum jelly to produce 20 g of 7.5% povidone Iodine ointment?

$$
\begin{array}{c}
10 \longrightarrow 7{\cdot}5 \\
\mid \quad 7{\cdot}5 \\
0 \longrightarrow 2.5 \\
\overline{\Sigma X_n = 10}
\end{array}
$$

Thus, 15 g of povidone iodine ointment of 10% w/w and 5 g of petroleum jelly should be mixed to produce 20 g of 7.5% w/w ointment.

Proprietary preparations: Povidone iodine ointment: 5%, 10%, Cream: 5%, Spray: 10%, Solution: 5%, 7.5%, 10%, Powder: 5% each w/w.

Exercise 20.5 In what proportion should 20%, 15% and 3% cetrimide solutions be mixed to get 8% cetrimide solution.

Rule 1: Link the composition containing higher concentration than desired concentration to the composition containing less concentration than the desired concentration.

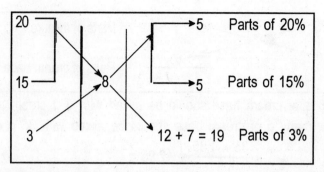

Proprietary preparations: Cetrimide solution, 3%, 5% and concentrated solutions 15% and 20% each w/v.

Exercise 20.6 In what proportion may a pharmacist mix 3%, 5%, 15% and 20%. cetrimide solutions to produce a 10% cetrimide solution.

Proportion : 1

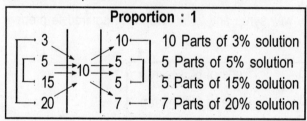

10 Parts of 3% solution
5 Parts of 5% solution
5 Parts of 15% solution
7 Parts of 20% solution

Rule 2 : Each low concentration composition is linked with high concentration composition. The two types of proportions are possible to prepare product of desired concentration.

Proportion : 2

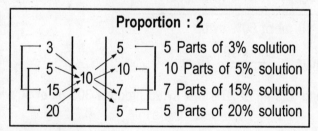

5 Parts of 3% solution
10 Parts of 5% solution
7 Parts of 15% solution
5 Parts of 20% solution

Exercise 20.7 How many grams of cream base should be mixed with 10 g of 4% w/w and 25 g of 8% w/w cream of quinidochlor to make 5% w/w cream.

$$
\begin{array}{rcl}
X_n \times P_c & & \\
10 \times 04 & = & 40 \\
+ \quad 25 \times 08 & = & 200 \\
\hline
\Sigma X_n = 35 & & \Sigma X_n P_c = 240
\end{array}
$$

Thus, $\dfrac{240}{35} = 6.85\%$ w/w

The mixing of these two cream results in 35 g of 6.85% w/w cream. This mixture should be diluted with cream base to produce 5% w/w cream.

Thus, 1.85 parts of cream base requires to mix with 5 parts of quinidochlor cream mixture. The total amount to mixture which is in hand is 35 g.

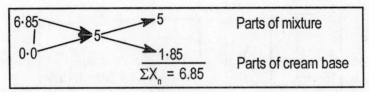

$$\Sigma X_n = 6.85$$

Parts of mixture

Parts of cream base

∴   1.85 g of cream base should be mixed with 5 g cream mixture.

∴   How many g of cream base should be mixed with 35 g of cream mixture.

$$\frac{35 \times 1.85}{5} = 12.95 \text{ g}$$

12.95 g of cream base and 35 g of cream mixture will produce 47.95 g of cream having 5% concentration.

Proprietary preparation: Quinidochlor, the antibacterial antifungal drug available in cream, 4% and 8% w/w.

Exercise 20.8 How many milliliters of 60% w/w syrup and 20% syrup are required to prepare 300 ml of 30% w/w syrup.

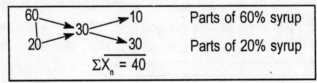

Parts of 60% syrup

Parts of 20% syrup

$$\Sigma X_n = 40$$

∴ 40 ml of 30% syrup requires 10 ml of 60% syrup.

∴ 300 ml of 30% syrup will require = $\dfrac{300 \times 10}{40}$ 75 ml

Thus, 75 ml of 60% w/w syrup and 225 ml of 20% w/w syrup produce 300 ml of 30% w/w syrup.

Exercise 20.9 How many grams of benzalkonium chloride (BAK) should be added to 1 litre of 25% w/v BAK solution to prepare an solution of 40% w/v.

```
BAK =      100          15  Parts of BAK
                   40
Solution = 25  %          60  Parts of 25% solution
              ΣXₙ = 75
```

$$\Sigma X_n = 75$$

Thus, 15 g of BAK and 60 ml of 25% w/v BAK solution produce 40% w/v solution. How many g of BAK should be required with 1 litre of 25% w/v solution.

$$\frac{1000 \text{ ml} \times 15 \text{ g}}{60 \text{ ml}} = 250 \text{ g of BAK}$$

Proprietary preparation: Benzalkonium chloride 40% w/v solution.

Pharmaceutical Calculations

VOLUME AND WEIGHT RELATION

Density: It is mass (m) per unit volume (v) of a substance, usually expressed as grams per ml.

$$D = m/v$$

Density of water is 1 g/ml at $4°$ C

Specific gravity or Relative density: It is the relation of the weight of any volume of subtance to the weight of an equal volume of a standard at 25°C. Water is standard for liquids and solids.

$$\text{Specific gravity} = \frac{\text{Weight of unit volume of liquid}}{\text{Weight of equal volume of water}}$$

In the metric system, both, density and specific gravity are numerically equal. According to IP, weight of 1 ml of water at $20°$ C is 0.99719 g and at $25°$ C it 0.99602 g.

Exercise 20.10 Calculate the weight of 80 ml of Dill oil whose density is 0.942 g / ml.

$$\text{Volume} = \frac{\text{Density}}{\text{Weight}} \quad 76.992 \text{ g} = \frac{0.9624}{80}$$

Exercise 20.11 Calculate the volume of 100 g of glycerin. The density of glycerin, IP is 1.257 g/ml.

$$\text{Volume} = \frac{\text{Weight}}{\text{Density}} \quad 79.55 \text{ ml} = \frac{100 \text{ g}}{1.257}$$

Exercise 20.12 An empty specific gravity bottle weighs 22 g and bottle filled with water weighs 47 g. When it is filled with honey it weighs 55. 95 g. Calculate specific gravity of the honey.

Weight of water = 47 - 22 = 25 g

Weight of honey = 55.95 - 22 = 33.95 $\quad \therefore \quad \dfrac{33.95}{25} = 1.358$ g

Exercise 20.13 What is the specific gravity of a 2 : 3 mixture of mentha oil and clove oil, and what will be the specific gravity of elixir if 10 ml of this mixture is mixed with 100 ml of an elixir with specific gravity of 0.950. The specific gravity of clove oil, IP is 1.038 and mentha oil is 0.892.

P_n x Pc		
2 x 0.892	=	1.782
+ 3 x 1.038	=	3.114
$\Sigma X_n = 5$	$\Sigma X_n P_c =$	4.896

$\therefore \quad \dfrac{4.896}{5} = 0.9738$ g

$\therefore$ Specific gravity of mixture of oil is 0.9738g

When 10 ml of mixture (sp. gr. 0.9738g) if mixed with 100 ml of elixir (sp. gr. 0.950).

P_n x Pc		
10 x 0.9738	=	9.738
+ 100 x 0.950	=	95.000
$\Sigma X_n = 110$	$\Sigma X_n P_c =$	104.738

$$\therefore \quad \frac{104.738}{110} = 0.9521 \text{ g/ml}$$

PERCENTAGE SOLUTIONS

Percentage means rate per 100. The different ways to express percentage are:

i) % of solid in liquid = % w/v

ii) % of solid in solid = % w/w

iii) % of liquid in liquid = % v/v and less frequently as % w/w

iv) % of liquid in solid = % v/w

Unless otherwise specified, the liquids in pharmacy are supplied as % w/v.

Exercise 20.14 How many grams of sodium chloride will be required to prepare 1liter of 2.5% solution.

2.5% means: 2.5 g in 100 ml $\quad \frac{2.5 \times 1000}{100} = 25$ g

$\therefore \qquad$? g in 1000 ml

Exercise 20.15 Calculate the quantity of sodium chloride required for preparing 500 ml I. V. infusion of 0.9% w/v concentration.

0.9% means: 0.9 g in 100 ml $\quad \frac{0.9 \times 500}{100} = 4.5$ g

$\therefore \qquad$? g in 500 ml

Exercise 20.16 What is the percentage strength (w/v) of solution of benzoic acid, if 70 ml contains 8 g?

$\therefore \qquad$ 10 g in 100 ml = 10% w/v

Thus, 7 g in 70 ml = 10% w/v

$\qquad$ 8 g in 70 ml = ? $\qquad \frac{8 \times 10}{7} = 11.42\%$ w/v

Check = 11.42 g in 100 ml = 11.42%

$\qquad$? g in 70 ml = 11.42% $\qquad \frac{11.42 \times 70}{100} = 7.994 = 8$ g

Exercise 20.17 How many milliliters of 5% amaranth solution can be made from 25 g of amaranth?

5 g in 100 ml produces 5%

25 g in ? ml produces 5% $\qquad \frac{25 \times 100}{5} = 500$ ml

Exercise 20.18 What is the percentage strength (v/v) of a solution of 12.5 g glycerin in water to make 100 ml. The sp. gr. of glycerin is 1.25.

Here the amount of glycerin is expressed in weight.

$$\therefore \quad \text{Volume} = \frac{\text{Weight}}{\text{Specific gravity}} = \frac{12.5}{1.25} = 10 \text{ ml}$$

∴   10 ml in 100 ml of water is 10% v/v solution

Exercise 20.19 How many grams of sugar is required to make 100 ml of 66.67% w/w solution having specific gravity of 1.31 g/ml

∴   100 x 1.31 = 131 g is the weight of sugar solution

∴   66.67% w/w means, 66.67 g sugar in 100 g of sugar solution.

∴   ? g of sugar is required for 131 g of sugar solution.

$$\frac{66.67 \times 131}{100} = 87.33 \text{ g}$$

i.e. 87.33 g sugar with 43.67 g of water will produce, 131 g of syrup which is equivalent to 100 ml.

Exercise 20.20 How to prepare 100 ml of 2.4% w/w solution of drug in glycerin. The Specific gravity of glycerin is 1.25.

$$\text{Volume} = \frac{\text{Weight}}{\text{Density}} \qquad 125 \text{ g} = 1.25 \text{ g} \times 100 \text{ ml}$$

i.e. 100 ml of glycerin is equal to 125 g.

2.4 g drug in 97.6 g of solvent is 2.4% w/w

∴   ? g drug in 125 g of solvent is 2.4% w/w = 3.073 g of drug.

Exercise 20.21 If 8 g of calamine is dispersed in 100 ml of water, what is the percentage strength (w/w) of the suspension.

100 ml water is equal to 100 g

Thus, 100 g of water + 8 g of calamine is 108 g

∴   108 g suspension contains 8 g calamine

100 g suspension should contain ?   = 7.407g i.e. 7.407% w/w

Exercise 20.22 Calculate percentage strength of a solution 1 : 300

The ratio strength 1 : 300 means, 1 part in 300 parts. The percentage means per 100 parts.

∴   1 in 300

        ? in 100 $\frac{100}{300} = 0.33\%$

Exercise 20.23 What is the ratio strength (w/v) of dispersion made by dispersing two paracetamol kid tablets, each contain 125 mg paracetamol, in enough water to make 250 ml.

    125 mg x 2 tablets = 250 mg of paracetamol.

∴ 1 g in 250 ml is 1 : 250

    Here, it is 0.25 g in 250 ml

∴   1 g in = ? ml = 1000 ml. ∴ Ratio strength is 1 : 1000

Exercise 20.24 How many grams of benzalkonium chloride should be used in preparing 400 ml of a 1 : 2500 ear drops and what is its % strength.

    1 : 2500 means   = 1 in 2500

    Thus, calculate % strength = ? in 100 = 0.04%

∴ 100 ml contains = 0.04 g

∴ 400 ml requires = 0.16 g

Exercise 20.25 What is ratio strength of 0.002% w/v phenylmercuric nitrate preservative solution. How many milligrams of phenylmercuric nitrate should be used to prepare 300 ml of such solution.

Exercise 20.26 If 400 ml of 40% v/v benzalkonium chloride concentrated solution for hospital is diluted to 1000 ml; what will the percentage strength of resulted solution?

  40% v/v means,   40 ml in 100 ml

  It means, we have 160 ml in 400 ml

  When diluted, it is 160 ml in 1000 ml

∴   ? ml in 100 ml

$$\frac{100 \times 160}{1000} = 16 \text{ ml} = 16\% \text{ v/v}$$

Table : Percentage strength and Ratio strength

Percentage strength		Ratio strength
1%	= 1 g in 100 ml	1 : 100
0.1%	= 100 mg in 100 ml	1 : 1,000
0.01%	= 10 mg in 100 ml	1 : 10,000
0.001%	= 1 mg in 100 ml	1 : 10,00,00
0.002%	= 2 mg in 100 ml	2 : 10,00,00
∴	= ? in 300 ml	∴ Ratio strength is
	= 6 mg in 300 ml	1 : 50,000

Exercise 20.27 In the preparation of concentrated extract by evaporation, if the extract containing 55% w/v non-volatile active constituents is evaporated to 80% of its volume, what is the percentage of strength of concentrated extract?

	55% w/v means,	55 g in 100 ml
∴	after evaporation,	55 g in 80 ml
∴		? g in 100 ml = 68.75 g
		That is, 68.75% w/v

PROOF SPIRIT

For the purpose of calculator, the strength of ethyl alcohol is expressed in terms of proof spirit. In India and Great Britain 57.1% v/v or 49.28 w/w ethyl alcohol is taken as proof strength, that is, it is 100 proof spirit. In U.S.A. 50% v/v alcohol is proof alcohol. The strength of alcohol above proof strength is expressed as over proof (o/p) and any strength below proof strength is expressed as under proof (u/p).

Concept Clear : Proof Spirit

- 57.1% v/v is 100 proof spirit
- 1% v/v ethyl alcohol is 1.753 proof spirit
- The strength below 57.1% v/v is u/p and above 57.1% v/v is o/p alcohol.

Exercise 20.28 What is the proof strength of 80% v/v and 45% v/v ethanol?

a)
$\qquad$ 1% v/v ethanol = 1.753 proof spirit

$\qquad$ 80% v/v ethanol = ? proof spirit

$\qquad$ 80 x 1.753 = 140.24 proof

∴ $\qquad$ Proof strength = 140.24 proof - 100 proof = 40.24° o/p

b)
$\qquad$ 1% v/v ethanol = 1.753 proof spirit

$\qquad$ 45% v/v ethanol = ? proof spirit

$\qquad$ 45 x 1.753 = 78.885 proof

∴ $\qquad$ Proof strength = 78.885 - 100 = 21.1° u/p

Exercise 20.29 Calculate percentage of strength of 40° o/p and 30° u/p

a) $\qquad$ 40° o/p is 140 proof spirit.

$\qquad$ Thus, 1% v/v = 1.753 proof spirit

$\qquad$? v/v = 140 proof spirit $\qquad\qquad \dfrac{140}{1.753}$ = 79.86% v/v

b) $\qquad$ 30° u/p is 70 proof spirit

Thus,   1% v/v = 1.753 proof spirit

?% v/v = 70 proof spirit $\dfrac{70}{1.753}$ = 39.93% v/v

Exercise 20.30 Calculate the proportion of 80% v/v ethanol and 30% v/v ethanol required to prepare 10 litre of 20° u/p alcohol.

The 20° u/p proof strength = 80 proof spirit

Thus, 1% v/v alcohol = 1.753 proof spirit

? % v/v alcohol = 80 proof spirit $\dfrac{80}{1.753}$ = 45.63% v/v

As per alligation method:

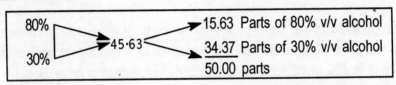

∴   50 litre of mixture of alcohol requires 15.63 litres of 80% v/v alcohol

∴   10 litre should require = ?

$$\dfrac{15.63 \times 10}{50} = 3.12 \text{ liters } 80\% \text{ v/v alcohol}$$

∴   10 liter - 3.12 liter = 6.88 litre of 30% v/v alcohol

Exercise 20.31 How many gallons of proof spirit are contained in 5 gallon of 80% v/v alcohol.

      1% v/v alcohol = 1.753 proof spirit

∴   80% v/v alcohol = 80 x 1.753 = 140.24 proof spirit

∴   Proof strength = 140.24 - 100 = 40.24 o/p

Therefore, 100 gallon 80% v/v alcohol = 100 + 40.24 = 140.24 gallon proof spirit

$$5 \text{ gallon of } 80\% \text{ v/v alcohol} = \dfrac{140.24 \times 5}{100} = 7.012 \text{ gallon of proof spirit.}$$

Thus, 5 gallons of 80% v/v alcohol are equivalent to 7.012 gallon of proof spirit.

ADJUSTMENT OF ISOTONICITY

Isotonic means the preparation having same osmotic pressure to that of blood or lachrymal secretions. If the preparation is not isotonic, it causes discomfort and irritation after administration. These effects are of two types.

1) Haemolysis of cells: If a hypotonic solution, i.e. the solution with lower osmotic pressure is used, it cause swelling or bursting of cells, leading to haemolysis. Means, blood cells are more osmotic and to achieve equilibrium, these take up fluid from hypotonic solution. The damage caused is irreversible

2) Shrinkage of cells: When hypertonic solutions having higher osmotic pressure, is administered, it leads to shrinkage of cells. To achieve equilibrium between hypertonic solution and cellular fluid, the cellular fluid comes out of the cell membranes. This damage is reversible. When osmotic pressure of body fluid and administered solution is made same, the shrunken cells regain their original size & shape. Therefore, injections, eye, nasal and rectal preparations, must be isotonic.

The osmotic pressure is a colligative property, which depends on number of 'particles' of solute in solution. The other colligative properties include vapor pressure, boiling point and freezing point. Human blood serum and lachrymal fluid have freezing point of –52°C. This property can be used to determine isotonicity, and the preparation having same freezing point is isotonic. The isotonicity of electrolyte and non-electrolyte substances is different. Electrolytes that ionise freely in solution, exert a greater osmotic pressure than the non-electrolytes with negligible dissociation.

Freezing Point Method

The freezing point of blood, and other body fluids is -52°C. The preparation containing drug and additives must have equal freezing point.

F.P. of body fluid - F. P. of drug solution of a particular strength.

F. P. of tonicity adjusting agent.

Table 20.2: Freezing Point of Some Commonly Used Substances (1% solution)			
Substance	**F. P.°C**	**Substance**	**F.P°C**
Atropine sulphate	- 0.074	Chlorbutanol	- 0.138
Borax	- 0.241	Dextrose anhydrous	- 0.101
Boric acid	- 0.288	Dextrose (monohydrate)	- 0.091
Benzalkonium chloride	- 0.046	Ephedrine HCl	- 0.165
Calcium chloride hydrous	- 0.200	Pilocarpine nitrate	- 0.132
Calcium gluconate	- 0.091	Potassium chloride	- 0.439
Sodium bicarbonate	- 0.380	Sodium citrate	- 0.178
Sodium metabisulphite	- 0.386	Sulphacetamide sodium	- 0.132
Thiamine HCl	- 0.139	Sodium chloride	- 0.576

Exercise 20.32 Calculate the amount of sodium chloride required to make a 5% dextrose solution isotonic. F. P. of 1% dextrose = 0.091°C, F. P. of 1% sodium chloride = 0.576°C

$$\therefore \quad \text{F. P. of drug solution is} = 5 \times 0.091 = -0.455°C$$

Thus, $\dfrac{0.52 - 0.455}{0.576} = \dfrac{0.065}{0.576} = 0.1128\%$

Alternatively, the ratio of F. P. of drug solution to the F. P. of 1 per cent sodium chloride solution can be taken as parameter to calculate isotonicity. The resultant ratio (sodium chloride equivalent) is subtracted from 0.9, which is concentration of sodium chloride that produces isotonic solution.

$$\left(\dfrac{5 \times 0.091}{0.576} \right) = 0.9 - 0.7899 = 0.110\%$$

Exercise 20.33 Prepare a potassium chloride injection containing 0.5% of drug. F.P. of 1% potassium chloride = 0.439. F.P. of 1% sodium chloride = 0.576

$$\therefore \quad \text{F.P. of drug solution} = 0.5 \times 0.439 = 0.2195$$

Thus, $\dfrac{0.52 - 0.2195}{0.576} = \dfrac{0.3005}{0.576} = 0.52\%$ or $0.9 - \left(\dfrac{0.2195}{0.576} \right) = 0.52\%$

An injection containing 0.5% Potassium chloride and 0.52%. Sodium chloride will be isotonic.

Sodium Chloride Equivalent Method

It is modification of freezing point method where ratio of freezing point depression, produced by a solution of medicament and Freezing point depressed by a sodium chloride of same strength is calculated as sodium chloride equivalent (E_{NaCl}) of that medicament. For example; sodium chloride equivalent of 1% potassium chloride is 0.76

$$\dfrac{0.439}{0.576} = 0.76$$

Table 20.3 : E_{NaCl} of same substance (1% solution)			
Substance	E_{NaCl}	**Substance**	E_{NaCl}
Ascorbic acid	0.18	Hyoscine HBr	0.12
Boric acid	0.50	Potassium chloride	0.76
Dextrose unhydrous	0.18	Silver nitrate	0.33
Ephedrine hydrochloride	0.30	Sodium chloride	1
Pilocarpine nitrate	0.22	Sodium metabisulphite	0.67

The percentage of sodium chloride required for adjustment to isotonicity can be calculated using the following formula.

% NaCl = 0.9 - [% strength of drug solution x E_{NaCl}]

Exercise 20.34 How much sodium chloride should be used in compounding 5 ml drops containing 2% pilocarpine nitrate.

$$\% \text{ NaCl required} = 0.9 - (2 \times 0.22)$$
$$= 0.46\%$$

Proprietary preparation :   PILOCAR Drops (FDC),
                             PILOPRESS (Centaur) : 1, 2 and 4%.

Exercise 20.35 Calculate the amount of dextrose anhydrous required to make a 1% solution of ephedrine hydrochloride isotonic?

a)   % NaCl required = 0.9 - (1 x 0.3) = 0.6

b)   To calculate amount of other isotonicity adjusting agent, divide the percentage of sodium chloride by E_{NaCl} of that agent.

$$\% \text{ Dextrose unhydrous required} = \frac{0.6}{0.18} = 3.3\%$$

Molecular Concentration Method

The osmotic pressure is proportional to molar concentration. The molar concentration is the gram per litre.

$$\text{Gram moles} = \frac{\text{Weight in gram per litre}}{\text{Molecular weight}}$$

This equation is applicable for non-ionisable substance. If substance is ionisable, then

$$\text{Gram moles} = \frac{\text{Weight in gram per litre}}{\text{Molecular weight}} \times n$$

Where, n is number of ions formed by dissociation of the substance. The n value is 2 for salt dissociating in 2 ions, 3 for salts, which dissociate in 3 ions, etc.

As discussed above 0.9 per cent sodium chloride is isotonic, thus on the basis of molar concentration, it can be explained as :

∴   0.9% sodium chloride = 9 g/litre of solution.

$$\text{Gram mole of NaCl isotonic} = \frac{9}{58.5} \times 2 = 0.31$$

Means, 0.31 gram molar solution of sodium chloride is isotonic.

Exercise 20.36 Prepare 2.5% dextrose injection. Make it isotonic by sodium chloride. Molecular weight of dextrose is 180.

∴   Calculate gram moles of dextrose, which is non-ionisable.

Modern Dispensing Pharmacy

2.5% dextrose = 25 g/litre.

$\therefore$ Gram moles of dextrose = $\dfrac{25}{180}$ = 0.139

Gram moles of NaCl - Gram moles of active ingredients = Required gram moles.

$\therefore$ 0.31 - 0.139 = 0.179

$\therefore$ The required concentration of sodium chloride is

$$\text{Gram moles} = \dfrac{X \text{ g / lit}}{58.5} \times 2 \qquad 0.179 = \dfrac{X \text{ g / lit}}{58.5} \times 2$$

$\therefore \dfrac{0.179 \times 58.5}{2}$ = 5.235 g / litre   Thus, required sodium chloride = 0.535%

The simple formula appears to calculate the % of isotonic adjusting agent:

$$= \left[0.31 - \left(\dfrac{\text{g / lit}}{\text{Mole. weight}} \times n \right) \text{of substance} \right] \times \left(\dfrac{\text{Mol. weight}}{n} \right) \text{ of an isotonicity adjusting agent.}$$

Exercise 20.37 Prepare 200 ml of 0.5% solution of procaine hydrochloride. Molecular weight of procaine HCl = 272.77.

$$\therefore \left[0.31 - \left(\dfrac{5}{272.77} \right) \times 2 \right] \times \left[\dfrac{58.5}{2} \right] = [0.31 - 0.0366] \times [29.25] = 7.99 \text{ g / lit} = 0.799\%$$

Thus, to make 100 ml solution 0.8 g and to make 200 ml, 1.6 g of sodium chloride is required.

WORKING FORMULA FOR COMPOUNDING OF PRODUCTS

Exercise 20.38 Compound and dispense 60 ml of chlorpheniramine maleate syrup, USP:

Ingredient	Master formula	Working formula
Chlorpheniramine maleate	400 mg	24 mg
Glycerin	25 ml	1.5 ml
Syrup	83 ml	4.5 ml
Sorbitol syrup	282 ml	17 ml
Sodium benzoate	1 g	60 mg
Alcohol	60 ml	3.6 ml
Water, to make	100 ml	to make 60 ml (33 ml approx)

The amount of vehicle prescribed to make final volume is not in exact amount but it is sufficient to fill up the volume to required level. Though it is not possible to calculate the exact quantity of water which is required, it is always better to calculate approximate amount of vehicle. In this case, the liquid ingredients other than water, are add up to 27 ml, therefore volume of water required is 60 - 27 = 33 ml approximately.

Exercise 20.39 Calculate the working formula for 120 ml of potassium citrate mixture NFI 1967:

In this prescription, the master formula gives quantities of ingredients for 15 ml. The product asked to be compounded is 120 ml, which is 8 times more than the master formula. The formula contains approximately 33 ml of other liquid ingredients and solid ingredients are

Ingredient	Master formula	Working formula
Potassium citrate	3.0 g	24 g
Citric acid	0.6 g	4.8 g
Syrup	4.0 ml	32 ml
Quillaia tincture	0.1 ml	0.8 ml
Chloroform water, to fill up to	15.0 ml	to fill up to 120 ml (58 ml)

29 g, which add up to 62 ml. Therefore, amount of chloroform water as vehicle is approximately : 120 - 62 = 58 ml.

Exercise 20.40 Check the equivalence in the formula of turpentine liniment, I.P and B.P.

Turpentine liniment I.P			Turpentine liniment B. P.		
Ingredient	Master formula	Working formula	Ingredient	Master formula	Working formula
Soft soap	90 g	2.7 g	Soft soap	75 g	2.7 g
Camphor	50 g	1.5 g	Camphor	50 g	1.8 g
Turpentine oil	650 ml	19.5 ml	Turpentine oil	650 ml	23.4 ml
Water,	to fill up to 1000 ml	to fill up to 30 ml	Water,	225 ml	8.1 ml
			Total		36.0 ml

In the turpentine liniment, I.P, the amount of vehicle, water, is prescribed to fill up the volume, whereas in B.P. preparation, the amount of vehicle is exact. Though the ingredients are expressed in mixed units of measure, that is, solids in grams and liquids in millilitres, the I.P. formula will yield 1000 ml liniment containing prescribed content of active ingredients. It contains 65 per cent v/v and 5 per cent w/v of turpentine oil and camphor, respectively. As discussed in previous example approximate amount of vehicle can be calculated and volume is made with it.

In B.P. formula, since amount of vehicle is exact and units of measure of ingredients are not same, mixing of these ingredients will not practically produce exact 1000 ml of turpentine liniment. Secondly, it will change the percentage content of the active ingredients. Therefores such formulas should be calculated, considering specific gravity of ingredients, or alternatively 20 per cent extra amount should be calculated. Practically, the later will produce near about 1000 ml of turpentine liniment, maintaining desired drug content.

Exercise 20.41 Write the working formula for camphor water 0.1% w/v.

Ingredient	Master formula	Working formula
Camphor	100 mg	100 mg
Alcohol	-	0.2 ml
Purified water,	to make 100 ml	to make 100 ml

Camphor is sparingly soluble in water and 500 mg / 1ml of alcohol 90 per cent.

Exercise 20.42 Write working formula for Zinc starch, dusting powder, NFI, send 25 g:

Ingredient	Master formula	Working formula
zinc oxide	50 parts	12.5 g
Starch powder	50 parts	12.5 g

Exercise 20.43 Interpret the master formulas for Macrogol ointment, B.P.C.

Ingredient	Master formula 1	Master formula 2
Macrogol 4000	35 g	35 g
Macrogol 300	65 g	to make 65 g

The master formula 1 contains 35 g and 65 g of the respective ingredients, making total 100 g of the final product, whereas formula 2 contains macrogol 300 sufficient to make 65 g of the final ointment. The working formula for it will be as follows.

Macrogol 4000 35 g   Macrogol 300   30 g

Exercise 20.44 Calculate the working formula for pain balm, 25 g.

Ingredient	Master formula	Working formula
Menthol	20% w/w	5.0 g
Eucalyptus oil	10% w/w	2.5 g
Emulsifying ointment	to fill up to, 100% w/w	17.5 g

Thus, menthol is 20% w/w, that is, 20 g per 100 g therefore, 25 g of product will contain.

$$\frac{20 \text{ g} \times 25 \text{ g}}{100 \text{ g}} = 5.0 \text{ g} \qquad \text{Eucalyptus oil} = \frac{10 \text{ g} \times 25 \text{ g}}{100 \text{ g}} = 2.5 \text{ g}$$

Emulsifying ointment = 25 g - (5.0 - 2.5) = 17.5 g

ELECTROLYTE CONCENTRATION

i) Milliequivalent:

Body requirements of individual ions are specific. Electrolytes ionise in the body and this ion concentration is important. The ionic concentration is expressed in terms of milliequivalent or millimoles. A milliequivalent (mEq) is one-thousandth part of the gram equivalent weight, it is expressed in milligrams. The gram equivalent weight of an ion is the ionic weight in grams divided by the valency of that ion.

$$mEq = \frac{\text{Gram mEq. wt}}{1000} \qquad \text{Gram Eq. wt.} = \frac{\text{Gram ionic weight}}{\text{Valency}}$$

mEq. wt. of a salt is amount in mg that provide 1 mEq of ion.

$$mEq. \text{ wt of salt} = \frac{\text{mol. weight}}{\text{Valency} \times \text{Number of ions}}$$

Every salt gives both cations and anions. Eg. $CaCl_2$ $2H_2O$ is commonly used divalent. It will provide Ca^{++} and 2 Cl^-.

Thus Eq wt. of Ca^{++} = $\frac{40}{2}$ = 20 g $\qquad$ Eq wt. of Cl^- = $\frac{35.5}{1}$ = 35.5 g

$\therefore$ $\quad$ mEq of Ca^{++} = $\frac{20}{1000}$ = 20 mg $\qquad \therefore$ $\quad$ mEq of Cl^- = $\frac{35}{1000}$ = 35 mg

The mEq of commonly used ions is as follows.

Table 20.4 : mEq (mg) of some ions

Ions	mEq.	Ions	mEq.
H^+	1	Cl^-	35.5
Na^+	23	HPO_4	48
K^+	39.1	HCO_3^-	61
Ca^{++}	20		

mEq (mg) of some ions

The amount of $CaCl_2$, which will provide 1 mEq each Ca^{++} and Cl^- is as follows.

$$\text{Weight of electrolyte (mg) which provide 1 mEq of ion} = \frac{\text{Mol Wt}}{\text{Valency} \times \text{no of ions in the molecule}}$$

$$\therefore \quad \text{mEq wt. for } CaCl_2. 2H_2O = \frac{147}{2} = 73.5 \text{ mg}$$

Some other example of weight of the salts which provide 1 mEq of ions are as follows.

1) Potassium chloride = 74.5 mg provides 1 mEq of K^+ and Cl^-
2) Sodium chloride = 58.5 mg provides 1 mEq of Na^+ and Cl^-
3) Sodium bicarbonate = 84 mg provide 1 mEq of Na^+ and HCO_3^-
4) Sodium citrate = 98 mg, provide 1 mEq of Na^+
5) Magnesium chloride = 101.5 mg provide 1 mEq Mg^{++}

Additional formulas to calculate mEq are as follows,

1) $mEq \text{ per litre} = \dfrac{\text{mg of salt / liter}}{\text{mEq. Wt. of salt}}$

2) $mEq \text{ per litre} = \dfrac{C \times 10,000}{\text{mEq. Wt. of salt}}$

Where, C is percentage strength w/v.

Exercise 20.45 Calculate milliequivalent of magnesium (Atomic wt of Mg^{++} is 24.30).

$$\text{Equivalent weight of } Mg^{++} = \frac{24.30}{2} = 12.15 \text{ g}$$

$$\text{mEq wt. of } Mg^{++} = \frac{12.159}{1000} = 12.15 \text{ mg}$$

Exercise 20.46 Calculate the milliequivalent weight of magnesium sulphate or calculate the weight in mg of magnesium sulphate containing on milliequivalent of Mg^{++}. The molecular weight of $MgSO_4.7H_2O$ is 246.

$$\text{Eq. wt. of } Mg^{++} = \frac{246}{2} = 123 \text{ g} \qquad \therefore \ mEq \text{ of } Mg^{++} = \frac{123}{1000} = 123 \text{ mg}$$

Exercise 20.47 Calculate the grams of KCl required to prepare a litre of solution containing 400 mEq of K^+. (mol. wt of KCl = 74.5).

$$mEq \text{ of } K^+ = \frac{\text{mg / litre}}{\text{MEq wt. of salt}} \quad 400 = \frac{\text{mg / litre}}{74.5} \quad \text{mg / litre} = 400 \times 74.5 = 29800 \text{ mg} = 29.800 \text{ g}$$

Pharmaceutical Calculations

Exercise 20.48 Calculate mEq of Na^+ of 1 liter of 0.86% w/v NaCl solution.

$$\text{mEq of } Na^+ \text{ per litre} = \frac{C \times 10,000}{mEq. \text{ Wt. of salt}} \quad 147 = \frac{0.86 \times 10,000}{58.8}$$

ii) Millimoles: Nowadays, electrolyte concentration is preferably written in terms of millimoles. A gram molecular weight of a drug in 1 liter of solution is defined as a 1 molar solution (1 mol). One-thousandth part of mole is called 1 millimole (mmol).

Sodium chloride ionises into Na^+ and Cl^-. The molecular weight of sodium chloride (mg) in one litre gives 1 mmole of Na^+ and 1 mmol of Cl^-. On this basis molecular weight (mg) of calcium chloride in one litre provides 1 mmole of Ca^{++} and 2 mmole of Cl^-. But non-electrolytes do not dissociate and their molecular weight (mg) in a liter produces 1 mmole concentration.

$$\text{Quantity of salt containing 1 mmol of a ion (mg)} = \frac{\text{molecular wt. of salt}}{\text{No. of ions that contained in salt}}$$

Formula to calculate millimole:

a) $$\text{mmole of ion per litre} = \frac{mg/ \text{ liter of salt}}{mg \text{ of salt containing 1 mmol of that ion}}$$

b) $$\text{mmole of ion per liter} = \frac{C \times 10,000}{mg \text{ of salt containing 1 mmole of that ion}}$$

Exercise 20.49 Calculate the amount of sodium chloride, which produces 1 liter of 1 molar solution and 1 litre containing millimoles (mol. wt. of NaCl is 58.5).
a) 1 molar solution (1 mole) of NaCl contains 58.5 g of NaCl in 1 litre of solution.

b) A 1 mmol of NaCl : $\dfrac{58.5 \text{ g}}{10,000}$ = 56 mg in a liter.

Exercise 20.50 Calculate the quantity of salt (mg) containing 1 mmol of ions : a) NaCl (mol wt. 58.5), b) $CaCl_2$ (147 mol. wt.).
a) Quantity of salt containing 1 mmol of $Na^+ = \dfrac{58.5}{1}$ = 58.5 mg and

$$\text{for 1 mmol of } Cl^- = \frac{58.5}{1} = 58.5 \text{ mg}$$

b) Quantity of salt containing 1 mmol of $Ca^{++} = \dfrac{147}{1}$ = 147 mg and

$$1 \text{ mmol of } Cl^- = \frac{147}{2} = 73.5 \text{ mg}$$

Exercise 20.51 Calculate the mmole of Na^+ and Cl^-, provided by 1 mg molecular weight of NaCl in 1 litre solution.

$$NaCl = Na^+ + Cl^- \qquad \therefore \quad 58.5 \text{ mg} = 23 \text{ mg} + 35.5 \text{ mg}$$

Exercise 20.52 Molecular weight of anhydrous dextrose is 180.2, what is the mmole of it.

$\therefore$ 1 mmol of a nonelectrolyte is the molecular weight in mg.

$\therefore$ 180.2 mg is 1 mmol of unhydrous dextrose.

Exercise 20.53 Calculate mole concentration of a solution containing 90 g of NaCl in 1 litre (mol. wt. 58.5).

$\therefore$ 58.5 g NaCl in 1 litre = 1 mole solution.

$$90 \text{ g NaCl in 1 litre} = \frac{90}{58.5} = 1.53 \text{ moles.}$$

Exercise 20.54 Calculate milligrams of KOH in 1 litre solution to give concentration of 10 mmol (atomic weights K : 39, O : 16, H : 1).

1 mmole of KOH = 56 mg

$\therefore$ 10 mmole of KOH = 560 mg in 1 litre.

Exercise 20.55 Calculate the amount of potassium chloride, which provides 5 mmole of Cl^-

$\therefore$ 74.5 mg KCl provides 1 millimole of K^+ and 1 millimole of Cl^-

$\therefore$ mg / litre of salt = 5 x 74.5 = 372 mg/litre

Exercise 20.56 Calculate the mmole of Mg^{++} and Cl^- provided by 1 g $MgCl_2$ solution in 1 litre. 203 mg of $MgCl_2$ provide 1 mmole of Mg^{++} and 2 mmol of Cl^-

a) 1,000 mg of $MgCl_2$ provide $= \dfrac{1000}{203} = 4.92$ mmol of Mg^{++}.

b) 1,000 mg of $MgCl_2$ provide $= \dfrac{1000 \times 2}{203} = 9.85$ mmol of Cl^-.

Exercise 20.57 Calculate number of mmol of Na^+ in 1 litre 0.9 % sodium chloride solution.

$$\text{mmol of } Na^+ = \frac{0.9 \times 10000}{58.5} = 154 \text{ mmol per litre.}$$

Exercise 20.58 Calculate the mmoles provided by oral rehydration salt (ORS A), I.P.

Sodium Chloride I.P	1.25 g
Potassium chloride I.P.	1.50 g

Sodium citrate I.P.	2.90 g					
Anhydrous Dextrose I.P.	27.00 g					
Excipients	q.s.					

35 g of ORS in 1 litre of water supplies electrolytes in the following concentration.

Electrolyte	Formula	Na⁺	K⁺	Cl⁻	Citrate	Glucose
Sodium chloride (mEq wt. = 58.5)	$=\dfrac{1250}{58.5}$	21.36	-	21.36	-	-
Potassium chloride (mEq wt. = 74.5)	$=\dfrac{1500}{74.5}$	-	20.13	20.13	-	-
Trisodium citrate (mEq wt. = 294)	$=\dfrac{2900}{294}$	9.86 x 3 29.60	-	-	9.86	-
Glucose (mEq wt. = 180)	$=\dfrac{27000}{180}$	-	-	-	-	150
Total mmoles		51.00	20	41	10	150

iii) Milliosmoles

Exercise 20.59 Calculate the osmolarity in milliosmol of the oral Rehydration salt (WHO-ORS) citrate. WHO-ORS citrate formula contains sodium chloride 3.5 g, sodium citrate 2.9 g, potassium chloride 1.5 g, glucose 20 g (Refer priscription No. 16.7).

$$\text{Milliosmole / litre (mOsm /l)} = \frac{\text{Substance g/litre}}{\text{Mol. Wt.}} \times \text{No. of ions} \times 1000$$

a) Sodium chloride $= \dfrac{3.5}{58.5}$ x 2 x 1000 = 119.66 mOsmol / litre

b) Potassium chloride $= \dfrac{1.5}{74.5}$ x 2 x 1000 = 40.26 mOsmol / litre

c) Sodium citrate $= \dfrac{2.9}{294}$ x 4 x 1000 = 39.45 mOsmol / litre

d) Glucose $= \dfrac{20}{180}$ x 1 x 1000 = 111.11 mOsmol /litre

Exercise 20.60 Calculate the gulcose: sodium molar ratio of the WHO-ORS-Bicarbonate.

WHO-ORS-Bicarbonate

Sodium chloride   3.5 g

Sodium bicarbonate   2.5 g

Potassium chloride   1.5 g

Glucose   20 g

Calculate molar concentration of Na^+ obtained from

a) Sodium chloride $= \dfrac{3500}{58.5} = 59.82$ mmoles

b) Sodium bicarbonate $= \dfrac{2500}{84.01} = 29.72$ mmoles

$\therefore$ Sodium ion $= 59.82 + 29.72 = 90$ mmoles

molar concentration of glucose $= \dfrac{20}{180} = 111$ mmoles.

$\therefore$ Glucose: Sodium ion molar ratio $= \dfrac{111}{90} = 1.23$ mmoles.

QUANTITY OF PRODUCT OF BE DISPENSED

Exercise 20.61 What will be the dose of amoxycillin per 5 ml, if dry powder containing 1.5 g of amoxycillin is reconstituted to 60 ml.?

60 ml reconstituted syrup contains 1.5 g amoxycillin.

5 ml reconstituted syrup will contain:

$$\dfrac{1500 \text{ mg} \times 5 \text{ ml}}{60 \text{ ml}} = 125 \text{ mg / ml.}$$

Exercise 20.62 What will be the dose of paracetamol syrup having strength 120 mg / 5 ml for a infant weighing 3 kg. (Dose : Under 3 months 10 mg / kg body weight) ?

$\therefore$ 3 kg x 10 mg = 30 mg

120 mg of paracetamol is in 5 ml

30 mg will be present in: $\dfrac{5 \times 30}{120} = 1.25$ ml

Therefore, 1.25 ml of paracetamol syrup can be given 3-4 times a day. It is advised to use calibrated dropper oral syringe to measure and administer the dose.

Exercise 20.63 The proprietary ampicillin syrups are available as 125 mg/5 ml in 30, 40 and 60 ml pack. Which pack should be dispensed if dose is 5 ml/t.i.d for 4 days?

∴   Dose per day 5ml x 3 = 15 ml.

        Dose for 3 day 15 ml x 4 = 60 ml.

Proprietary product: CAMPICILIN (Cadila pharma)

Exercise 20.64 Simple Linctus Paediatric is prepared by diluting simple linctus 1.25 ml upto 5 ml with syrup. If dose of simple linctus paediatric is 5 ml q.i.d. for 3 days. Calculate the dilution.

Amount of simple linctus paediatric:

5 ml x 4 times x 3 days = 60 ml

Dilution calculations: 1.25 ml is diluted upto 5 ml

                           ? is diluted upto 60 ml

$$\therefore \frac{1.25 \times 60}{5} = 15 \text{ ml}$$

Therefore, 15 ml of simple linctus should be diluted to 60 ml with syrup to produce simple linctus paediatric.

THERMOMETRIC SCALE

Fahrenheit and centigrade are commonly used thermal scales. The difference is as follows. Freezing point of water = 32°F or 0°C Boiling point of water = 212°F or 100°C.

The Reaumur scale has freezing point 0°R and boiling point 80°R for water.

Conversion of thermometric scales = °C $= \frac{5}{9}$ (°F - 32) ,   °C $= \frac{5}{4}$ °R.

INDEX

Eye ointment   246, 372, 374

F
Family Pharmacists   7, 10, 48, 56, 69, 70, 128
Family physician   7, 57, 69, 70, 128, 133
Fasting plasma glucose (FPG)   371
FDA (Food and Drug Administration)   3, 22, 36-7, 66
FDC   120, 131, 179, 318, 325, 374, 399
Fibrous food   236-7, 241, 315
Filled capsules   337-8
Film coating   344
Filter   51, 146, 154-5, 157, 159, 164, 166-7, 171, 180, 183, 187-9, 191-2, 194, 365-6
Filter paper   146, 235, 292, 296
Filtrate   146, 152
Filtration   115, 146, 152, 158, 204, 365
Fine powder of drug   145, 203
Fine powders   112, 184, 204, 213-5, 218, 227, 249, 254, 283, 318, 328, 330, 355
Flavouring agents   110, 114, 135-6, 138, 145, 147, 153, 159, 187, 203, 206-8, 210, 216, 235, 237, 241-2
Flavours   72-3, 106, 111, 136, 138-9, 144, 148, 150-1, 153, 168, 187-8, 191-2, 198-9, 205-6, 210, 212 [4]
Fluted bottles   167, 169-72, 181, 192, 205, 233, 239
  coloured   148, 174, 176, 182, 184, 193
Food and Drug Administration, see FDA
Format   18-9, 40, 67, 69
Formation   72, 109, 111, 114, 137, 145, 154, 169, 203-4, 222, 231, 233, 241, 259, 287-8, 292 [4]
Formulation, parenteral   362
FPG (Fasting plasma glucose)   371
Fraction   44, 81, 83, 147, 163, 189, 191
Freezer   53, 76, 370
Freezing point   75, 397-8
Friction   27, 113, 182-4, 215-6, 219, 311, 318, 342
Fruit juice   235-6, 309
Fusion method   245, 250-1, 255, 257, 269, 300

G
Gargles   25, 113, 116, 141, 147-8, 164-6, 171, 192, 356
Gelatin   229, 263, 265, 285-6, 295, 297, 332, 334-5, 351, 363
  solubility of   334

Gelatin capsules   278-9, 382, 384
Gels   95, 97, 121, 209, 215, 244, 264-7, 270-1, 320, 351
  aluminum hydroxide   126, 209-10, 227
Generic   17, 35, 37, 123
GI ulcer   91, 97-9, 101, 317
Glass   25, 29, 62, 152-3, 186, 295, 298, 301, 304, 314, 363-4, 373
Glass bottles   152, 160, 364, 371
  coloured fluted   180, 183-5, 238
Glass containers   108, 121, 210, 362, 372
Glass of water   43, 91, 95, 97-8, 100, 312, 323, 344
Glass pestle   169, 171, 176, 192-3
Glass rod   152-5, 157, 159, 161-5, 167-9, 171, 178-81, 183, 185-7, 189-94, 208, 216-8, 239-42, 263-4, 273-6, 297-8 [14]
Glidants   136, 309, 327, 335, 342
Globules   220-2, 224, 230, 234
Glucose   139, 309, 324-5, 371, 407-8
Glycerin   137-9, 142-5, 158-60, 167-72, 176-8, 186-8, 191-3, 200, 215-6, 236-7, 261-3, 265-8, 285, 296-8, 351, 393 [21]
  anhydrous   174-5, 261
  weight of   169, 171
Glycerin-alcohol mixture   218
Glycerin solutions   170
Glycerin suppositories   285, 289, 297, 304-5
Glycerin suppository bases   285
Glycerites   169-71
Glycerol-gelatin mass, warm   263
Good Dispensing Practices   13, 52, 54, 78
Good Pharmacy Practices (GPP)   50, 52, 54, 56, 58, 60, 62-4, 66, 68, 70-1
GPP, see Good Pharmacy Practices
Grains   20, 33, 109, 312-3
Granulation   319, 322-3, 326, 342-3
  wet   320, 322
Granules   25, 28, 115, 122, 146, 212, 306-7, 309, 313, 319-23, 326-7, 333-5, 342, 377
  effervescent   309, 321-3, 327
Gravity   150, 152-3, 198, 289, 391, 393, 402
Grittiness   73-4, 253, 258
Groups   6, 51-2, 131, 340, 342
Gum powder   232
Gums   169-70, 231-3, 237, 242, 346

H

Hand homogenisers   230

Hand rolling   278-9, 286, 288, 301-2

Handling precaution   155, 163, 167-8, 180-1, 190, 192, 216, 219, 254-5, 264, 274, 329

Hard gelatin capsules   307, 312, 317, 319, 333-7, 377

Hard Gelatin Capsules, *see* HGC

Hard soaps   227, 330

Headache   8, 36, 43, 276, 371

HealthCare Provider   2, 4, 6, 8, 10, 12, 14

Heating   151, 201, 252, 255, 284-5, 296, 302-3, 321

Hectorite   202, 228, 265

Hemorrhoids   236, 269, 280-1, 294-5

Hepatic functions   79, 80, 155, 160, 162, 191, 350

HGC (Hard Gelatin Capsules)   307, 312, 319, 333-7, 377

High dose drugs   308-9

Hospital Pharmacist   2, 3, 358

Hospital prescription   18, 21

Hospitals   2, 4, 5, 8, 10-1, 46-7, 66, 179, 384, 394

Housekeeping   51-4

Hydrates, chloral   109, 125, 194, 282, 292

Hydration, water of   322-3

Hydroalcoholic   140, 199

Hydroalcoholic solutions   203, 334

   flavored   158

   flavoured   159

Hydrocolloids   135, 200-1, 227, 230, 232, 262-3, 265

Hydrolysis   73, 113, 117, 300, 317, 362

Hygroscopic   25, 170, 174, 272, 275, 288, 297, 300, 309, 312-3, 315, 321

Hygroscopic nature   285-7, 325

Hyperacidity   207, 343, 345, 367-8

Hypersense   98, 100-2

Hypertension   4, 44-5, 88, 91, 94, 98-100, 127, 132

Hypnotic   104, 162-3, 179, 194, 281

Hypoglycemia   44, 371

Hypotonic solutions   361, 396-7

I

Ibuprofen   113, 120-1, 205, 266

IDT (Individualization of Drug Therapy)   8

Immiscible liquids   220, 222-3, 225, 230

Implants   342, 346, 348

Improvement   55, 105-6, 116-7, 218

Improvisation   115-7

In-patients   1, 2

Incompatibilities   22, 52, 103-4, 106-7, 111-2, 114, 116-7, 224

Incomplete patient information   123, 125

Incorporation method   245, 249-50, 252

Indiffusible suspensions   112, 199

Individual dose   126, 307, 312, 316

Individualization of Drug Therapy (IDT)   8

Infections   2, 116, 126-7, 169, 174-5, 208, 240, 252, 255, 281, 328, 379

Information   5-7, 9, 12-3, 18, 24, 42-3, 47, 51, 55-7, 59, 62-3, 66-7, 103, 128-9, 193-4, 346-7 [11]

Inhalations   25, 27, 44, 88, 100, 110, 155-6, 197, 199, 205, 212-4, 381-2

   benzoin   212

Inhalers   37, 88, 121, 124, 172, 379-80, 382-3

   metered dose   44, 379

Injection site   369-70

Injections   74, 80, 101-2, 105, 119, 135, 226, 358-64, 367-70, 372, 397-8

   single dose   364, 367

Inpatient prescription   18, 21

Insertion   27, 278-82, 286-7, 294-5, 298, 300-1, 304, 346-7

Insolubility   107-8, 117, 125, 217, 282, 377

Insoluble drug   108, 110, 115, 141, 197-8, 200, 240, 249, 251-2, 288, 292, 300, 307

Insoluble medicaments   272, 291, 296, 300, 302-3

   powdered   291

Insoluble powders   263, 359

   oral   308

Inspiration   379-80, 382, 384

Instillation   174-5, 373

Instructions   7, 16-7, 43, 47, 64, 101, 120, 124, 148, 236-43, 295, 383

Insufflations   28, 109, 308-9, 318

Insulin   45, 76-7, 102, 104, 359, 368-71

Insulin injection   359, 368-71

Intention   36, 39, 106, 116, 118, 126, 129, 290

Interactions, product-container   107

Interfacial films   213, 223, 226-8

   multi-molecular   227-8, 231

Interfacial tension   223, 232, 259

reducing 200, 226-8, 233

Internal phase 220-1, 225, 231, 233-5, 257

Intestine 80, 127, 324, 344

Iodine 114, 154-5, 167-8, 170, 179, 194-5, 250, 252, 261, 273-4

Iodine ointment 238, 262, 273

  povidone 388

Iodine resistant containers 51, 155, 168

Iodine solutions 154-5, 168

Ions 116, 252, 399, 403-5, 407

IPA (Indian Pharmaceutical Association) 11, 50, 70

Iron 120, 145, 163, 188-90, 236

Isotonic solution 149, 398, 324-25

Isotonicity 361-2, 396-7, 399

Ispaghula husk 326-7

J

Jar, capped 293, 295, 298, 301, 304

Jellies 25, 27, 172, 264-6

K

Kaolin 104, 109, 115, 197, 203, 216-7, 263, 267, 308-9, 311-2, 314, 318, 353

  heavy 267

Kaolin poultice 267

KCl 404, 406

Keratolytic 182, 185, 218, 253, 260, 274

Knoll 371

L

Label 12-3, 16, 23-6, 28-9, 36-7, 39-41, 160-2, 165-9, 171-4, 179-86, 192-5, 205-6, 216-9, 236-43, 275-6, 328-9 [28]

  bulk pack 41

  container's 62

Label preparation 24, 26

Lactation 68, 86-102, 155

Lactation pregnancy 86, 93

Lactose 109, 134-6, 309, 311-2, 320-1, 326, 335, 339-42, 348-50, 382

Lakes 203, 249

Lanolin 136, 245, 247, 249, 255-6, 284, 372

Large doses of insoluble drugs 197

Laxatives 110, 122, 126, 134, 157, 207, 209, 211, 226, 236-7, 241, 280-1, 297, 308, 320-1, 326-7 [3]

Left hand pan (LHP) 30

Lemon oil 144, 153, 156-7, 183

Lemon syrup 112, 138, 150, 153

Lemongrass oil 183

Length 33-4, 219, 257, 279, 302, 337, 354, 356

Levigation 108, 200, 249-50, 263, 303

LHP (left hand pan) 30

Life, shelf 26, 74, 138, 211, 246, 361

Light magnesium carbonate 108, 186, 197, 206, 212-4

Linctus 27, 140, 147, 154, 160-1

  codeine 161-2

  simple 160-1, 409

Linctuses 140, 148, 160-1

Liniments 25, 27, 37, 140-1, 182, 185, 197, 221, 237

  alcoholic 182

Liquefaction 107, 109, 117, 213, 328

Liquid base 332, 335

Liquid dosage forms 73, 135, 138, 147, 189, 221, 245, 307, 341, 348

Liquid emulsions 221, 256-7

Liquid excipients 353-4

Liquid extracts 73, 146, 148, 308, 311-2

Liquid glucose 351, 353, 355

Liquid ingredients 146, 401

Liquid orals 105, 143, 147-9

  monophasic 144-5

Liquid paraffin 37, 92, 104, 213, 226, 228, 231, 236-7, 241, 246, 258-9, 265, 272, 289, 295-6, 338 [1]

Liquid paraffin 10.2per cent 271

Liquid phase 196, 220, 222, 226, 255

Liquid phenol 215-6

Liquid preparations 32, 109, 137, 140-1, 143, 197, 200, 212, 239, 309, 348

Liquids

  diluted 147, 162-3

  dilution of 147

  granulating 320-2

  paediatric 142-4, 159

  viscous 25, 31, 115, 146, 149-50, 292, 350

Liquorice 111, 155-6, 356, 388

Liver diseases 80, 90, 92, 95, 98, 126

Liver dysfunction 92, 95-6, 101

Liver impairment 86-7, 89, 91, 93, 95-9, 101-2

Locking 337-9

6

Metered Dose Inhalers, *see* MDI

Methyl cellulose   202, 320, 332, 351

Methyl salicylate   15, 51, 115, 165, 176, 252-3, 255-6, 261, 267, 273-4, 318, 330

Micro-emulsions   221

Microbial growth   73, 137, 143-4, 148, 150, 164, 221, 228, 246, 248, 267, 286-7, 307

Microcapsules   377-8

Milk   44, 62, 88, 90, 92, 96-8, 127, 154-5, 209, 235-6

Milk of magnesia   209-10, 241

Mix powders   304, 310, 327

Mixing   23-4, 29, 51-2, 103, 106-9, 112, 117, 148, 200, 209, 250, 252, 310-1, 313, 321-2, 387 [13]

Mixture   26-7, 108-9, 111-2, 140, 143-5, 150-2, 157-9, 196-7, 201-2, 208, 214-8, 235-9, 241-4, 271-2, 296, 389-91 [24]

   cream   390

Mixtures Solutions Syrup Draught Drops   140

Moist   73, 318-9, 321, 323, 329, 349, 352, 355

Moisture   24, 70, 72-3, 170, 174, 267-8, 275, 293, 297, 300, 311, 314-5, 334-5, 341, 343, 348 [1]

Molecular weight   248, 286, 399, 404-6

Moles   405-6

Monomolecular interfacial films   227-8, 233

Monophasic Liquids   140-4, 146, 148, 150, 152, 154, 156, 158, 160, 162, 164, 166, 168, 170, 172, 203 [11]

Monovalent soaps   223, 225, 227, 230, 238, 243, 256

Mortar   31, 190, 204, 206, 208-9, 211, 214, 216, 218, 239-43, 250, 259, 310, 313-5, 319, 340 [7]

Motivation   11, 14, 48, 52, 54

Mould cavities   288, 292, 296, 300, 349-50

Mould lubrication   284, 286, 288-9, 295-6, 299, 300

Mould plate   349

Moulded tablets   343, 347-8

Moulding   279, 287-8, 293, 297, 300, 341, 348-9

Moulds   223, 279, 282-6, 288-93, 295-300, 302, 304, 349

   lubricated   291, 295, 297, 301

Mouth bottles, wide   253-4, 264, 273-5

Mouthfeel effect, better   138-9, 150-1, 158, 164

Mouthpiece   380-4

Mouthwashes   25, 27, 141, 147-8, 165-7, 169-71, 192

N

Narcotic drugs   36, 81

Nasal bougies   278-9

Nasal solutions   172, 175

Nasal Solutions   172-3

National Health Policy (NHP)   13-4

NDPS   36

Nebulisers   173, 379, 384

NHP (National Health Policy)   13-4

Niacinamide   340-1

Non-aqueous solvents   142-4, 158-9, 164

Non-effervescent type   306, 314

Non-staining iodine ointment   273-4

Non-steroidal anti-inflammatory drugs, *see* NSAID

Non-sugar syrups   150-1

Novel Drug Delivery Systems (NDDS)   106, 121, 375-6, 378-80, 382, 384, 386

Nozzle   266, 269-70, 318, 373, 380

NSAID (non-steroidal anti-inflammatory drugs)   43, 89, 91, 94-5, 126, 266, 294, 320, 344, 374, 378-9

O

Occlusive   249, 261-2, 271, 274

Oil-in-water   220

Oil phase   109, 220-1, 224, 226, 228-32, 234, 237, 251, 256-7

Oil soluble drugs   143, 221, 226, 272

Oils   110, 112, 143, 150, 153, 172, 214, 220-1, 224-8, 233-5, 241-2, 247-8, 259, 271-2, 281, 353-4 [8]

   arachis   183, 226, 239, 273, 289, 295-6

   mentha   168, 170, 267, 391

   theobroma   283-4, 295, 303-4

Ointment bases   244-7, 252, 262, 271, 273, 277, 372

   emulsifying   230, 272

   water-soluble   272

Ointment slab   250, 253-5, 264, 271, 274-5, 295, 301

Ointment tube   269

Ointments   15, 25-7, 37, 74, 86, 98, 105, 116, 121, 244-53, 256-7, 260-3, 269, 271-4, 372-3, 387-8 [3]

   simple   245, 253-4, 272-3

Oleaginous bases   136, 245-7, 249, 283

Oleic acid   183, 239, 243

Oleoresins   231-3, 268

Ophthalmic   135, 137, 145, 265

Ophthalmic preparations   138, 145, 372, 374

Refresher courses 11, 13

Refrigerators 45, 53, 76-8, 102, 111, 157, 205, 233, 294, 296-7, 325, 369-71

Relief 161, 172, 213, 215, 255, 260, 344

Removal of Medicines 39, 46

Renal 86-7, 89-91, 93, 95-102

Renal impairment 86-90, 92, 95, 97, 99, 100, 102, 241

Repeated administration of drugs 281

Repetature 15-6, 18, 20

Reproducibility 33

Resins, ion exchange 343, 377-8

Resistant 154, 202, 246-7, 287

Resorcinol 261, 274-5, 290, 303-4

Respiratory tract 155-6, 172-3, 379

Return Medicine Records 65, 71

Review 8, 55, 57, 128-9

RHP (right hand pan) 30

Riboflavin 74, 112, 138, 144, 340

Right hand pan (RHP) 30

Ringworms 253-4

Rinse 31, 154-5, 159, 164, 167, 180, 183, 188-9, 191-2, 194, 206, 208-9, 216, 218

Roller 351-4

Rolling 175, 292-3, 300, 302, 338

Rotahaler 379, 382-4

Route 56, 118, 199, 200, 358, 360, 362-3, 375
primary 359-60

Route of administration 12, 16, 105, 140-1, 203, 229, 294, 306, 312

Rubber 107, 162-3, 259, 268

Rubber stoppers 363-4

Rubbing 238-9, 255, 373

Rubefacient 144, 182-4, 238, 242-3, 261

S

Sachets 121-2, 321, 325, 327

Safety 2, 3, 24, 28, 36, 103-4, 362

SALA (Sound Alike Look Alike) 119-20

SALA medicines 123-4

SALA Medicines 119, 122

Salicylic acid 114, 180-1, 185, 250, 253-5, 260, 264, 268, 318, 328-9

Salts 108, 111, 142, 191, 227, 288, 325, 399, 403-6

Sealing plate 337-9

Sediment 108, 197-9, 209

Self-medication 18, 21, 43-4, 59

Self-preservative activity of syrup 149, 151

Semisolid dosage forms 73, 121, 135, 244-6, 248, 252-3

Semisolid preparations 244-5, 249, 270

Semisolids 226, 244-6, 248, 250, 252, 254, 256-8, 260, 262, 264, 266, 268, 270, 272, 274, 332 [5]

Sensitivity 32-3, 89

SGCs (Soft Gelatin Capsules) 333, 335

Shaking 124, 196-7, 223-4, 243, 265, 274, 338

Shape 105-7, 261, 278-9, 282, 293, 324, 333, 341

Shelves 23, 39, 53, 64, 77

Shelves pharmacists 124

Side effects 12, 42-3, 47, 66, 103, 116-8, 126, 188, 245, 379, 384

Sieves 117, 214, 249, 253-4, 295, 301, 304, 314-5, 317, 319, 321, 323, 325, 327-30, 340-1, 349

Simple linctus paediatric 409

Single dose 31, 86, 88, 96, 122, 162, 191, 331, 334, 363, 375, 384

Sip 160-2

Size reduction 250, 309-10, 313

Skin 144, 172, 179-80, 214-5, 218-9, 237-40, 244-6, 248, 255-6, 259-62, 265, 296, 318-9, 358-9, 370, 385-6 [7]
broken 27-8, 146, 182, 229, 246, 254-5, 257, 273-4, 308, 318-9, 329
dry 116, 144, 229, 237, 239, 252, 257, 271-2, 326, 371
intact 105, 184, 238-9, 243, 308, 317, 385-6
unbroken 182-5, 227, 257

Skin infections 260

Skin penetration 238, 262, 276

Skin surface 117, 184-5, 252, 318

Small volume parenterals (SVP) 359, 364

Smooth dispersion 169, 171, 192, 204, 208, 211, 217, 232, 249, 267

Soap 180, 182-3, 230, 232, 243, 257, 259, 269-70, 285, 304, 369

Soap emulsifying agents 227, 229

Soap emulsions 230, 238, 242

Soap formation 226-8

Soap glycerin base 296

Soap glycerin suppositories 289, 296

Sodium alginate 136, 202-3, 207, 227, 229, 262, 265

Tragacanth mucilage 197, 201, 203, 351, 353
Tragacanth Powder 207, 236, 267
Training 4, 6, 11-2, 52, 54
Triglycerides 283-4
Triturate 32, 157, 166, 171, 192, 206, 217-8, 235, 237, 295, 312-3, 321, 326, 340-1, 350, 352-3 [11]
Trituration 232-3, 240, 249-50, 253-4, 263, 267, 310-1, 313, 315, 317, 326, 329
Trituration method 31, 117, 263
TT base 349-50
Tumbling 310-1, 313
Turpentine liniment 182, 238, 242, 401
Turpentine oil 177, 193, 226, 231, 238, 242-3, 401

U

Ulcers 87-8, 94-5, 165, 350
Unit Dosage Forms 105, 331-2, 334, 336, 338, 340, 342, 344, 346, 348, 350, 352, 354, 356
Unit dose of powder 307
Unit volume 292, 391
Units 26, 32, 39-41, 52, 64, 66, 73, 100, 102, 121, 123-5, 146, 341, 347-8, 402
Urethral bougies 278-9
Urine 81, 93, 96
USP, oral solution 145, 156
UV light 234

V

Vaccines 76, 78, 104, 358-9
Vagina 270, 278, 280-1, 287, 298-9, 318, 346
Vanillin 164, 236-7, 320
Vaporisation 213-4, 356
Vapours 27, 150, 212-4, 276
Vegetable oils 135-6, 175, 180, 183, 226-7, 285
Vegetables 295, 298, 301, 305
Vehicle 16, 31, 78, 108, 110, 113, 115-6, 122, 135-6, 142-7, 158, 160-1, 174-5, 199, 200, 202-6, 214 [15]
  amount of 146-7, 401-2
  approximate amount of 401
  non-aqueous 143, 362
Vessel 146, 274
Veterinary prescription 19, 21
Vial 102, 148, 363-4, 367-9, 373
Viscosity 73, 108, 135, 143, 158, 163-5, 167, 169-71,

174, 198, 201, 205, 213, 215, 224, 227 [8]
  low 201, 230-1, 354
Viscous 138, 143, 146-7, 149, 151, 160-1, 169, 171, 184, 199, 201, 210, 213, 215, 224, 238-9 [1]
Viscous colloidal solution, producing 320
Vitamin B2 340-1
Vitamin B6 340-1
Vitamin B12 340-1
Vitamin B12 340-1
Vitamins 74, 112, 152, 154, 159, 163, 214, 221, 242, 340-1, 351, 362, 365
Volatile 110, 114, 137, 206, 208, 217, 242, 251-2, 255, 274, 310, 312-3, 334
Volatile oils 51, 110, 135-6, 138, 144-5, 156, 183, 193, 199, 210, 213, 230-1, 233, 237, 292, 309 [6]
Volatile substances 213, 252, 308, 318, 328-9, 352, 356-7
Volume 31, 33, 146, 161, 163, 166-7, 176-8, 208-9, 216-9, 237-8, 335-6, 346, 359, 391, 393, 401 [21]
  equal 192, 243, 311, 391
  final 31, 146-7, 153-5, 157-8, 160, 162, 164, 167-8, 174, 176, 180, 183, 185-94, 203-4, 211, 239-40 [3]
Volume adjustment 146-7, 204
Volume parenterals, large 359-60, 364

W

Warm water 148, 165-7, 176, 192, 210-1, 240, 264, 269-70, 298, 308, 315, 318
Wash 64, 117, 208, 211, 240, 248-9, 269-70, 299, 369, 373
Water 108-11, 141-3, 147-52, 154-69, 183-95, 200-3, 205-6, 208-11, 214-8, 234-8, 246-50, 271-4, 286-8, 294-302, 319-27, 343-5 [56]
  amount of 122, 251, 296, 320
  anise 144, 161
  boiled 157, 328
  cinnamon 110, 207-8, 235
  cold 163, 202, 263
  cooled 116, 142, 145, 165, 193, 212, 226, 259, 327-8
  draught of 28
  drink 160-2, 168-9, 352
  drinking 154
  evaporation of 215, 287, 324
  excess 236-7, 315